TOWARD A HUMAN-FRIENDLY ASSISTIVE ENVIRONMENT

Assistive Technology Research Series

Volume 14

Previously published in this series

Vol. 13. H. Mollenkopf, F. Marcellini, I. Ruoppila and M. Tacken (Eds.), Ageing and Outdoor Mobility – A European Study
Vol. 12. M. Mokhtari (Ed.), Independent Living for Persons with Disabilities and Elderly People
Vol. 11. G.M. Craddock, L.P. McCormack, R.B. Reilly and H.T.P. Knops (Eds.), Assistive Technology – Shaping the Future
Vol. 10. C. Marincek, C. Bühler, H. Knops and R. Andrich (Eds.), Assistive Technology – Added Value to the Quality of Life
Vol. 9. M. Mokhtari (Ed.), Integration of Assistive Technology in the Information Age
Vol. 8. H.-W. Wahl and H.-E. Schulze (Eds.), On the Special Needs of Blind and Low Vision Seniors
Vol. 7. N. Katevas (Ed.), Mobile Robotics in Healthcare
Vol. 6. C. Bühler and H. Knops (Eds.), Assistive Technology on the Threshold of the New Millennium
Vol. 5. L.H.V. van der Woude, M.T.E. Hopman and C.H. van Kemenade (Eds.), Biomedical Aspects of Manual Wheelchair Propulsion
Vol. 4. I. Placencia Porrero and E. Ballabio (Eds.), Improving the Quality of Life for the European Citizen
Vol. 3. G. Anogianakis, C. Bühler and M. Soede (Eds.), Advancement of Assistive Technology
Vol. 9. M. Mokhtari (Ed.), Integration of Assistive Technology in the Information Age
Vol. 2. K. Cullen and S. Robinson, Telecommunications for Older People and Disabled People in Europe
Vol. 1. I. Placencia Porrero and R. Puig de la Bellacasa (Eds.), The European Context for Assistive Technology

ISSN 1383-813X

Toward a Human-Friendly Assistive Environment

ICOST'2004

2nd International Conference On Smart homes and health Telematics

Edited by

Daqing Zhang

Context Aware Systems Department
Institute for Infocomm Research
Singapore

and

Mounir Mokhtari

GET/INT Institut National des Télécommunications
Telecommunication Network and Services Department
Handicap Engineering & Communication Lab.
Evry, France

IOS Press

Amsterdam • Berlin • Oxford • Tokyo • Washington, DC

Published in cooperation with NATO Scientific Affairs Division

ISBN 1 58603 457 X
Library of Congress Control Number: 2004111370

Publisher
IOS Press
Nieuwe Hemweg 6B
1013 BG Amsterdam
The Netherlands
fax: +31 20 620 3419
e-mail: order@iospress.nl

Distributor in the UK and Ireland
IOS Press/Lavis Marketing
73 Lime Walk
Headington
Oxford OX3 7AD
England
fax: +44 1865 750079

Distributor in the USA and Canada
IOS Press, Inc.
4502 Rachael Manor Drive
Fairfax, VA 22032
USA
fax: +1 703 323 3668
e-mail: iosbooks@iospress.com

PRINTED IN THE NETHERLANDS

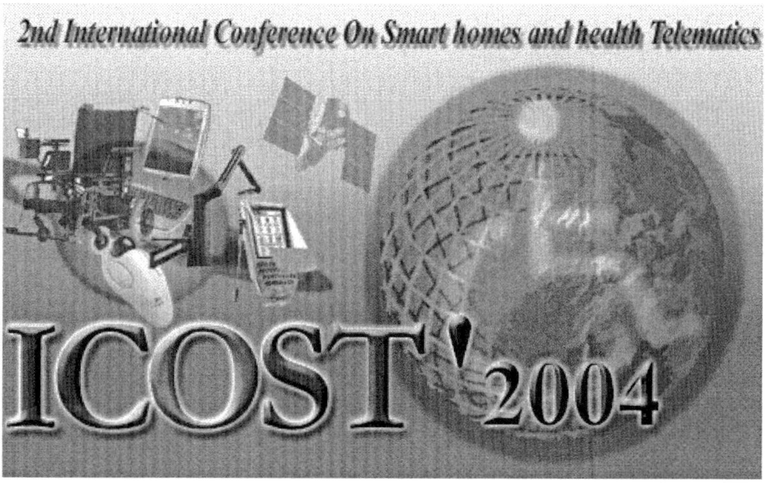

ICOST'2004 home page: http://icost2004.i2r.a-star.edu.sg

The organizers of ICOST'2004 gratefully acknowledge the following organizations for their contributions to the conference:

Sponsored by:

- Institute for Infocomm Research, Singapore
  - Context Aware Systems Department
- Institut National des Télécommunications (INT), France
  - Handicom Lab., Telecommunications Networks and services Department (RST)
- Groupe des Ecoles des Telecommunications (GET)
  - Scientific Direction (DS/GET)

ICOST'2004 Committees members

Conference Chairs

Dr. Daqing ZHANG,
Acting Manager
Context Aware Systems Department
Institute for Infocomm Research
21 Heng Mui Keng Terrace
Singapore 119613
Tel: +65 6874 7860 Fax: +65 6775 5014
E-mail: daqing@i2r.a-star.edu.sg

Dr. Mounir Mokhtari, Ph.D., Associate Professor
GET/INT Institut National des Télécommunications-INSERM (U.483)
Telecommunication Network and Services Department
9, rue Charles Fourier
91011 Evry Cedex, France
Tel: +33-1-60-76-47-55 Fax: +33-1-60-76-42-91
Email: Mounir.Mokhtari@int-evry.fr

International Scientific Committee

Chair: **Prof. Sumi Helal**, University of Florida, USA

- **Prof. Christian Roux**, ENST Bretagne, France
- **Prof. Gregory D. Abowd**, Georgia Institute of Technology , USA
- **Prof. Jadwiga Indulska**, University of Queensland, Australia
- **Dr. Machiel van der Loos**, VA Palo Alto, USA
- **Prof. Pung Hung Keng**, National University of Singapore, Singapore
- **Dr. Pang Hwa Hwee**, Institute for Infocomm Research (I^2R), Singapore
- **Prof. Sylvain Giroux**, University of Sherbrooke, Canada
- **Dr. Thijs Soede**, IRV. The Netherlands
- **Prof. Toshiyo Tamura**, Chiba University, Japan
- **Dr. Yves Burnod**, INSERM U. 483, Paris, France
- **Prof. Zen Bien**, Korea advanced institute of science and technology, Korea
- **Prof. Zhou Xingshe**, Northwestern Polytechnical Univ., P.R. China

Technical Program Committee

Chair: **Dr. Jit Biswas**, Institute for Infocomm Research (I^2R), Singapore

- **Prof Adel Ben Mnaouer**, Nanyang Technology University, Singapore
- **Dr Alvin Kam**, Institute for Infocomm Research (I^2R), Singapore
- **Dr. Bessam Abdulrazak**, GET/INT, Handicom Lab. France
- **Dr. Chris Nugent**, University of Ulster at Jordanstown, United Kingdom
- **Prof Debashis Saha**, Indian Institute of Management (IIM) Calcutta, India
- **Dr. Dimitar Stefanov**, University of Wales, United Kingdom
- **Dr Edwige Pissaloux**, University of Paris, France
- **Dr. Ismail Khalil Ibrahim**, University of Linz, Austria
- **Dr. Juan C. Augusto**, University of Ulster at Jordanstown, United Kingdom
- **Prof Keith Chan**, Hong Kong Polytechnic University, Hong Kong
- **Asst Prof Lim Ee Peng**, Nanyang Technology University, Singapore
- **Prof. Liu Xiang**, Beijing University, P.R. China
- **Dr Lonce Wyse**, Institute for Infocomm Research (I^2R), Singapore
- **Dr. Matthew Ma**, Panasonic, USA
- **Prof Miao Kejian**, Northwestern Polytechnical Univ., P.R. China
- **Dr. Ronnie Lee**, Infocomm Development Authority (IDA), Singapore
- **Dr Steven Miller**, Singapore Management University, Singapore
- **Prof Teo Yong Meng**, National University of Singapore, Singapore

Local Organizing Committee

- **Dr. Yang Rong Huan**, Singapore Polytechnic, Singapore
- **Dr. Cheng Heng Seng**, I2R, Singapore
- **Chin Chung Yau**, I2R and NUS, Singapore
- **Zheng Song**, I2R and NUS, Singapore
- **Wang Xiaohang**, I2R and NUS, Singapore
- **Casey Ong**, I2R, Singapore
- **Cheong Yu Chye,** IDA, Singapore
- **Patricia Loh**, I2R, Singapore
- **Ni Xiao,** I2R, Singapore
- **Gu Tao**, NUS and I2R, Singapore
- **Tan Joo Geok**, I2R, Singapore

Keynote Speakers

The Aware Home Research Initiative: Balancing Technology and Applications Research
Presenter: Prof. Gregory D. Abowd (no paper submitted for this Proceedings)

Health Monitoring in an Agent-Based Smart Home by Activity Prediction
Presenter: Prof. Sajal K. Das

Research Challenges on 4G Mobile Communications for the Next Generation of m-health Systems
Presenter: Prof. Robert S. H. Istapanian

Preface

Riding on the success of the inaugural ICOST'2003 in Paris, we are honored to welcome you to the ***2nd International Conference On Smart homes and health Telematics*** (ICOST'2004) in Singapore.

Recent years have witnessed rapid advances in the enabling technologies such as wireless communication, smart sensors/actuators, robotics and smart devices/services. As the pervasive computing technologies become more and more mature, people in both academia and industry are thinking of how to deploy those technologies to enhance the quality of life for all the world citizens and maintain independent living for elderly and disabled people. With the goal of using assistive technology to help elderly and disabled people carry out daily living activities, socialize, and enjoy entertainment and leisure activities, ICOST2004 continues focusing on "**smart home and health telematics**" and choosing again "**independent living for persons with disabilities and elderly people**" as the theme of the conference. It has to be clarified that smart home techniques are not only limited to home environment, but can also be deployed into other environments such as hospitals, offices, schools, or even train stations.

ICOST intends to provide a forum for researchers, practitioners, business leaders and policy makers to exchange ideas and experiences in the smart home and health care domain. Three keynote speechs and more than 30 papers from 15 countries worldwide have been planned. On behalf of ICOST'2004 organising committee, we would like to thank the International Scientific Committee for their technical guidance, the International Program Committee for their in-depth and timely review of the papers, the Local Organising Committee for their continuous efforts, and more importantly the authors and attendees for their contributions and participation. Last but not least, we would like to express our gratitude to the official sponsors of this event: Institute for Infocomm Research, A-Star, Singapore, Institut National des Télécommunications and DS/GET, France.

Thank you for joining us, and wishing you a great experience and enjoyable stay here in Singapore.

Daqing Zhang and Mounir Mokhtari

ICOST'2004 Conference Chairs

Contents

Chapter 4. Communications for Health Telematics

Chapter 5. Personal Assitive Devices and Robotics

Keynote Speeches

Toward a Human-Friendly Assistive Environment
D. Zhang and M. Mokhtari (Eds.)
IOS Press, 2004

Health Monitoring in an Agent-Based Smart Home by Activity Prediction

Sajal K. Das and Diane J. Cook
Center for Research in Wireless Mobility and Networking (CReWMaN)
Department of Computer Science Engineering
The University of Texas at Arlington
{das, cook}@cse.uta.edu

Abstract

To many people, home is a sanctuary. For those people who need special medical care, they may need to be pulled out of their home to meet their medical needs. As the population ages, the percentage of people in this group is increasing and the effects are expensive as well as unsatisfying. We hypothesize that many people with disabilities can lead independent lives in their own homes with the aid of at-home automated assistance and health monitoring. In order to accomplish this, robust methods must be developed to collect relevant data and process it dynamically and adaptively to detect and/or predict threatening long-term trends or immediate crises. The main objective of this paper is to investigate techniques for using agent-based smart home technologies to provide this at-home health monitoring and assistance. To this end, we have developed novel prediction algorithms that will determine common activities of an inhabitant and report significant activity anomalies that may indicate health crises. Specifically, we address the following technological challenges: 1) developing secure situation- or context-aware methods to collect at-home health and activity data, 2) learning patterns from the collected data, 3) identifying long-term trends of increasing or deteriorating health, 4) detecting and responding to anomalies in the data, and responding to predicted health problems, and 5) providing reminder and automation assistance to promote independent living at home. The proposed solution approaches are being tested in simulation and with volunteers at the UTA's MavHome site, an agent-based smart home project funded by NSF.

1 Introduction and Motivation

We live in an increasingly connected and automated society. We are investigating monitoring and automation assistance in our most personal environment: *the home*. In particular, we will investigate methods of adapting such a smart home environment to perform health monitoring and assistance for persons with disabilities and for aging adults. This integration of engineering and life science builds upon UTA's MavHome project [9], a home environment that perceives the state of the home through sensors and intelligently acts upon the environment through controllers.

As Lanspery and Hyde [17] state, "For most of us, the word 'home' evokes powerful emotions [and is] a refuge". They note that older adults and people with disabilities want to remain in their homes even when their conditions worsen and the home cannot sustain their safety. In a national survey, researchers found that 71% of the respondents felt strongly that they wanted to remain in their current residence as long as possible, and another 12% were somewhat likely to remain there [1]. Nearly 1/4 of the respondents expected that they or a member of their household would have problems getting around their house in the next five years. Of these respondents, 86% stated that they had made at least one modification to their home to make it easier to live there, and nearly 70% believe that the modifications will allow them to live in the current homes longer than would have otherwise been possible. A separate study supported these results and found that the most common modifications were an easy-to-use climate control system and a personal alert system.

Zola [26] maintains that the problems of aging and disability are converging. Improvements in medical care are resulting in increased survival into old age, thus problems of mobility, vision, hearing, and cognitive impairments will increase [19, 20]. As the baby boomers enter old age, this trend will be magnified. By 2040, 23% will fall into the 65+ category [17]. An AARP report [1, 2] strongly encourages increased funding for home modifications that can keep older adults with disabilities independent in their own homes.

While use of technology can be expensive, it may be more cost effective than the alternative [13]. Nursing home care is generally paid either out-of-pocket or by Medicaid. Typical nursing home costs are about $40,000 a year, and the $197 billion of free care offered by family members comes at the sacrifice of independence and job opportunities by the family caregivers.

In this paper, our goal is to assist the elderly and individuals with disabilities by providing home capabilities that will monitor health trends and assist in the inhabitant's day to day activities in their own homes. The result will save money for the individuals, their families, and the state. We are seeking to meet this goal using the MavHome smart home environment. MavHome is equipped with sensors that record inhabitant interactions with many different devices, medicine-taking schedules, movement patterns, and vital signs. We have developed novel algorithms that learn patterns of activities from this data. We will apply these capabilities to health monitoring in the following steps: (i) Perform secure, situation (or context)-aware collection of inhabitant health and activity data; (ii) Use our data mining and prediction techniques to learn patterns in collected data; (iii) Identify trends that could indicate health concerns or a need for transition to assisted care; (iii) Detect anomalies in regular (monitored) patterns that may require intervention; and (v) Provide reminder and automation assistance for inhabitants.

We will report experimental results on simulated data and on data collected from student volunteers in smart apartments (MavPad) on UTA campus. By investigating these issues we can offer the community an intelligent system with learning algorithms that not only perform their individual tasks well, but also form a synergistic whole that is stronger than the parts. We will show the benefits that can be derived from these algorithms in intelligent environments and other learning-driven situations for aging adults and persons with disabilities.

The rest of the paper is organized as follows. Section 2 gives an overview of the MavHome project while Section 3 explains how to identify significant episodes in smart homes. Section 4 deals with prediction of inhabitants' mobility and activities. Section 5 summarizes the capabilities of MavHome to assist the elderly and disabled.

2 Overview of the MavHome Smart Home

We define an intelligent environment as one that is able to acquire and apply knowledge about its inhabitants and their surroundings in order to adapt to the inhabitants and meet the goals of comfort and efficiency [7]. These capabilities rely upon effective prediction, decision making, robotics, wireless and sensor networking, mobile computing, databases, and multimedia technologies. With these capabilities, the home can adaptively control many aspects of the environment such as climate, water, lighting, maintenance, and multimedia entertainment. Intelligent automation of these activities can reduce the amount of interaction required by inhabitants, reduce energy consumption and other potential wastages, and provide a mechanism for ensuring the health and safety of the environment occupants [6].

Compared to existing smart home research projects and/or prototypes, MavHome is unique in combining technologies from artificial intelligence, machine learning, databases, robotics, and multimedia computing to create a smart home that acts as an intelligent agent, as shown in Figure 1. MavHome's smart home capabilities are organized into an agent-based software architecture that seamlessly connects needed components while allowing improvements to be made to any of the supporting technologies. that are separated into four cooperating layers. The *Decision layer* selects actions for the agent to execute. The *Information layer* collects information and generates inferences useful for decision making. The *Communication layer* routes information and requests between agents. The *Physical layer* contains the environment hardware including devices, transducers, and network equipment. The MavHome software components are connected using a CORBA interface.

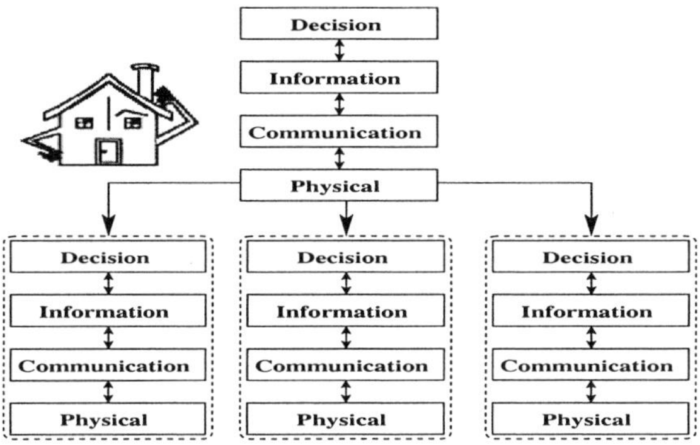

Figure 1: MavHome agent architecture.

Because controlling an entire house is a very large and complex learning and reasoning problem, the problem is decomposed into reconfigurable subareas or tasks. Thus the Physical layer for one agent may in actuality represent another agent somewhere in the hierarchy, which is capable of executing the task selected by the requesting agent.

Perception is a bottom-up process. Sensors monitor the environment (e.g., lawn moisture level) and, if necessary, transmit the information to another agent through the Communication layer. The database records the information in the Information layer, updates its learned concepts and predictions accordingly, and alerts the Decision layer of the presence of new data. During action execution, information flows top down. The Decision layer selects an action (e.g., run the sprinklers) and relates the decision to the Information layer. After updating the database, the Communication layer routes the action to the appropriate effector to execute. If the effector is actually another agent, the agent receives the command through its effector as perceived information and must decide upon the best method of executing the desired action. Specialized interface agents allow interaction with users, robots, and external resources such as the Internet. Agents can communicate with each other using the hierarchical flow shown in Figure 1.

3 Learning to Identify Significant Episodes

In order to maximize comfort, minimize cost, and adapt to inhabitants, a smart home must rely upon tools from artificial intelligence such as data mining and prediction. Prediction can be used to determine the inhabitant's next action. Specifically, MavHome needs to identify repetitive tasks performed by inhabitants that establish a baseline for learning trends in behaviors, detecting anomalies, and determining repetitive tasks worthy of automation by the home. The home can make this prediction based solely on previously-seen inhabitant activities and the current state of the inhabitant and the house.

A smart home inhabitant performs various routine activities, which may be considered as a sequence of events, with some inherent pattern of recurrence. This repeatability leads us to the conclusion that the sequence can be modeled as a stationary stochastic process. We can then perform inhabitant action prediction by first mining the data (using episode discovery techniques) to identify sequences of actions that are regular and repeatable enough to generate predictions, and by second using a sequence matching approach (LeZi-update or Active LeZi) to predict the next action in one of these sequences.

Our Episode Discovery (ED) data mining algorithm is based on the work of Srikant and Agrawal [23] for mining sequential patterns from time-ordered transactions. We move an examination window through the history of events or inhabitant actions, looking for episodes (sequences) within the window that merit attention, or *significant episodes*. Each candidate

Table 1: Scenario prediction results.

Scenario	1	2	3	4	5	Average
Events	12958	12884	12848	13058	12668	12883
Significant Episodes	13	13	13	13	13	13
IPAM Percentage Correct	39%	42%	43%	40%	41%	41%
IPAM+ED Percentage Correct	77%	84%	69%	73%	65%	74%
BPNN Percentage Correct	62%	64%	66%	62%	64%	64%
BPNN+ED Percentage Correct	84%	88%	84%	84%	88%	86%
ED Processing Time (secs)	11	9	10	9	9	10

episode is evaluated using the Minimum Description Length (MDL) principle [21]. The MDL principle favors patterns that can be used to minimize the description length of a database by replacing each instance of the pattern with a pointer to the pattern definition. A detected regularity factor (daily, weekly, or other time frame) further compresses the data because the sequence can be removed without storing a pointer to the sequence definition, and thus increases the value of a pattern. Deviations from the pattern definition in terms of missing events, extra events, or changes in the regularity of the occurrence add to the description length because extra bits must be used to encode the change, thus lowering the value of the pattern. The larger the potential amount of description length compression a pattern provides, the greater the impact that results from automating the pattern.

Our ED algorithm successfully identified daily and weekly patterns in synthetic data based on the MavHome scenario described earlier. We also used ED to mine data that was collected in the MavHome environment from six students during 2003. These students indicated in advance their likely daily and weekly activities, although the timing, regularity, and order of events would vary throughout the semester. The dataset contains 618 interactions that are members of patterns occurring once a week, multiple times a week, and randomly. ED successfully identified the patterns of three of the inhabitants as weekly significant episodes, and marked which of the 618 interactions contributed to the significant episodes [14].

The knowledge that ED obtains by mining the user action history can be used in a variety of ways. First, the mined patterns provide information regarding the nature of activities in the home, which can be used to better understand lifestyle patterns and aid in designing homes and devices for the home. Second, the significance of a current event as a member of a discovered pattern can be used in controlling the home, to determine whether this task is worth attempting to automate. Third, knowledge of the mined sequences can improve the accuracy of predicting the next action, by only performing prediction for events known to be part of a common pattern. We demonstrate the ability of ED to perform the third task, improving the accuracy of prediction algorithms, by adding the mined results as a preprocessor to two simple prediction algorithms. Action sequences are first filtered by the mined sequences. If a sequence is considered significant by the mining algorithm, then predictions can be made for events within the sequence window.

To test the filtering capabilities of ED, we coupled it with the IPAM sequential predictor [24] and a back-propagation neural network (BPNN). We created a sequence of 13,000 actions based on five randomly-generated scenarios, a situation in which these algorithms by themselves may not perform well. ED discovered 14 episodes in the data sets, and appreciably improved the accuracy of both algorithms across all five scenarios, as can be seen in Table 1. By using ED, we improve the accuracy of the prediction algorithms by reducing the total number of incorrect predictions, leading to inaccuracies in learned health trends, detected anomalies, and automated patterns.

4 Learning to Predict Inhabitant's Mobility and Actions

Prediction is an important component in a variety of domains in artificial intelligence and machine learning, that allows intelligent systems to make more informed and reliable decisions. Certain domains require that prediction be performed on sequences of events that can typically be modeled as stochastic processes. Especially common is the problem of sequential prediction: given a sequence of events, how do we predict the next event based on a limited known history? This is true, for example, when predicting inhabitant actions in a smart environment such as MavHome. Prediction can be performed of upcoming inhabitant movement activities based on observed past movement/activity patterns.

The fundamental framework due to Bhattacharya and Das [3, 4] demonstrate how optimal, on-line learning and prediction algorithms can be designed for user mobility in a wide area cellular network. This adaptive framework is based on the fundamental hypothesis that *a good leaner is a good predictor*, thus applying information theoretic concepts and Lempel-Ziv (LZ78) family of text compression techniques [25], on the mobility profiles collected over time. We have also shown how to adapt this framework for managing indoor mobility and context-aware resource management in smart home environments [22].

We have recently extended this framework and designed an algorithm, named *Active LeZi (ALZ)*, for sequential action prediction from an information theoretic standpoint. For any sequence of events that can be modeled as a stochastic process, this algorithm employs the power of Markov models to optimally predict the next symbol in any stochastic sequence. Inhabitant action prediction, similar to other prediction problems, requires that the prediction algorithm be capable of incrementally gathering information and deliver real time, "online" predictions. Active LeZi is based on the LZ78 data compression algorithm, which employs incremental parsing, thereby addressing this requirement. The smart home provides a ready environment for employing sequential prediction algorithms such as ALZ. The home will have to make inhabitant predictions based only on previously-seen inhabitant actions.

Consider a sequence of events being generated by an arbitrary deterministic source, which can be represented by the stochastic process $X = \{x_i\}$. The sequential prediction problem can then be stated as follows. Given the sequence of symbols $\{x_1,\ x2,\ \ldots\ x_i\}$, what is the next symbol x_{i+1}? Well-investigated text compression methods, such as LZ78, have also been established as good predictors [4, 11]. According to information theory, a predictor that builds a model whose entropy approaches that of the source achieves greater predictive accuracy. Also, it has been shown that a predictor with an order that grows at a rate approximating the entropy rate of the source is an optimal predictor [11]. Another motivation to look to the field of text compression is that such algorithms are essentially incremental parsing algorithms, providing a basis for online processing. ALZ addresses this prediction problem based on the above-mentioned motivations.

The LZ78 data compression algorithm due to Lempel and Ziv [25], is a dictionary-based text compression algorithm that performs incremental parsing of an input sequence and, as a result, gradually changes the Markov order at the appropriate rate. This algorithm parses an input string $x_1,\ x_2,\ \ldots,\ x_i$ into c(i) substrings $w_1,\ w_2,\ \ldots,\ w_{c(i)}$ such that for all j¿0, the prefix of the substring w_j (i.e., all but the last character of w_j) is equal to some w_i for $1 < i < j$. Because of this prefix property, parsed substrings can efficiently be maintained in a trie.

Consider the sequence of input symbols $x^n = aaababbbbbaabccddcbaaaa$. An LZ78 parsing of this string would yield the following set of phrases: $a, aa, b, ab, bb, bba, abc, c, d, dc, ba, aaa$. This algorithm maintains statistics for all contexts seen within the phrases. For example, the context a occurs 5 times (at the beginning of the phrases a, aa, ab, abc, aaa), the context bb is seen 2 times (bb, bba), etc. These context statistics are stored in a trie.

LZ78 suffers from two drawbacks: in any LZ parsing of an input string, all the information crossing phrase boundaries is lost. In most situations, there might be significant patterns crossing phrase boundaries that affect the next symbol in the sequence. Second, although

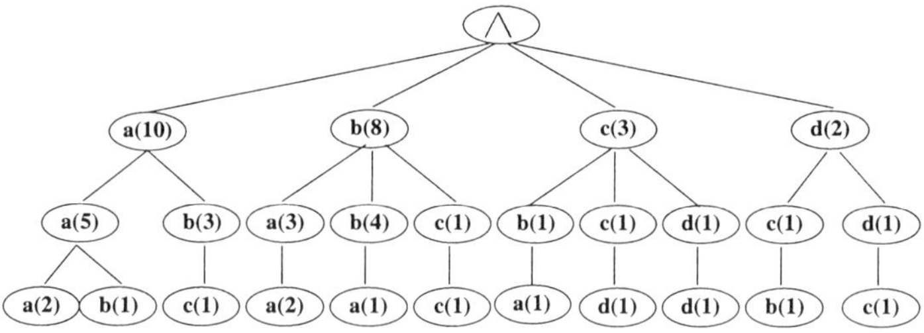

Figure 2: Trie formed by the ALZ parsing of the string *aaababbbbbaabccddcbaaaa*.

LZ78 asymptotically approaches optimal predictability, its convergence rate is slow [11].

Our Active LeZi (ALZ) algorithm is an enhancement of LZ78 that addresses these drawbacks. As the number of states in an input sequence grows, we can see that the amount of information being lost across the phrase boundaries increases rapidly. Our solution to this problem involves maintaining a variable length window of previously-seen symbols. We choose the length of the window at each stage to be equal to the length of the longest phrase seen in a classical LZ78 parsing of the symbol history. The reason for selecting this window size is that the LZ78 algorithm is essentially constructing an (approximation to an) order-(k-1) Markov model, where k is equal to the length of the longest LZ78 phrase seen so far, which builds a better approximation to the order-k Markov model. Therefore, we gain a better convergence rate to optimal predictability as well as greater predictive accuracy. Figure 2 shows the trie formed by the ALZ parsing of the input sequence aaababbbbbaabccddcbaaaa, which results in an order-2 Markov model.

In order to predict the next event of the sequence for which ALZ has built a model, we calculate the probability of each next action (symbol) occurring in the sequence, and predict the one with the highest probability. For sequential prediction, to achieve good convergence rates to optimal predictability, the predictor must "lock on" to the minimum possible set of states that is representative of the sequence being considered by using a "mixture" of all possible order models in assigning the next symbol its probability estimate. For this goal, we employ the Prediction by Partial Match (PPM) family of predictors.

PPM algorithms combine weighted different-order Markov models to build a probability distribution. In our predictive scenario, ALZ builds an order-k Markov model. The window maintained by ALZ represents the set of *contexts* used to compute the probability of the next symbol. In our example sequence aaababbbbbaabccddcbaaaa, the last phrase aaa (which is also the current ALZ window) is used. Within this phrase, the contexts that can be used are all suffixes within the phrase, except the window itself (i.e., aa, a, and the null context).

Suppose the probability that the next symbol is an a is being computed. From Figure 2 we see that an a occurs two out of the five times that the context aa appears, the other cases producing two null outcomes and one b. Therefore, the probability of encountering an a at the context aa is 2/5, and we now fall back (escape) to the order-1 context (i.e., the next lower-order model) with probability 2/5. At the order-1 context, we see an a five out of the ten times that we see the a context, and of the remaining cases, we see two null outcomes. Therefore we predict the a at the order-1 context with probability 5/10, and escape to the order-0 model with probability 2/10. At the order 0 model, we process an a for 10 out of 23 symbols seen so far, and we therefore predict a with probability 10/23 at the null context. The blended probability of seeing an a as the next symbol is therefore $\frac{2}{5} + \frac{2}{5}\{\frac{5}{10} + \frac{2}{10}(\frac{10}{23})\}$. This blending strategy assigns greater weight to higher-order models, while lower-order models are suppressed owing to the null context escape probability. This is in keeping with the advisability of making the *most informed* decision.

Figure 3 shows the performance of ALZ tested on data obtained from a Synthetic Data

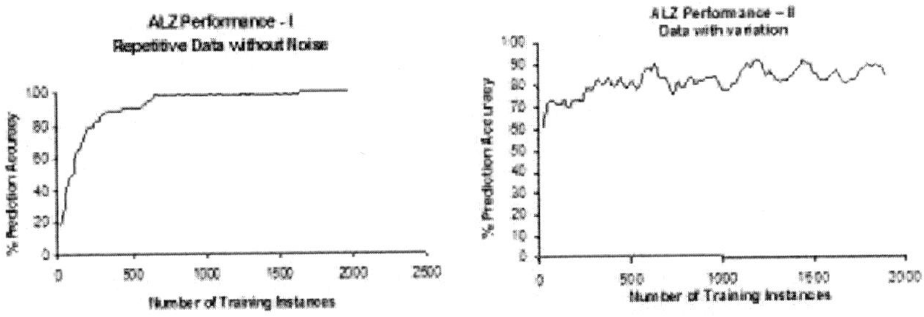

(a) (b)

Figure 3: ALZ learning curve on data a) without noise and b) with noise.

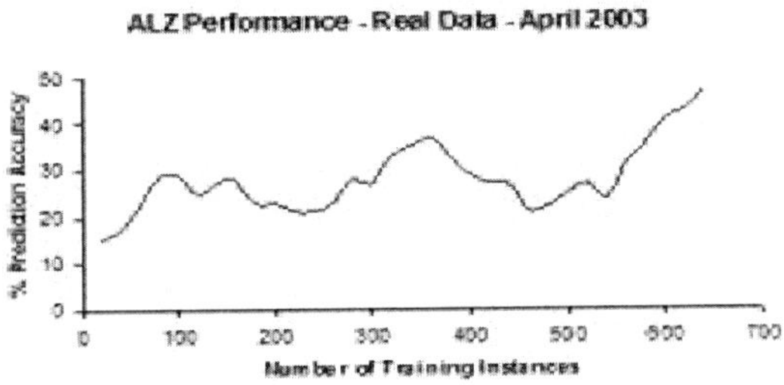

Figure 4: ALZ performance on real data from April, 2003.

Generator containing in the first case a high degree of repetitiveness and little noise, and containing in the second case a lower percentage of repeated events and more noise. The ALZ learning curves were plotted by testing the number of correct predictions from the next 100 events, while increasing the training data set. ALZ's performance converges quickly to 100% in the first experiment (Figure 3a), and eventually converges to 86% accuracy in the second experiment (Figure 3b).

In addition to the tests performed on the simulated data, ALZ was also tested on data collected in an actual smart home environment - the UTA MavHome Lab. This data was collected from monitoring the interactions of six different participants with devices, based on regular daily and weekly patterns of activity. These represent data that will typically be seen in a home environment – with all the associated randomness and noise within the system. As we can see from Figure 4, the algorithm converges to about 47% accuracy on one month of data consisting of 750 data points.

We have also enhanced ALZ to learn a Gaussian distribution representing relative time intervals between actions in the observed sequences, each characterized by a mean μ and standard deviation σ. Here, the relative frequency counts of the various phrases are stored as before in the trie and used to incrementally build Gaussians that represent the observed normal distribution of the relative time of occurrence of the last event in the corresponding phrase. As with the prediction of the event itself, information stored at various orders of the trie are blended to strengthen the resulting prediction. This enhancement was tested using synthetic data consisting of a smart home scenario with repeating events, where the order of events was constant, but the time difference between successive events were drawn from different distributions depending on the context in which that event was taking place. Results from this test show that in 92% of the cases, the next event occurred within the mean +/- 2 standard deviations of the predicted time.

As an additional experiment, we use ED to filter data for prediction by ALZ using actual collected MavHome activity data. Based on one month of collected data with an extremely large amount of noise (there are 20 students and 50 devices in the environment), ALZ achieves a predictive accuracy of 30%, while ALZ with ED achieves an improved predictive accuracy of 44%. These results show that even a powerful predictor such as ALZ benefits from being combined with the results of a data mining algorithm.

5 Using a Smart Home to Assist Elderly and Disabled

The data mining, prediction, and multiagent technologies available in MavHome can be employed to provide health care assistance in living environments. Specifically, models can be constructed of inhabitant activities and used to learn activity trends, detect anomalies, intelligently predict possible problems and make health care decisions, communicate with caregivers, and provide automation assistance for inhabitants with special needs.

A variety of approaches have been investigated in recent years to automate caregiver services. Many of the efforts offer supporting technologies in specialized areas, such as using computer vision techniques to track inhabitants through the environment and specialized sensors to detect falls or other crises. Some special-purpose prediction algorithms have been implemented using factors such as measurement of stand-sit and sit-stand transitions and medical history, but are limited in terms of what they predict and how they use the results. Remote monitoring systems have been designed with the common motivation that learning and predicting inhabitant activities is key for health monitoring, but very little work has combined the remote monitoring capabilities with prediction for the purpose of health monitoring. Some work has also progressed toward using typical behavior patterns to provide reminders, particularly useful for the elderly and patients suffering from various types of dementia [12, 15, 18].

Our approach differs from these earlier explorations in that we are combining capabilities in the areas of data collection, remote monitoring, prediction, data mining, and knowledge engineering to provide predictive health monitoring assistance for inhabitants with disabilities and caregivers. Instead of designing one specialized component, we demonstrate here that a smart environment can accomplish all of the tasks needed to identify patterns indicating or predicting a sudden or slow change in health status, to supply caregivers with periodic or emergency information, and to provide inhabitants with needed automation assistance.

5.1 Capability 1: Perform Secure, Context-Aware Data Collection

The first capability we are developing is that of remote collection of long-term activity and health status data. Data will consist of monitored inhabitant activities, vital signs, and interactions with the environment, and will be collected using context-aware technology.

Our smart home environment is currently equipped to gather the following types of information: 1) inhabitant usage of any electrical device in the home, 2) usage of water in the home and amount, 3) temperature settings, 4) inhabitant weight, 5) inhabitant movement throughout the home, 6) prescribed and actual medicine dispensing schedule, 7) time, duration, and intensity of exercise, and 8) use of food items in kitchen. Active sensors including wearable vital sign monitors can be integrated to further refine the model.

We have designed efficient algorithms for collecting real-time data that are context- and/or situation-aware. For example, the inhabitant's current activity (e.g., cooking vs. watching television) or location in the environment (e.g., bedroom vs. navigating the stairs) can affect the choice of sensors to use, and thus represent a defined context. Our data mining and prediction algorithms are highly scalable, a desirable feature when numerous tiny, portable sensor devices are involved. Furthermore, the algorithms create personal profiles and hence provide customized solutions to individual patients. There may also be a need for ad hoc collaboration of various entities as the emergency need arises. These problems can be elegantly tackled with the help of pervasive computing and communications technology [10, 16].

Use of sensors in smart homes and on elderly or people with disabilities is critical for collecting, storing, and processing appropriate data intelligently and in a timely manner. Data collection and processing needs to be backed by an infrastructure that allows anytime, anywhere reliable access to data sources (e.g., national data bases or vital records). This is crucial for the purpose of data mining, intelligent decision making and profiling. Privacy of the information is highly required since personal information will be collected during the monitoring phase.

5.2 Capability 2: Identify Trends in Long-Term Data

The second health monitoring capability uses our data mining and prediction techniques to identify trends in long-term data. Trends in time-varying data can be discovered and predicted using the same data mining and prediction techniques described earlier. Instead of capturing individual events and readings to store in the trie and use for prediction, changes in these values over varying periods of time are captured, stored, and predicted. In particular, for each feature of interest, the qualitative change in value (increase, decrease, same) and quantitative relative change (numeric difference) is recorded. Because the chosen time steps are limitless in value and yet critical to learning trends, we allow the user to determine the time step of choice (e.g., daily, weekly, monthly) and use auto-correlation techniques to automatically determine the time step most indicative of a temporal trend in the data.

The user can select features to monitor for trend analysis, including 1) change in mobility (schedule, time, room location, total movement), 2) change in amount of exercise, 3) change in deviation from prescribed medicine schedule, 4) change in amount of smart home requested assistance (reminders or automation assistance), 5) change in nutrition (types of food, number of calories), and 6) change in amount and types of activities.

Using the ED algorithm, long-term trends can be discovered from the raw data. The algorithm can also be used to search for changes of a type of duration indicated by the user. In addition, the prediction algorithm can be used to predict the upcoming changes in these features for the next time step. Finally, we can use data from individuals assessed by practitioners to learn classes of patient types, such as patients who require a move to an assisted care facility. Time-varying data captured for a particular individual can then be classified based on the learned models.

The result of this technology can be used in a number of ways. For patients recovering from an illness or accident, the algorithms can be used to determine whether they are regaining strength and vitality at an acceptable rate. For patients at risk of various types of accidents and health risk situations, the trends can be used to determine the current health risk and predicted short term health risk. These analyses can aid a caregiver in deciding whether the individual requires a change in medication, activity schedule, care scheduling, or environment.

5.3 Capability 3: Detect Anomalies in Current Data

A direct outcome of our work in data mining prediction is the ability to detect anomalies in collected data. For this purpose, we use the intuitive notion of an anomaly as *a surprising or unusual occurrence*. With this notion in mind, the anomaly value of each monitored activity or captured feature value can be collected and used to provide health status information.

An important consideration in any anomaly-detection system is the regularity, or predictability, of the data. Generally, the more predictable the data, the easier it is to detect anomalies. As a result, the anomaly value of each data point is influenced first by the degree of membership of the current state in a significant episode, second by the significance value of the episode itself, and third by the deviation of the observed activity from the predicted activity given the known episode.

The degree of membership of the current state in any of the discovered significant episodes is calculated as the probability of occurrence of the episode given the immediate history of observed activities. A probability is returned for each episode. This probability is then multiplied with the significance of the episode itself to calculate the regularity of the data context. The episode yielding the highest regularity value, episode i, represents the baseline for the anomaly calculation. Once membership in episode i is established, the ALZ trie is used to provide the probability of the next predicted event e. If the event that actually occurs has a very low probability given the context, the resulting event constitutes an anomaly. If the regularity of the context is high and the probability of the observed event is low, this event should be flagged as an anomaly. Thus the anomaly value of observed event e can be calculated as $A = \frac{(Member(e, Episode_i) * Significance(Episode_i))}{P(e|Episode_i, ImmHistory(e))}$.

Anomalies can be be handled in a manner appropriate to the nature of the event and anomaly value. The criticality of events can be set by the user. For example, an anomaly in predicted interactions with the house will typically have a low criticality and thus simply be recorded as an anomaly or prompt a reminder of the inhabitant of their normal routine. For a more critical anomaly, such as a sudden disruption in vital signs, the home will first attempt to contact the inhabitant. If contact cannot be made, the home will contact the caregiver. Web cameras placed throughout the house can be used by the caregiver to check on the inhabitant in such a situation and intervene with a medical difficulty.

5.4 Capability 4: Design Reminder Assistance System

An additional benefit that our smart home data mining and prediction capabilities can offer is to provide a reminder system for inhabitants. Reminders can be triggered by two situations. First, if the inhabitant queries the home for his/her next routine activity, the activity with the highest probability will be given based on the ALZ prediction. Second, for episodes with a high degree of significance and criticality, if the inhabitant deviates from the normal routine (creates an anomaly), the house will initiate contact with the inhabitant to remind him/her of the next expected activity. Such a reminder service will be particularly beneficial for individuals suffering from dementia. The reminder can enable the individual to feel secure about performing daily activities, and prevent accidents such as forgetting to turn off the water in the bathtub or keeping the doors unlocked when leaving the house.

5.5 Capability 5: Provide Automation Assistance

Intelligent automation of home activities can reduce the amount of manual home interaction required by inhabitants. Earlier we developed a decision-making algorithm to automate activities in the house [8]. Selection of actions for the house to take is based on suggestions from a reinforcement learning algorithm, which minimizes necessary manual intervention with the house and reduces actions with costly effects. The decision maker relies on input from ALZ to suggest the typical next inhabitant action, and uses results from the ED data mining algorithm to segment the learning space and improve the quality of the learned results.

Users can specify specific activities they would like the house to automate (temperature control, control of hard-to-reach devices, etc.). MavHome will then automate the activities based on learned preferences and action patterns. In addition, if the inhabitant does not respond to a reminder of a critical event, MavHome will automate an activity to ensure safety of the individual. Such actions include shutting off the bathwater, turning off the stove, or locking up the house when it is empty.

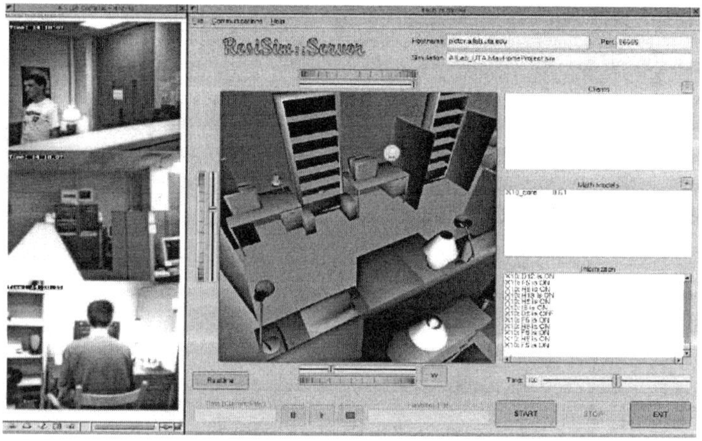

Figure 5: MavHome environment and interface.

6 Conclusion

Initial algorithms are in place for data mining, mobility and action prediction, decision making, and automation. These capabilities are being used in the MavHome lab (MavLab) and apartment (MavPad). Figure 5 shows lights in the entryway (top left) and on Ryan's desk (bottom left) turning on in reaction to inhabitant activities (these automated actions are also reflected in the simulator). We are collecting health-specific data and testing using volunteers living in MavPad and MavHome, as well as recruited residents of the C.C. Young Retirement Community in Dallas, Texas.

Acknowledgments: This work is supported by US National Science Foundation under ITR grant IIS–0121297.

References

[1] AARP, "Fixing to Stay: A National Survey of Housing and Home Modification Issues," 2000.

[2] AARP, "These Four Walls ... Americans 45+ Talk About Home and Community," 2003.

[3] A. Bhattacharya and S. K. Das, "LeZi-update: An information-theoretic approach to track mobile users in PCS networks," *Proc. Ann. Int'l Conference on Mobile Computing and Networking*, August 1999, pp. 1-12.

[4] A. Bhattacharya and S. K. Das, "LeZi-update: An information-theoretic approach for personal mobility tracking in PCS networks," *ACM-Kluwer Wireless Networks* (WINET), vol. 8, no.2, pp.121-137, 2002.

[5] M. Chan, C. Hariton, P. Ringeard, and E. Campo, "Smart House Automation System for the Elderly and the Disabled," *Proceedings of the IEEE International Conference on Systems, Man and Cybernetics*, pp. 1586-1589, 1995.

[6] D. J. Cook and S. K. Das, "Health Monitoring in an Agent-Based Smart Home," To be presented at the *International Conference on Aging, Disability and Independence* (ICADI), Washington, DC, Dec 2003.

[7] D. J. Cook and S. K. Das (Eds.), *Smart Environments: Architectures, Protocols and Applications*, John Wiley, to appear, Sept 2004.

[8] D. J. Cook, M. Huber, K. Gopalratnam, and E. Heierman, "Learning to Control a Smart Home Environment," *IEEE Transactions on Systems, Man and Cybernatics*, to appear.

[9] S. K. Das, D. J. Cook, et al., "The Role of Prediction Algorithms on the MavHome Smart Home Architectures," *IEEE Wireless Communications* (Special Issue on Smart Homes), Vol. 9, No. 6, pp. 77-84, Dec 2002.

[10] S. K. Das, M. Kumar, and B. Shirazi, "Pervasive Community Computing (PCC) Paradigm with Application to Health care," *Proc. International Conference on Ubiquitous Computing* (Keynote Talk), Seoul Korea, Oct 2003.

[11] M. Feder, N. Merhev, and M. Gutman, "Reflections on 'Universal Prediction of Individual Sequences'," *IEEE Information Theory Society Newsletter*, 1994.

[12] T. T. Fulmer, et al. "An Intervention Study to Enhance Medical Compliance in Community-Dwelling Elderly Individuals," *Journal of Gerontological Nursing*, 25(8): 6-14, 1999.

[13] P. J. Grayons, "Technology and Home Adaptation," In S. Lanspery and J. Hyde (Eds.), *Staying Put: Adapting the Places Instead of the People*, pp. 55-74, Baywood Pub. Co., 1997.

[14] E. Heierman and D. J. Cook, "Improving Home Automation by Discovering Regularly Occurring Device Usage Patterns," *Proceedings of the International Conference on Data Mining*, 2003.

[15] H. Kautz, L. Arnstein, G. Borriello, O. Etzioni, and D. Fox, "An Overview of the Assisted Cognition Project," *Proceedings of the AAAI Workshop on Automation as Caregiver*, 2002.

[16] M. Kumar, S. K. Das, et al, "PICO: A Middleware Framework for Pervasive Computing," *IEEE Pervasive Computing*, Vol. 2, No. 3, pp. 72-79, July-Sept 2003.

[17] S. Lanspery and J. Hyde (Eds.), *Staying Put: Adapting the Places Instead of the People*, Introduction, pp. 1-22, Baywood Pub. Co., 1997.

[18] M. E. Pollack, et al., "Autoreminder: A Planning, Monitoring, and Reminding Assistive Agent," *Proceedings of the International Conference on Intelligent Autonomous Systems*, 2002.

[19] J. Pynoos, "Neglected Areas in Gerontology: Housing Adaptation," In *Panel Presentation at the Annual Scientific Meeting of the Gerontological Society of America*, 2002.

[20] J. Pynoos and V. Regnier, "Design Directives in Home Adaptation," In S. Lanspery and J. Hyde (Eds.), *Staying Put: Adapting the Places Instead of the People*, pp. 41-54, Baywood Pub. Co., 1997.

[21] J. Rissanen, *Stochastic Complexity in Statistical Inquiry* World Scientific Pub. Co., 1989.

[22] A. Roy, S. K. Bhaumik, A. Bhattacharya, K. Basu, D. J. Cook, and S. K. Das, "Location Aware Resource Management in Smart Homes," *Proceedings of First IEEE International Conference on Pervasive Computing and Communications* (PerCom'03), Ft Worth, Texas, pp. 481-488, Mar 2003.

[23] R. Srikant and R. Agrawal, "Mining Sequential Patterns: Generalizations and Performance Improvements," *Proceedings of the Fifth International Conference on Extending Database Technology*, 1996.

[24] M. C. Torrance, "Advances in Human-Computing Interaction: The Intelligent Room," *Proceedings of the Working Notes of the CHI'95 Research Symposium*, 1995.

[25] J. Ziv and A. Lempel, "Compression of Individual Sequences via Variable Rate Coding," *IEEE Transactions on Information Theory*, Vol. 24, pp. 530-536, 1978.

[26] I. K. Zola, "The Convergence of Aging and Disability," In S. Lanspery and J. Hyde (Eds.), *Staying Put: Adapting the Places Instead of the People*, pp. 25-40, Baywood Pub. Co., 1997.

Wireless Challenges for Mobile Robotic Tele-Echography System

F. Courreges*, R.S.H Istepanian*, Salem A. Garawi *

*MINT Research Centre, School of Computing and Information Systems, Kingston University, Kingston Upon Thames, UK

Keywords: 2.5/3G, GPRS, Telemedicine, Telerobotics, multimedia medical application, OTELO project.

Abstract In this paper we describe the 3G challenges for future m-health applications. M-health represents the new generation of wireless telemedicine system that deals with emerging mobile network systems for healthcare systems.
We also describe some of the limitations of existing 2.5G mobile system for a mobile robotic tele-echography system (OTELO - m**O**bile- **T**ele-**E**chography using an ultra-**L**ight r**O**bot). The aim is to search the best way to exploit the GPRS link for the OTELO medical application. The link capability and Quality of Service (QoS) issues are investigated for tele-robotic control and tele-echography image transmission over GPRS. This study correlated with some results of transmission of ultrasound still images, enabled us to define adapted operating modes of the OTELO system over GPRS.

1 Introduction

The next generation of "m-health technologies" is a new and evolving topic in the areas of telemedical and telecare systems. These technologies involve the exploitation of mobile telecommunication and multimedia technologies to provide better access to healthcare personnel on the move, by removing the key disadvantage of trailing wires in current systems. These technologies provide equal access to medical information and expert care by overcoming the boundaries of separation that exist today between different users of such medical information [1]. A great benefit to all users will be a more efficient use of resources and far greater location independence.

OTELO (m**O**bile- **T**ele-**E**chography using an ultra-**L**ight r**O**bot) is a European IST funded project [3] that develops a fully integrated end-to-end mobile tele-echography system for population groups that are not served locally, either temporarily or permanently, by medical ultrasound experts. It comprises a fully portable tele-operated robot allowing a specialist sonographer to perform a real-time robotised tele-echography to remote patients [2] [4]. Fig 1 shows the main operational blocks of the system. This Tele-echography system is composed of three main parts [3]:

- An « Expert » site where the medical expert interacts with a dedicated patented pseudo-haptic fictive probe instrumented to control the positioning of the remote robot and emulates an ultrasound probe that medical experts are used to handle, thus providing a better ergonomy.
- The communication media. We developed communication software based upon IP protocol to adapt to different communication means (ISDN, ADSL, LAN, Satellite, mobile…).
- A « Patient » site made up of the 6 degrees of freedom (DoF) light weight robotic system and its control unit -Fig 2.

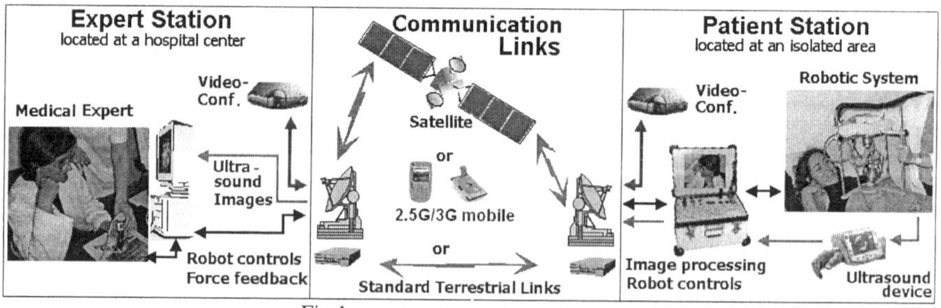

Fig 1 **The OTELO Mobile Robotic System**

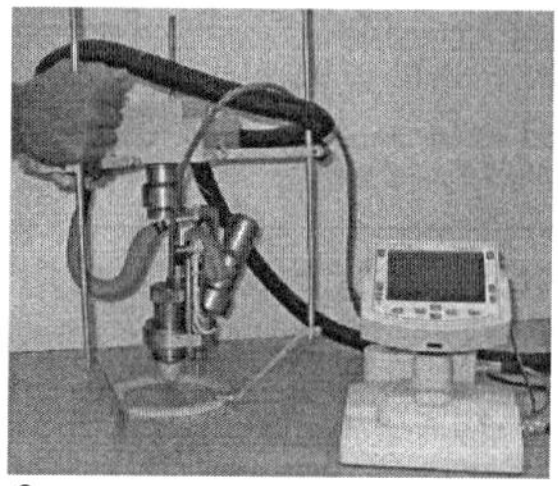
Fig 2 **OTELO Robot with the echograph Unit**

In this paper we specify medical operational modalities of OTELO and discuss the performance of the existing GPRS that can comply with mobile telemedical requirements of such system. The OTELO functional modalities and data flows requirements are explained in the following section. Section three presents briefly the QoS classes for GPRS and UMTS so as to identify how to fulfil the OTELO requirements. The fourth section presents some of the experimental results with ultrasound still images transmission over GPRS Channel, the final section is discussing the results.

2 OTELO functional modalities

2.1 Physical set-up on UMTS

OTELO is a mobile multimedia telemedicine application with different data traffic with different classes of QoS requirements. These have to be transmitted simultaneously. Figure 3 shows the physical settings of the OTELO system and the interface requirements with UMTS/UTRA.

The OTELO Expert Station may either link from the IP Multimedia Network or through the ISDN/ADSL.

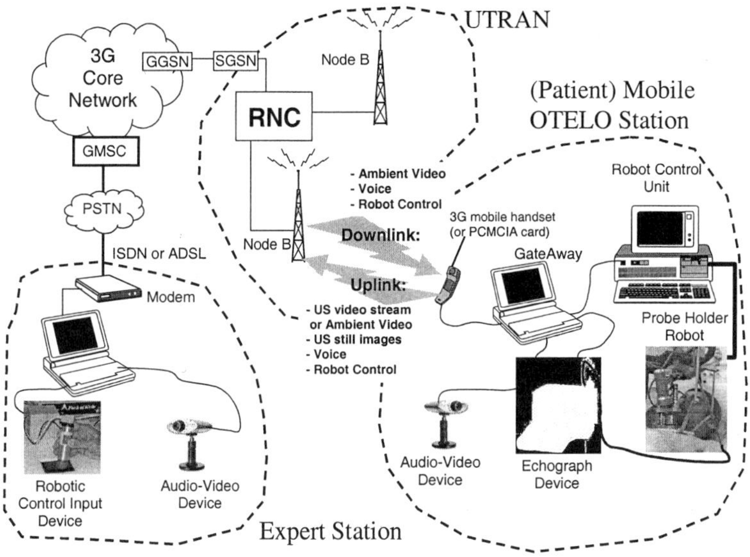

Figure 3 OTELO Scheme with UMTS, scenario with a fixed expert station and a mobile patient station

To support packet switching, two new nodes are required to modify the existing GSM network to support GPRS and UMTS radio packets [5]:

Serving GPRS Support Node (SGSN); This keeps track of the individual Mobile Station (MS) location, performs security functions and performs access control.

Gateway GSN (GGSN); Provides interworking with external packet-switched networks and connected with SGSN's via IP-based GPRS backbone networks. The data rates for OTELO system are shown in Table 1;

Table 1 OTELO medical data requirements and corresponding data rates

	Ultrasound video stream	Ultrasound still images	Ambient video stream	Voice	Robot control data
Flow direction	Simplex: Patient to Expert	Simplex: Patient to Expert	duplex	duplex	duplex
Transport protocol	RTP/UDP/IP	TCP/IP	RTP/ UDP/IP	RTP/UDP/IP	UDP/IP
Speed requirement	Real-time	Non Real-time	Real-time	Real-time	Real-time
Payload data rate requirement over the air-interface (without protocol headers)	15 frames/s @ 210 kbit/s Uplink	1 frame/ 10s Uplink	1 to 15 frame/s symmetricall y	9.0 kbit/s symmetrically	4.0-8.0 kbit/s symmetrically

As the ultrasound images are mostly transferred from the robot probe to the OTELO Master Station, the air interface, Uu, between the OTELO Patient Station and the Radio Network Controller (RNC) bears an asymmetric traffic load. The ultrasound image, ambient video & audio stream and robot control feedback data are sent over the uplink channel, whilst only the latter three types of data are transmitted over the downlink channel.

2.2 Robot Real-Time Control

Data rate for robot control indicated in table 1 is not related to a force reflected control [6], but to a unilateral position control. It means that thanks to an instrumented fictive probe, the position (3 angles and 3 Cartesian co-ordinates) of the medical expert hand is grabbed and sent periodically to the robot control unit as position set-points that are to be tracked by the robot., and no feedback control is provided through th communication link.
Since the change in orientation of the robot probe must be done in a continuous mode, and the velocity of these movements must be adjustable from the operating centre, the robot control data is very sensitive to time delay jitters [7].

In addition to be sensitive to jitters bilateral control is sensitive to time delay. Indeed recent researches show that a time delay of no more than 20ms remains acceptable for the teleoperation of a robot over the Internet [6]. It is important to promise a constant data rate for robot feedback control. If the robot control data is sharing the bandwidth with other types of data, such as videoconferencing images, etc. about 50% of the connection bandwidth should be assigned to robot control to keep the control loop active in case of haptic feedback. In comparison with TCP, connectionless protocols such as UDP, RTP (Real Time Protocol) or E-UDP (Enhanced UDP) are best suited to provide quicker data delivery. UDP has been chosen for the first prototype of OTELO.

2.3 Ultrasound Video Stream

Based on the quality of the received information, the expert controls the remote probe holder robot by using a dedicated input device and. This information is mainly ultrasound images, the position of the robot on the patient's body and the current position of his/her input device. The resulting hand-to-eye coordination enables the specialist to propose a pre-diagnosis.
Ultrasound images sequences can be processed following two approaches:

1) When the expert is searching for a specific organ (liver, kidney,...), high quality images may not be required: simple compression methods or lossy techniques can be applied. Therefore we use the H.263 (provisional ITU-T standard) video compression algorithms allowing streaming over low bit-rate link and using motion compensation.The lowest data rate acceptable to medical experts is 210kb/s with a frame update of 15 fps.
2) When the organ of interest is found and small displacements of the robot are appealed, it may be necessary to consider lossless compression techniques that would bring higher image quality to the expert. This lossless compression can be applied on the whole image or on the Region Of Interest (R.O.I.). This choice depends also on the characteristics of the chosen communication link. This option is still under work [8].

It shall be also taken into account that the round trip delay from the expert station between the robot commanded position and the received corresponding image should not exceed 300 ms for an ergonomic purpose.

Since the ultrasound video stream carries the medical information and it has the biggest need in throughput, it represents the most critical data flow for this application.

2.4 Ultrasound still images

During a second phase of examination, when the expert has found an accurate US slice to study, high-resolution ultrasound still images are needed. According to the available bandwidth on the communication link, a lossy (JPEGLS, JPEG-2000) or lossless reversible compression technique (e.g. Wavelets-LZH) is applied.
The size of the medical images varies from 256x256 pixels up to 512x512 pixels while the gray level of each pixel can be saved up to 16 bits. Files are encapsulated in a DICOM (Digital Imaging & Communications in Medicine) format for file storage and interoperability.

2.5 Videoconferencing

This information mainly deals with the ambient video and audio information and patient's reflex and video feedback to the OTELO video operation during the medical diagnosis procedure. The suggested frame rate for video transmission is 15 frame/s to minimum 1 frame/s. Color or B/W video can be chosen in transmission. Interactive compression standards, H.263 is considered here to transmit the real-time video.

3. OTELO Performance evaluation on Mobile Link

3.1 GPRS data rate and QoS

Theoretical maximum speeds of up to 171.2 kilobits per second (kbps) are achievable with GPRS using all eight timeslots at the same time. This is about three times as fast as the data transmission speeds possible over today's fixed telecommunications networks (eg. ISDN 64kbps) and ten times as fast as current Circuit Switched Data services on GSM networks. By allowing information to be transmitted more quickly, immediately and efficiently across the mobile network, GPRS may well be a relatively less costly mobile data service compared to SMS and Circuit Switched Data.

Achieving the theoretical maximum GPRS data transmission speed of 172.2 kbps would require a single user taking over all eight timeslots without any error protection. Clearly, it is unlikely that a network operator will allow all timeslots to be used by a single GPRS user. Additionally, the initial GPRS terminals are expected be severely limited- supporting only one, two or three timeslots. The bandwidth available to a GPRS user will therefore be limited. As such, the theoretical maximum GPRS speeds should be checked against the reality of constraints in the networks and terminals. The reality is that mobile networks are always likely to have lower data transmission speeds than fixed networks.

The Quality of Service QoS requirements of typical mobile packet data applications are very diverse (e.g., consider real-time multimedia, Web browsing, and e-mail transfer). Support of different QoS classes, which can be specified for each individual session, is therefore an important feature. GPRS allows defining QoS profiles using the parameters service precedence, rcliability, dclay, and throughput [9].

- The service precedence is the priority of a service in relation to another service. There exist three levels of priority: high, normal, and low.
- The reliability indicates the transmission characteristics required by an application. Three reliability classes are defined, which guarantee certain maximum values for

the probability of loss, duplication, mis-sequencing, and corruption (an undetected error) of packets.

- The delay parameters define maximum values for the mean delay and the 95-percentile delay. The delay is defined as the end-to-end transfer time between two communicating mobile stations or between a mobile station and the Gi interface to an external packet data network. This includes all delays within the GPRS network, e.g., the delay for request and assignment of radio resources and the transit delay in the GPRS backbone network. Transfer delays outside the GPRS network, e.g., in external transit networks, are not taken into account.
- The throughput specifies the maximum/peak bit rate and the mean bit rate.
  Using these QoS classes, QoS profiles can be negotiated between the mobile user and the network for each session, depending on the QoS demand and the current available resources.

4. Simulation results

Theoretical simulation based on approximating Vodafone GPRS network which is deploying at the present time CS-2 (coding scheme 2) has been carried out.
Ultrasound medial images compressed with JPEG2000 with different compression ratio are transmitted over the simulated GRPS channel to study and analyse the objective performance of the GPRS Up-link communication channel in terms of the transmission time delay and the average throughput in different bandwidth and channel conditions.

Two bandwidth setting has been experimented; first at 53.6 Kbps (equivalent to four Time Slot) as shown in Fig 4 and 13.4 Kbps (equivalent to one Time Slots) as in Fig 5 below;

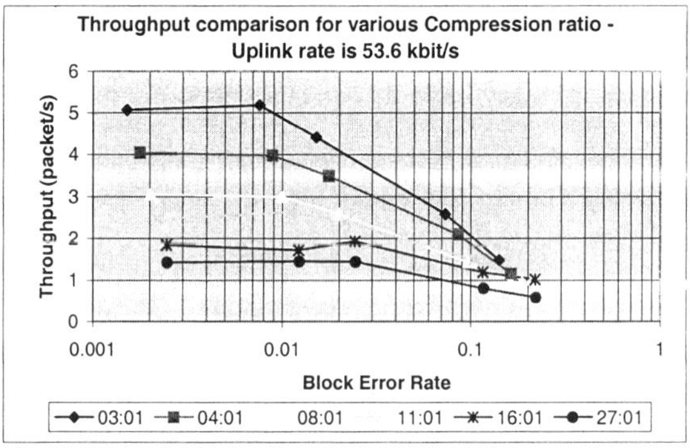

Figure 4 the Packet throughput with respect to the Block Error Rate (BLER) on 53.6 Kbps Uplink Channel

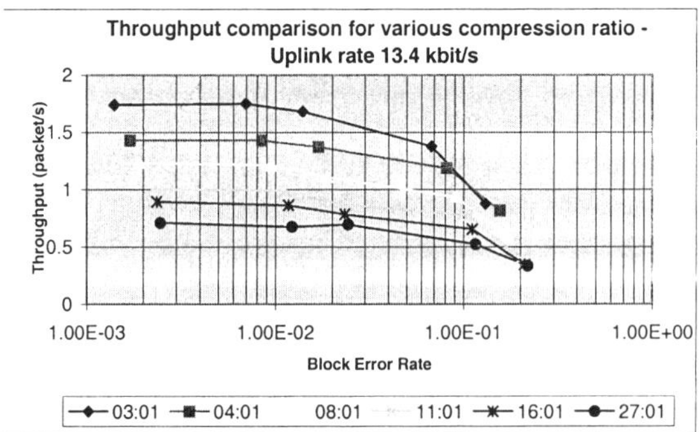

Figure 5 the Packet throughput with respect to the Block Error Rate (BLER) on 13.4 Kbps Uplink Channel

The simulated results show that;

- Compression ratio of the transmitted Images is directly effecting the transmission time, average throughput and the ratio of the TCP number of packets needed to complete the transmission.
- Higher data rate achieved at lower compression ratio.
- Increasing the data rate of the channel to 53.6 Kbps (4 timeslots), enhance the possibility of justifying further investigation of the GPRS capability to fulfil OTELO end-to-end user requirements.
- The issue of (ROI) Region of Interest within the Ultrasound image, can be considered to reduce the transmitted image size. About 200 x 200 pixels might be enough for clinical diagnosis.

In order to overcome the limitation of the Uplink bandwidth, the Ambient video data and the Ultrasound Data produced by the Patient station, should not be transmitted simultaneously.

5. Discussion

The following conclusions about adopting GPRS as a communication link for OTELO system are:

1. From the simulation studies we can conclude that GPRS system is capable of transmitting good quality still US images up to data rate of 53.6kbps with proper JPEG2000 compression ratios.
2. For the ambient information (videoconferencing stream), the current data rates WILL NOT be suitable for acceptable performance. One possible method is to transmit the robot control data and good quality still US image with GPRS whilst transmitting videoconferencing stream with HSCSD.
3. Although technically the OTELO GPRS scheme is feasible, financially, the tariff the network operators make will be vital for adopting OTELO GPRS scheme. According to current tariffs that most of the network operator released in UK, the cost of using GPRS network will be even more expensive than using satellite links which will definitely not be competitive.

If we need and have no choice but to deal with the existing or available communication network infrastructure for the rural areas, which is the heart idea of OTELO project, then mobile link through GPRS network might be able to do the job or part of it until UMTS services and coverage become reality and beyond the commercial barrier.

Acknowledgment
We are grateful to the European Union for support for this project (EU IST-2001-32516 project “OTELO: Integrated, end-to-end, mobile tele-echography system”). We are also

grateful to D. Phil Gousset and Mr. Haris Zisimopoulos of Vodafone Research (UK) for providing access to their Labs and facilities for examining our test matrix.

References

[1] R. Istepanian, C.S.Pattichis, E.Kyriacou, S. Voskarides, "Wireless Telemedicine Systems: an overview," *IEEE Antenna's Propagation Magazine,* Vol. 44, No. 2, April 2002.

[2] G. Kontaxakis, G. Sakas, S. Walter, "Mobile Tele-Echography Systems – TELEINVIVO: Acase study," *co ngnitive Computing and Medical Imaging, Fraunhofer Institute for Computer Graphics (IGD), Fraunhoferstr. 5, Darmstadt, Germany D-64283, E-mail:* gsakas@igd.fhg.de.

[3] OTELO Project, "Description of scientific/technology objectives & work plan," Part–B. OTELO Project internal paper, OTELO Proposal No. IST-2001-32516, April 2001.

[4] Vilchis, J. Troccaz, P. Cinquin, F. Courreges, G. Poisson, and B. Tondu: *Robotic Tele-Ultrasound System (TER) : Slave Robot Control.* 1st IFAC Conference on Telematics Application in Automation and Robotics, Weingarten, Allemagne 24-26 **2001**, pp95-100.

[5] Pavlopoulos, S.; Kyriacou, E.; Berler, A.; Dembeyiotis, S.; Koutsouris, D., A novel emergency telemedicine system based on wireless communication technology-AMBULANCE, *IEEE Transactions on Information Technology in Biomedicine, Vol. 2 NO. 4 DECEMBER 1998, pp 261-267.*

[6] Robertto Oboe, "Web-Interfaced, Forced-Reflecting Teleoperation Systems," *IEEE Transactions on Industrial Electronics,* Vol. 48, No. 6, pp. 1257-1265, Dec. 2001.

[7] K. Masuda, E. Kimura, K. Ishihara, N. Tateishi, Y. Suzuki, "Robotic Tele-diagnosis System of Echography & Wireless Experiment for Mobile Telemedicine," *in Proceeding of the second joint EMBS/BMES Conf.* Houston, TX USA, pp. 23-26, October 2002.

[8] Consortium Otelo, *OTELO : mObile Tele-Echography using an ultra-Light rObot,* http://www.bourges.univ-orleans.fr/otelo/, 2001-2004.

[9] R.Gilabert, M. Vannoni, F. Courreges, C. Delgorge, C. Novales, G. Poisson, P. Vieyres, C. Bru, *Clinical Validation of a tele-operated mobile ultrasound scanner using a leight weight robot (OTELO project).* ECR 2004, European Congress of Radiology, Poster, Vienna, Austria, 5-9 mars **2004.**

Chapter 1

Human-Machine Interface

User Profile Merging Based on Total Distance Minimization

Zhiwen YU[1], Xingshe ZHOU[1], Yanbin HAO[2], and Jianhua GU[1]
1. School of Computer Science, Northwestern Polytechnical University
Xi'an, P.R.China, 710072
yuzhiwen77@yahoo.com.cn, zhouxs@nwpu.edu.cn, gujh@nwpu.edu.cn
2. Management School, Northwestern Polytechnical University, Xi'an, P.R.China, 710072
haoyanbin-000@sohu.com

Abstract. For more and more programs today's television can receive, and the reality that television is often viewed by groups of people, such as a family or a student dormitory, smart TV that can recommend programs for multiple viewers is required eagerly. In this paper, we propose a recommendation scheme that merges individual user profiles to form a common user profile, and then generates common recommendation according to the common user profile. The user profile merging strategy is based on total distance minimization. We are the first to introduce distance concepts into measure difference among user profiles. The total distance minimization guarantees that the merged result could close to most users' preferences. The experimental results proved that the merging result actually reflects most members' preferences of the group.

1. Introduction*

The rapid growth of communication technologies and the invention of set-top-box (STB) and personal digital recorder (PDR) have enabled today's television to receive and store tremendous programs. The abundance of TV programs precipitates a need for smart "recommenders" to help people obtain programs that they really want to watch. To fulfill this requirement, many personalized TV systems have been built to assist individual users in filtering and recommending programs by adapting to their respective personal preferences.

However, for social custom and economic reasons, television is often a common equipment in both private and public areas, e.g., a family or a student dormitory. The television is usually viewed by multiple members of the groups sitting together. So the TV recommendation system should not only provide personalized programs for individuals, but also can recommend programs to multiple viewers taking care of most members' preferences, in the case the viewers are watching TV at the same time, and in the same spot. The existing TV recommendation systems have not proposed solutions to address this issue. A possible solution is to merge individual user profiles to form a common user profile, then generate common recommendation according to the common user profile. This paper proposes an user profile merging algorithm that is based on total distance minimization.

The rest of this paper is organized as follows. Section 2 discusses previous relevant work with this paper. Section 3 describes the user profile merging scheme, which is based on total distance minimization. The evaluation methodology and results are presented in

* This work was supported by the National Science Foundation of China, and the Doctorate Foundation of Northwestern Polytechnical University of China.

Section 4. Finally, Section 5 concludes the paper.

2. Relevant Work

Much work has been done in the area of TV program personalization. Several personalized TV systems have been built in recent years to help users deal with the overabundant TV programs, such as TV3P[1], multi-agent TV recommender [2], TV-Advisor [3], PTV [4], P-EPG [5]. But none of them have proposed solutions to recommend programs for multiple viewers. A possible solution is to merge individual user profiles to form a common user profile, then generate common recommendation according to the common user profile. For user profile merging, existing related research work were "merge knowledge bases" and "information fusion".

"Merge knowledge bases" means how to merge different sources of information in the fields of databases and artificial intelligence, which is called by Liberatore and Schaerf as *arbitration*. In [6] they proposed a set of postulates and actual operators for arbitration. Alchourron, Gärdenfors and Makinson [7] proposed AGM postulates that any operator revising a knowledge should satisfy. Katsuno and Mendelzon [8] introduced KM postulates to model the process of updating a knowledge base. In general, the objective of above research is to seek principles for guarantee completeness and consistency during the merging process. Although these theories are partially mature, they are rarely adopted in real applications.

Another related research subject is "information fusion", which means knowledge or information fusion from multiple data sources, eg., multi-sensor data. There are several techniques for this fusion operation, such as Baysian Inference, Dempster-Shafer, Neural Network, Fuzzy Logic, etc. These algorithms are mainly applied in fault detection and diagnosis [9], prognostics and health management [10], and decision making [11], etc.. These techniques are computationally expensive. They are not practical to implement in television systems with limited sources and capability.

Our merging strategy is based on total distance minimization. We are the first to introduce distance concepts into measure difference among user profiles. The total distance minimization guarantees that the merged result could close to most users' preferences.

3. User Profile Merging Algorithm

The user profile merging algorithm merges individual profiles so as to form a common user profile, trying to reflect most and consistent preferences of the group. In this section, we first describe the merging scheme, then in the end, we give an example to demonstrate the merging process.

3.1 Universal Vector Representation

In each user profile, there are many features. We gather all the features from user profiles by alphabet as a lexicon, and represent it as a vector.

$$Lexicon = (feature_1, feature_2, \dots, feature_n) \tag{1}$$

With the lexicon vector, we can define each user profile universally as a vector V :

$$V = (f_1, f_2, \dots, f_n) \tag{2}$$

V is a vector with n (total number of terms in above lexicon) items, where f_i is the value assigned to corresponding $feature_i$ $(1 \le i \le n)$ in the lexicon vector. Supposing user's feature weight belongs to [-1, 1], of which '–1' means dislike at most, '1' means like at most, the value f_i is assigned complying with the following rules:

- Rule (i): if $feature_i$ is included in the user profile and its weight is positive or zero, then f_i=1;
- Rule (ii): if $feature_i$ is included in the user profile and its weight is negative, then f_i=-1;
- Rule (iii): if $feature_i$ is not included in the user profile, then f_i=0.

3.2 Definition of Merging Result

In [12], Dalal proposed distance concept for belief revision. We adopt Dalal distance to measure the inconsistentness between two user preferences, and define the merging result.

Definition 5: Distance between two bits (x and y), d(x, y), $x \in \{1, 0, -1\}$, $y \in \{1, 0, -1\}$, d(1, 0)=d(0, 1)=d(0, -1)=d(-1, 0)=1, d(1, 1)=d(0, 0)=d(-1, -1)=0, d(1, -1)=d(-1, 1)=2.

Definition 6: Distance between two user profiles (U_i and U_j), $D_u(U_i, U_j)$, $D_u(U_i, U_j)=D(V_i, V_j)=\sum_{k=1}^{n} d(a_k, b_k)$, $a_k \in V_i$, $b_k \in V_j$, V_i and V_j denote respective vector of U_i and U_j.

Definition 7: Ψ_n is the set of all vectors composed of n elements, each of them belongs to {1, 0, -1}.

Definition 8: Suppose that $V_1, V_2, \ldots, V_N$, and $V \in \Psi_n$, the merging result of $V_1, V_2, \ldots, V_N$ is V. It satisfies $\forall B\{B \in \Psi_n\}$, $\sum_{i=1}^{N} D(V_i, V) \le \sum_{i=1}^{N} D(V_i, B)$, that is the total distance is minimum.

3.3 Merging Procedure

The merging procedure consists of two steps. The first step is feature selection, whose task is to determine whether a feature should be included in the target common user profile. As we know, each user profile may have a lot of features. The total number of features occur in all user profiles may be very large. So we should select part of them to represent common interest. The second step is weight assignment, which means how much weight should be assigned to a selected feature. The schematic structure of profile merging is shown as Fig. 1.

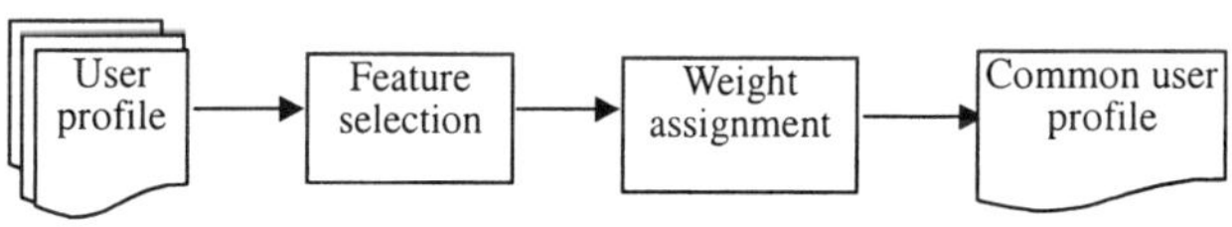

Fig. 1. Schematic structure of profile merging

3.3.1 Feature Selection

Feature selection is based on total distance minimization. For each element of the target vector (merging result), choosing which one from {1, 0, -1} as its value depends on whether it makes the total distance minimum.

Theorem 1: Given N user profile vectors. Each vectors has only one element, $V_i=\{a_i\}$, (i=1, 2, ..., N, $a_i \in \{1, 0, -1\}$). We define c_1 as the total times of '1' occurs in the vectors; c_0 as the total times of '0' occurs in the vectors; c_{-1} as the total times of '-1' occurs in the vectors. Under Definition 5-8, the merging result of the N vectors is:

$$\text{Merging result (V)}=\begin{cases} 0 & \text{if } c_1+c_{-1}<c_0+2c_1 \text{ and } c_1+c_{-1}<c_0+2c_{-1} \\ \pm 1 \text{ or } 0 & \text{if } c_1+c_{-1}=c_0+2c_1=c_0+2c_{-1} \\ 0 \text{ or } -1 & \text{if } c_1+c_{-1}=c_0+2c_1 \text{ and } c_1+c_{-1}<c_0+2c_{-1} \\ 0 \text{ or } 1 & \text{if } c_1+c_{-1}<c_0+2c_1 \text{ and } c_1+c_{-1}=c_0+2c_{-1} \\ \pm 1 & \text{else} \end{cases} \quad (3)$$

Proof: According to Definition 5, the total distance of '1' to the N vectors is c_0+2c_{-1}; the total distance of '0' to the N vectors is c_1+c_{-1}; and the total distance of '-1' to the N vectors is c_0+2c_1. If $c_1+c_{-1}< c_0+2c_1$ and $c_1+c_{-1}< c_0+2c_{-1}$, according to Definition 8, the merging result whose total distance should minimize, is 0. Similarly, if $c_1+c_{-1}= c_0+2c_1= c_0+2c_{-1}$, the merging result is ± 1 or 0; if $c_1+c_{-1}= c_0+2c_1$ and $c_1+c_{-1}< c_0+2c_{-1}$, the merging result is 0 or -1; if $c_1+c_{-1}< c_0+2c_1$ and $c_1+c_{-1}= c_0+2c_{-1}$, the merging result is 0 or 1; else the merging result is ± 1. □

In the cases of $c_1+c_{-1}= c_0+2c_1= c_0+2c_{-1}$, $c_1+c_{-1}= c_0+2c_1$ and $c_1+c_{-1}< c_0+2c_{-1}$, $c_1+c_{-1}< c_0+2c_1$ and $c_1+c_{-1}= c_0+2c_{-1}$, the result is not certain. For these cases, we set the merging result as ± 1. So Theorem 1 can be revised as:

Theorem R1: Given N user profile vectors. Each vectors has only one element, $V_i=\{a_i\}$, (i=1, 2, ..., N, $a_i \in \{1, 0, -1\}$). We define c_1 as the total times of '1' occurs in the vectors; c_0 as the total times of '0' occurs in the vectors; c_{-1} as the total times of '-1' occurs in the vectors. Under Definition 5-8, the merging result of the N vectors is:

$$\text{Merging result (V)}=\begin{cases} 0 & \text{if } c_1+c_{-1}<c_0+2c_1 \text{ and } c_1+c_{-1}<c_0+2c_{-1} \\ \pm 1 & \text{else} \end{cases} \quad (4)$$

Theorem 2: Given N user profile vectors. Each vectors has K elements, $V_i=\{a_1, a_2, \ldots, a_j, \ldots, a_K\}$, (i=1, 2, ..., N, $a_j \in \{1, 0, -1\}$). V is the merging result of these N vectors. Each element of V is the merging result of corresponding element of $V_1, V_2, \ldots, V_N$.

Proof: The K-element vectors $V_1, V_2, \ldots, V_N$ are represented as follows:

V_1: $\{a_{11}, a_{12}, \ldots, a_{1j}, \ldots, a_{1K}\}$
V_2: $\{a_{21}, a_{22}, \ldots, a_{2j}, \ldots, a_{2K}\}$
...
V_N: $\{a_{N1}, a_{N2}, \ldots, a_{Nj}, \ldots, a_{NK}\}$
V: $\{a_1, a_2, \ldots, a_j, \ldots, a_K\}$

a_{ij} denotes the j-th element of the i-th vector. V is the merging result.

Now, calculate the total distance (TD) of vector V to $V_1, V_2, \ldots, V_N$:

$$TD=\sum D(V_i,V) = D(V_1, V) + D(V_2, V) + \ldots + D(V_i, V) + \ldots + D(V_N, V) \quad (i=1,2\ldots N)$$
$$=\sum d(a_{1j},a_j)+\sum d(a_{2j},a_j)+\ldots+\sum d(a_{Nj},a_j) \quad (j=1,2\ldots K)$$
$$=\sum d(a_{i1},a_1)+\sum d(a_{i2},a_2)+\ldots+\sum d(a_{iK},a_K) \quad (i=1,2\ldots N)$$

Obviously, if we make $\sum d(a_{ij},a_j)$ minimum, TD can be minimum. $\sum d(a_{ij},a_j)$ is the total distance of the j-th element in V to corresponding element (that is, the j-th element) in $V_1, V_2, \ldots, V_N$. So Theorem 2 is proofed. □

We can select features to form the common user profile according to Theorem R1 and Theorem 2. If the value of the j-th element of V is ± 1, we mean selecting the corresponding feature (the j-th feature in the lexicon vector). If the value of the j-th element of V is 0, we mean discarding the corresponding feature. In Section 3.4, we will give an example to illustrate the selection process.

3.3.2 Weight Assignment

We should not assign weight to a selected feature by simply doing sum of all weights of it in individual user's profile. The reason is that the same weight value in different user's profile often means different importance. For instance, 0.8 in Tom's profile means the feature is the favorite feature, but in Jack's profile, it is just so so, not implying very interesting. In other words, weights in different user profiles are not obtained with universal measurement. So we should do normalization for them firstly.

(1) Weight normalization

For each user profile,

First, find out the weight, whose absolute value is maximum in the user profile,

$$w_{\max} = \max\ (|\ w_1\ |, |\ w_2\ |, \ldots, |\ w_i\ |, \ldots, |\ w_j\ |) \tag{5}$$

where j is total number of features in the user profile; w_i is feature_i's weight.

Then, the original weight can be *normalized* to its normalized value,

$$w_i' = \frac{w_i}{w_{\max}} \tag{6}$$

where w_i' is the normalized value of w_i. Such normalized value is always on a standard universe, say [-1, 1].

(2) Weight calculation

For each selected feature,

$$Weight_i = \frac{\sum_{j=1}^{m} w_{ij}'}{m} \tag{7}$$

where $Weight_i$ is the weight assigned to $feature_i$ in the target user profile, w_{ij}' is the normalized weight value of $feature_i$ in the j-th user profile. There are totally *m* user profiles containing $feature_i$. The *m*-mean makes the weight values of selected features into the range [-1, 1].

3.4 Example

Supposing there are 5 user profiles, named U_1, U_2, U_3, U_4, and U_5, the profiles are shown as Table 1. The merging process is as follows.

Step 1: First, represent user profiles as (feature, weight) vectors.

U_1=((A, -0.3), (C, 0.8), (D, -0.7), (E, -0.6), (H, 0.9), (I, -0.2), (J, 0.6), (N, 0.4), (P, 0.3))

U_2=((A, 0.7), (B, -0.9), (D, 0.3), (E, 0.5), (F, -0.8), (K, -0.2), (N, 0.5), (O, -0.3))

U_3=((A, 0.3), (D, -0.4), (E, 0.2), (H, 0.5), (J, 0.7), (K, -0.1), (L, -0.4), (M, 0.8))

U_4=((A, 0.2), (D, -0.3), (E, 0.6), (H, 0.8), (I, -0.3), (J, 0.5), (K, 0.7), (M, -0.3))

U_5=((C, 0.7), (E, -0.8), (F, 0.4), (G, 0.8), (J, -0.2), (K, -0.2), (L, -0.4), (N, 0.7), (O, 0.6))

Step 2: Construct the lexicon.

Lexicon={A, B, C, D, E, F, G, H, I, J, K, L, M, N, O, P}

Table 1: User profile examples

U_1		U_2		U_3		U_4		U_5	
Feature	Weight	Feature	Weight	Feature	Weight	Feature	Weight	Feature	Weight
A	-0.3	A	0.7	A	0.3	A	0.2	C	0.7
C	0.8	B	-0.9	D	-0.4	D	-0.3	E	-0.8
D	-0.7	D	0.3	E	0.2	E	0.6	F	0.4
E	-0.6	E	0.5	H	0.5	H	0.8	G	0.8
H	0.9	F	-0.8	J	0.7	I	-0.3	J	-0.2
I	-0.2	K	-0.2	K	-0.1	J	0.5	K	-0.2
J	0.6	N	0.5	L	-0.4	K	0.7	L	-0.4
N	0.4	O	-0.3	M	0.8	M	-0.3	N	0.7
P	0.3							O	0.6

Step 3: Construct the universal vector for each user profile, shown as Table 2.

Table 2: Universal vector

	A	B	C	D	E	F	G	H	I	J	K	L	M	N	O	P
V_1	-1	0	1	-1	-1	0	0	1	-1	1	0	0	0	1	0	1
V_2	1	-1	0	1	1	-1	0	0	0	0	-1	0	0	1	-1	0
V_3	1	0	0	-1	1	0	0	1	0	1	-1	-1	1	0	0	0
V_4	1	0	0	-1	1	0	0	1	-1	1	1	0	-1	0	0	0
V_5	0	0	1	0	-1	1	1	0	0	-1	-1	-1	0	1	1	0

Step 4: Select feature

According to Theorem R1 and Theorem 2, for feature A, $c_0=1$, $c_1=3$, $c_{-1}=1$, since $c_1+c_{-1}>c_0+2c_{-1}$, merging result of feature A, V(A)= ± 1. For feature B, $c_0=4$, $c_1=0$, $c_{-1}=1$, since $c_1+c_{-1}<c_0+2c_1$ and $c_1+c_{-1}<c_0+2c_{-1}$, merging result of feature B, V(B)=0. Similarly, we can get V(C)=0, V(D)=± 1, V(E)=± 1, V(F)=0, V(G)=0, V(H)=± 1, V(I)=0, V(J)=± 1, V(K)=± 1, V(L)=0, V(M)=0, V(N)=± 1, V(O)=0, V(P)=0. That is, the merging result V=(± 1, 0, 0, ± 1, ± 1, 0, 0, ± 1, 0, ± 1, ± 1, 0, 0, ± 1, 0, 0). So the target common user profile contains the following features: A, D, E, H, J, K, and N.

Step 5: Normalize the weight

For U_1, since feature A, D, E, H, J, and N are included in the target user profile, we should normalize the weights of these features. In U_1, the weight whose absolute value is maximum is 0.9, so

$w'(A)$ =-0.3/0.9=-0.3333

$w'(D)$ =-0.7/0.9=-0.7778

$w'(E)$ =-0.6/0.9=-0.6667

$w'(H)$ =0.9/0.9=1

$w'(J)$ =0.6/0.9=0.6667

$w'(N)$ =0.6/0.9=0.6667

Similarly, we can do normalization for U_2, U_3, U_4, and U_5.

Step 6: Calculate the target weight

For feature "A" in the target user profile, it occurs in U_1, U_2, U_3, and U_4.

$$Weight(A) = \frac{-0.3333 + 0.7778 + 0.375 + 0.25}{4} = 0.2674$$

Similarly, we can obtain $Weight(D) = -0.3299$, $Weight(E) = -0.0222$, $Weight(H) = 0.875$, $Weight(J) = 0.4792$, $Weight(K) = 0.2778$, $Weight(N) = 0.6991$.

Step 7: Generate the target common user profile

So the common user profile, U_{Common}=((A, 0.2674), (D, -0.3299), (E, -0.0222), (H, 0.875), (J, 0.4792), (K, 0.2778), (N, 0.6991)).

4. Experimental Results

Since there is no existing similar systems before, and no benchmark for performance testing, evaluation of this system is very difficult. In order to test the efficacy of our system, we have designed an evaluation method and made corresponding experiments. The evaluation methodology is depicted as follows.

(i) Get a group of viewers;

(ii) Merge their profiles to generate a common user profile;

(iii) Show programs to the group, and use a learning approach to capture the group's preferences.

(iv) Compare the results (feature weights merged and feature weights learned) by using standard deviation (SD) indicated as formula (8). The smaller SD is, the better performance the strategy has.

$$SD = \sqrt{\frac{1}{n}\sum_{i=1}^{n}(weightMerged_i - weightLearned_i)^2} \quad (8)$$

The interface for multiple viewers to login to the system is shown in Fig. 2. In this scenario, five members of the family intended to login and watch TV together.

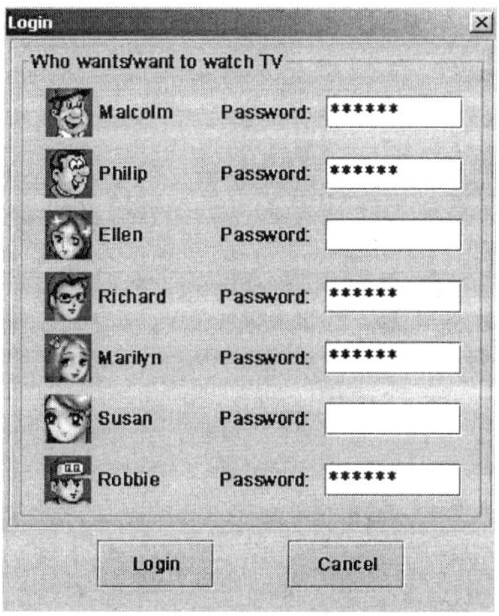

Fig. 2: Interface for multi-user login

We took top 10 features in the merged common user profile, and compared with corresponding weights in the learned profile. The results are shown in Table 3. The value of SD is 0.2648. From the results, we can see that the weights of top 4 features in the merged common user profile are very close to those in the learned user profile, while the weights of last features vary largely. The reason is that in the learning process, no program involves the feature "Discovery" and "Robert Zemeckis". We believe that if the period of learning process is sufficient, and the number of testing programs is as large as possible, the performance could be fine.

Table 3: Experimental results

Feature name	Weight merged	Weight learned
Soccer	0.9996	0.9547
Stephen Chow	0.9354	0.8751
Diego Maradona	0.8788	0.97
Comedy	0.725	0.6593
Tom Hanks	0.7216	0.5082
Zinedine Zidane	0.70	0.9371
Romance	0.6667	0.4893
Discovery	0.538	0.0
Britney	0.5112	0.3601
Robert Zemeckis	0.4875	0.0

5. Conclusion

In this paper, we presented an user profile merging algorithm that is based on total distance minimization, which guarantees that the merged result could close to most users' preferences. Two theorems are proposed and proved for feature selection, which simplifies the process of finding the target vector, and leads the system feasible and efficient. The experimental results are encouraging, which proved that the merging result actually reflects TV program watching preferences of the group.

References

[1] Zhiwen Yu and Xingshe Zhou. "TV3P: An Adaptive Assistant for Personalized TV". *IEEE Transactions on Consumer Electronics*. Vol. 50, No. 1, Feb. 2004, pp. 393-399

[2] K. Kurapati, S. Gutta, D. Schaffer, J. Martino and J. Zimmerman. "A Multi-Agent TV Recommender". In *Proceedings of the User Modeling 2001: Personalization in Future TV Workshop*, Sonthofen, Germany, 2001.

[3] Das, D. and ter Horst, H. "Recommender Systems for TV". In *Proceedings of AAAI*, 1998.

[4] Cotter, P., and Smyth, B., "PTV: Personalised TV Guides". In *Proceedings of the 12th Conference on Innovative Applications of Artificial Intelligence, IAAI 2000*, Austin, Texas, 2000.

[5] M. Ehrmantraut, T. Härder, H. Wittig and R. Steinmetz. "The Personal Electronic Program Guide --Towards the Pre-selection of Individual TV Programs". In *Proceedings of 5th International Conference on Information and Knowledge Management (CIKM'96)*, Rockville, MD., 1996, pp. 243-250.

[6] P. Liberatore and M. Schaerf. "Arbitration (or How to Merge Knowledge Bases)". *IEEE Transactions on Knowledge and Data Engineering*. 1998, vol 10(1): 76-90

[7] Alchourron, C., Gardenfors, P., & Makinson, D. "On the logic of theory change: Partial meet contraction functions and their associated revision functions". *Journal of Symbolic Logic*, vol 50: pp510-530, 1985.

[8] H. Katsuno and A. Mendelzon. "On the difference between updating a knowledge base and revising it". *In Proceedings of 2nd International Conference on Principles of Knowledge Representation and Reasoning* (KR' 91), pp387-394, 1991.

[9] Qinzu Xu and Zhanghong Yue. "Information fusion method in fault detection and diagnosis". In *Proceedings of the IEEE International Conference on Industrial Technology*, pp. 472 – 475, 5-9 December, Guangzhou China, 1994

[10] Roemer, M.J., Kacprzynski, G.J., and Orsagh, R.F. "Assessment of data and knowledge fusion strategies for prognostics and health management". In *Proceedings of the IEEE Conference on Aerospace*, Vol (6): 2979 - 2988, 10-17 March, Big Sky, MT USA, 2001

[11] Yongmian Zhang, Qiang Ji, and Looney, C.G. "Active information fusion for decision making under uncertainty". In *Proceedings of the Fifth International Conference on Information Fusion*, vol.1, pp. 643 – 650, 8-11 July 2002

[12] M.Dalal. "Updates in propositional databases". Technical report, Rutgers University, 1988.

Using Vehicular Communication to Support Older Drivers at Road Intersections: A Feasibility Study

Nahid SHAHMEHRI, Ioan CHISALITA, Johan ABERG,
Dennis MACIUSZEK, Marie HELLQVIST
Department of Computer and Information Science
Linköping University, S-581 83, Linköping, Sweden

Abstract. More and more people are living to old age, and it is usually a desire among elderly to sustain mobility. Unfortunately, the crash rate of older adults is much larger than for other drivers. Older drivers are also more likely to get serious injuries that lead to disability or death. Therefore, technological contributions for improving traffic safety and preserve mobility of older people are important. One new promising approach is to use traffic safety systems based on vehicular communication, where vehicles exchange warning messages. This paper evaluates the feasibility of using such vehicular communication for supporting older drivers in road intersections, which is the most common accident setting for older drivers. Using a temporal reasoning systems (ECAM) this accident setting is analyzed in depth, and the potential for accident avoidance is quantified, while taking into account several relevant factors such as speed, driver reaction time, and transmission delay for warning messages. The results indicate the high potential of vehicular communication, and highlights requirements on transmission delay.

1. Introduction

Due to societal improvements in health-care, living standards, and socio-economic status, more and more people are living to old age [21]. It is usually a desire among elderly to sustain mobility and continue with their daily activities, such as driving, and thus remain independent [18]. However, statistics show that the crash rate of older adults is considerably larger than that of other drivers [9]. Older drivers are also more likely than other drivers to get serious injuries that lead to disability or death [15]. Therefore there are great opportunities for technological contributions with respect to improving traffic safety while preserving the mobility of older people.

In this paper we focus on a particular accident type of great importance, namely the road intersection accident, which is the most common accident type for drivers of old age [10]. We analyze in depth to what extent traffic safety systems based on vehicular communication can help to avoid this type of accident. Using warning messages sent between nearby vehicles or from base stations located at the side of the road, these safety systems has the potential of overcoming the limitations of safety systems relying only on sensors placed on the vehicle. More specifically, we use a temporal reasoning system (ECAM) for analyzing the impact of information transfer properties (transmission delay of warning messages), driver characteristics (reaction time), and accident scenario characteristics (e.g. speed), on collision avoidance. The results indicate the strong potential of safety systems based on vehicular communication for helping older drivers maintain safe driving in road intersections.

The rest of this paper is structured as follows. In section 2 we analyze older drivers and the accident risks they face. In section 3 we give an overview of traffic safety systems, followed by a detailed description of the road intersection accident scenario in section 4. In section 5 we describe our simulation experiments and present the results. This is followed by a discussion in section 6. In section 7 we describe related work on traffic simulators, and in section 8 we conclude the paper.

2. Older drivers and accidents

Accident statistics reveal that the accident risk for elderly drivers is higher than for other age groups [20]. These statistics indicate that most of the accidents involving older drivers happen in complex traffic situations such as road intersections [4]. People of old age are a highly heterogeneous group. Still, there is general agreement that several functions important for driving behavior tend to degenerate with increased age among older people. These functions are related to cognitive and motor capabilities [4]. Cognitive functions affect a person's intellectual abilities including perception, memory, problem solving ability, space orientation, information management, and attention. Research on driving-related problems has focused on perception, which has been shown to have a strong relationship to accident occurrences [4,19]. In addition, older drivers are slower at handling information when it comes to making difficult decisions. They have difficulties maintaining all the needed information for making decisions due to deterioration in attention and memory. When they act on the information they have gathered, they are slower than what the situation may demand. When it comes to visual perception, it has been found that older people have increased difficulties to perceive impulses from their surroundings. For traffic situations, they have difficulties determining speed and distances. The decay of motor capabilities for older people implies a decrease in movement range, and reaction time [16]. This causes problems for head movements for gathering visual information from the sides, and for handling of pedals, steering wheel, gears, but also for making the coordination work.

To help old people maintain safe driving, it is important to investigate the development of traffic safety systems for accident avoidance.

3. Traffic safety systems

Safety systems can be classified into *passive* and *active* systems [12]. Passive systems, such as anti-lock breaks and seat belts, react to dangerous situations, trying to help the driver avoiding an accident, or reducing the consequences of an accident. However, such passive systems are inherently limited in the sense that they are not designed to hinder a dangerous situation to develop in the first place.

Active systems, such as adaptive cruise control, are designed to proactively prevent vehicles from colliding with each other or with other objects. They collect and analyze information extracted from the local environment surrounding a vehicle, through sensors or video cameras to identify dangers in traffic [1, 3]. The active safety systems act towards avoiding accidents by warning the driver about a potential danger, and can eventually employ automatic actions such as emergency braking. Such systems can be categorized according to the type of support provided to the driver as [11]:

- *Information delivery systems*: These systems present the driver with information that can increase his/her situation awareness and let the driver take the appropriate measures.

- *Automatic control systems*: These systems aim at providing more support to the driver by employing automatic actions. However, attention needs to be given to the transfer of tasks from humans to vehicles, since unknown problems may arise.

Three technologies were mainly considered for implementing active safety systems: radar and laser sensor systems, computer vision, and communication systems [12]. Active safety systems that employ sensors usually use radar and lidar devices (i.e. sensor based on laser) for detecting obstacles that exist around a vehicle and may interfere with its travelling path. Active safety systems that employ computer vision also perform detection of possible dangerous obstacles existing around a vehicle by using stereo cameras. These systems are also employed for monitoring the movement of a vehicle by analyzing its position with regard to road elements such as lane markers. However, relying on data from local sensors or cameras is an inherent drawback of these systems. This severely limits their utility for detecting objects that are not in line of sight, such as vehicles entering an intersection [17]. A potential solution to many of the limitations of such active safety systems is to equip vehicles with communication capabilities, allowing the exchange of safety related information. Using communication, a vehicle can then obtain data about vehicles that are not detected by sensors or computer vision systems. Consequently, the perception of the vehicle is improved and the possibility for the active safety systems installed in it to detect dangers in complex traffic situations is enhanced. For example, two vehicles entering an intersection from perpendicular paths could become aware of each other's presence through communication.

We illustrate in figure 1 an active safety system that employs communication between vehicles. This system integrates in-vehicle sensors (e.g. positioning devices, speedometer) and a communication system that provides information used in traffic analyses. In this example, the vehicles are able to exchange messages that contain safety-related information such as the front seat data of a vehicle (e.g. speed, heading, position) or messages that indicate events in traffic (e.g. accident, traffic jam). The active safety system analyzes this data and the data describing the subject vehicle for determining threats in traffic. For instance, a threat is determined if two vehicles are in danger of crashing at an intersection [17], or if a vehicle is too close to another vehicle [13]. When such dangerous situations are detected, the system reacts by issuing warnings that are presented to the driver.

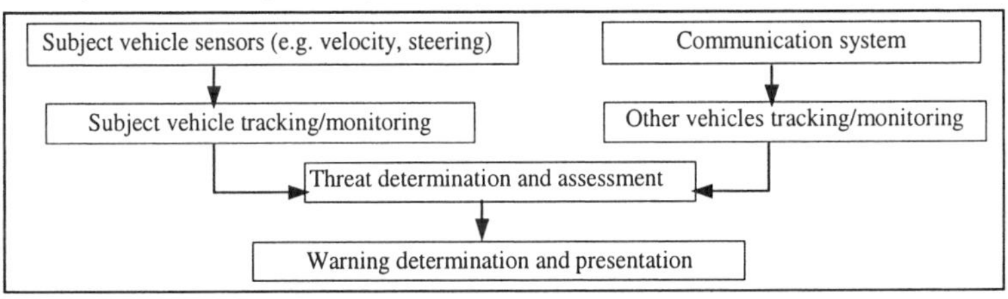

Figure 1 Active safety system using communication.

However, even if vehicular communication is generally thought to have a high potential for supporting active safety systems (e.g. [1, 17]), it may not be effective in all traffic situations. For example, communication may have little impact in helping avoiding lane departure accidents. In our previous work, we have proposed vehicular communication solutions, and analyzed their performance (in terms of message delay, etc). Now, we investigate to what extent these solutions, based on their performance, can help to avoid road intersection accidents involving elderly drivers.

4. Road intersection accidents

Studies have indicated that a large majority of accidents involving elderly drivers take place at intersections [10]. The main difficulties elderly drivers face at intersections are [4, 7, 22]:

- Estimation of a safe gap and the estimation of velocity of other vehicles.
- Fast execution of driving maneuvers (e.g. turning).
- Failure to sense and comprehend traffic signals and signs.
- Inability to perceive and process information about high traffic volumes.

We illustrate in figure 2 an intersection collision involving an elderly driver by the use of an intersection crash with perpendicular path scenario. This type of accident accounts for more than 30% of the total number of accidents that appear each year at intersections [19]. It is also considered to be of very high risk for elderly drivers [20].

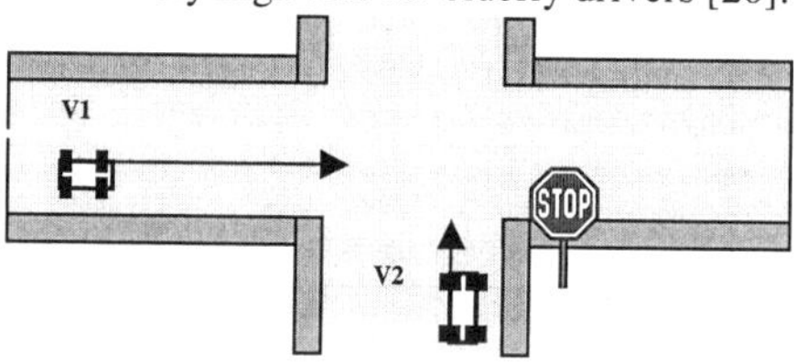

Figure 2 Intersection crash with perpendicular path

The scenario contains two vehicles that approach an intersection. The driver in vehicle V2 is an elderly driver (e.g. over 65) and the driver in V1 is a mid-age driver (e.g. 40-49). Vehicle V1 is travelling on the priority road. Vehicle V2 is initially stopped at the STOP sign and plans to cross the intersection. When V2 starts to cross, its acceleration is low as the elderly driver tends to drive carefully. Let us consider that V2's driver is not able to notice the presence of V1 perhaps because the driver fails to make a correct estimate of V1's distance and velocity. The driver in vehicle V1 is misled by the maneuver of V2 and considers that V2 will not pass the intersection or will pass it in time. At some later time, V1's driver realizes that these assumptions are not valid and intends to brake for stopping. However, due to a small separation distance between vehicles, V1 crashes into V2.

Now, the question is how to avoid this type of accident.

5. Simulation experiments

5.1 Simulation goals and environment

The main goal of our study was to investigate the feasibility of using vehicular communication for supporting older drivers at road intersections. The specific issues that we addressed were:

- Investigate requirements on information transfer that need to be fulfilled by vehicular communication systems.
- Quantify the impact of the accident scenario conditions and information transfer properties on accident avoidance.

In previous work we developed ECAM, a temporal reasoning system for modeling and analyzing accident scenarios [5]. This system constituted the simulation environment that we used within our study for analyzing the possibility of avoiding intersection accidents by the use of communication. A brief description of this system is provided in the following. Details on the design, functionality, and implementation of the system can be found in [5]. ECAM is a formal framework that provides a reasoning engine for studying the time evolution of traffic accidents. It is based on a well-known logical formalism, the Event Calculus [14], and it is implemented using logic programming (i.e. Prolog). This system gives the possibility of investigating the relations between events that occur in traffic and their possible consequences. It is thus able to model changes that take place when different actions happen in a traffic situation. For performing analyses, the system can be questioned to determine if and when certain traffic conditions related to vehicles involved in a scenario become valid. For instance, we can determine if and when a collision between two vehicles has occurred within a traffic scenario. Further, by modifying different parameters in the scenario (e.g. initial speed of vehicles) or by introducing new actions that modify the development of the scenario (e.g. a heavy braking) we can investigate changes in the scenario behavior. For instance, by performing such analyses we can determine if and how a collision can be avoided.

5.2 Experiments and results

As a case study, we have employed ECAM for studying the intersection accident previously introduced. As mentioned before, our focus has been to evaluate to what extent vehicular communication can help to avoid this accident. Therefore, in our experiments we assumed that an active safety system based on communication is installed in each vehicle. This system can present the driver with warnings about dangers in traffic and can also employ automatic actions if it is set in an automatic mode. Further, we based our investigation on a number of assumptions, which are presented in figure 3.

Assumptions:

- When vehicle V2 starts to cross the intersection a warning message is sent to vehicle V1.
- The active safety system in V1 receives the warning message and reacts to it, either by notifying the driver that V2 has started to cross the intersection, or by braking automatically.
- The driver in V1 reacts to the notification and starts to brake heavily after a driver reaction time has passed (a reaction time of 0 indicates automatic braking).
- The acceleration of V2 when entering the intersection is fixed, and fairly low (i.e. 1.5 m/s^2). This assumption is based on the fact that many older drivers drive slowly, as a compensatory measure for their limited cognitive abilities [10].
- The distance of vehicle V2 from the entry point into the intersection is fixed and is set to 4 meters.
- Vehicle V2 starts crossing the intersection at 1 second after the beginning of the scenario.
- A maximum deceleration of 9 m/s^2 is considered for vehicle V1.
- The width of a road lane is set to 4 meters.

Fig. 3. Assumptions made within the experiments.

The avoidance of the accident between V1 and V2 can be achieved due to the heavy braking maneuver performed by V1 when it receives the warning message sent by V2. Therefore, our interest was to investigate the maximum delay for the warning message sent by V2 that can still assure the accident avoidance. We performed our experiments by varying the scenario conditions and dynamics, represented by the variation of the reaction times of the driver and of the initial speed of vehicle V1. Figure 4 summarizes these independent variables. In our experiments, we have used the *cut-off distance* for V1 as the dependent variable. We defined this parameter as the minimum distance from the entry point into the intersection at which V1 needs to be positioned when V2 issues the warning message, for the collision between V1 and V2 to be avoided.

In figure 5 we present the results obtained by modifying the initial speed of vehicle V1 (i.e. the speed until V1 performs the braking due to the warning message), when we employed a 1.5 seconds reaction time of the driver. We note that we use dotted lines for marking the *accident range* in the figure, which is the distance range where the initial collision between V1 and V2 occurs (i.e. when no active safety system is used). Thus, if V1 is initially situated at distances below and above these dotted lines, the accident will not occur. (Note that the accident range increases in size with increased speed of V1.) Further, by representing the cut-off distance for V1 as a function of V2's warning message delay we divided the representational space into accident and non-accident areas. Thus, the area above the separating (continuous) curve represents the cases where a collision was avoided, while the area below the curve represents the situations where, in spite of an emergency braking, a collision still occurs.

Independent Variables:

- *Delay of V2's warning message* - varied between 0.6 msec and 2.3 seconds. The values for delay were selected based on realistic results for simulation of communication between vehicles that we obtained in earlier work [5, 6].
- *Speed of V1* – varied between 10 m/s (i.e. 36 km/h) and 25 m/s (i.e. 90 km/h).
- *Driver reaction time (DRT)* – varied between 0 and 3 seconds based on research in collision avoidance (e.g. [13]). We note that a DRT of 0 seconds corresponds to an automatic active safety system. For the overall population, a DRT of 1.5 seconds is an upper limit for simple reactions [13, 8]. However, we have adopted this value as a normal value, since it is known that older people tend to have longer reaction times. A DRT of 3 seconds is an extreme upper bound that rarely occurs in real cases [8].

Fig. 4. Independent variables used within the experiments.

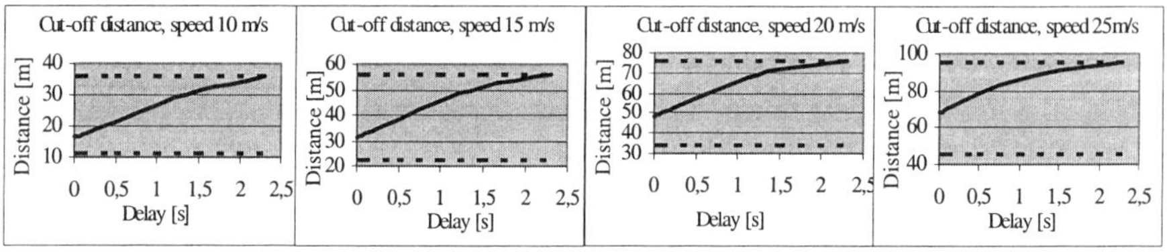

Fig. 5. Cut-off distance as a function of communication delay. Speed values from 10m/s to 25 m/s.

Further, in figure 6 we present the results obtained for using the other two representative values for the driver reaction times (DRT):

- DRT = 0 seconds. This corresponds to the active safety system in V1 set to the automatic mode and performing a heavy braking without any delay when the warning message from V2 is received.
- DRT = 3 seconds. This is an extreme upper bound that rarely occurs in real cases [8].

The graphs in the figure illustrate the results for an initial speed of V1 of 15 m/s and 20 m/s. Observe that a considerable portion of the accidents in the accident range for DRT of 0 seconds can be avoided due to vehicular communication. On the other hand, with a DRT of 3 seconds, very few accidents can be avoided.

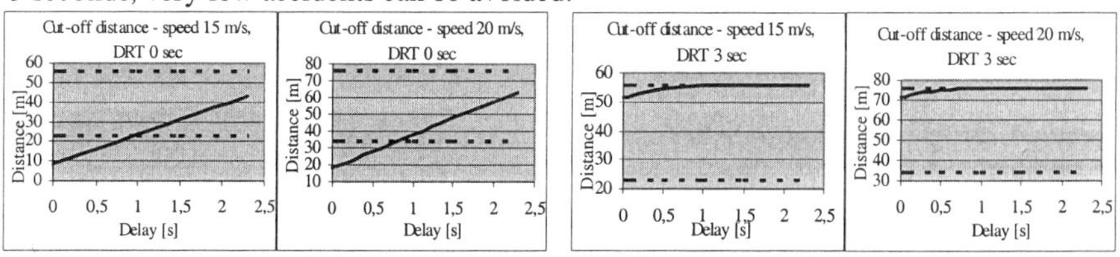

Fig. 6. Cut-off distance and communication delay. Speed values: 15m/s and 20 m/s. DRT: 0 sec and 3 sec.

A peculiarity with the cut-off distance curves for DRT of 0 seconds is that the curve continues below the lower part of the accident range (where accidents are not supposed to happen). The explanation for this is that the automatic braking performed when the warning message arrives actually can lead to accidents if the message is received when V1 is too close to the intersection. If V1 had not started to brake, and continued with normal speed, V1 would have passed the intersection before V2 had entered, and thus the accident would have been avoided.

From the graphs in figure 5 we note that delays above approximately 2.3 seconds mean that no accidents can be avoided. With a DRT of 3 seconds, the corresponding maximum delay is around 1 second. The maximum delay for a DRT of 0 seconds cannot be determined directly from figure 6, but in further experiments we have determined the maximum delay to be around 3.8 seconds.

6. Discussion

From the experiments we saw that transmission delay has a fairly large influence on collision avoidance. Hence, it is of great importance to minimize the transmission delay. Fortunately, our initial experiments with vehicular communication protocols show that small delays are feasible in many realistic traffic scenarios [5, 6]. However, minimizing delay may not be of much help for people with very long reaction times. In these cases, an automatic system may be the only feasible solution. Still, note that even though an accident may not be entirely avoided, its consequences can be limited due to braking in response to a warning message (e.g. by reducing the speed at collision time).

Traffic safety systems that take automatic action show the best potential for accident avoidance. But such systems need to be more complex than information delivery systems that leave the driver in control. As we saw in the results, automatic braking in response to a warning message may actually introduce an accident. This indicates that further analysis (e.g. continuing the work started in this paper) is needed for the eventual realization of fully dependable automatic active safety systems. Such automatic systems cannot just react to warning messages, but must be deliberative and reason about potential consequences of their actions.

7. Related traffic simulators

A large number of traffic simulators exist. In [2], 57 different simulators are analyzed and compared. The authors conclude that only 3 of the evaluated simulators are event based, “where the states of objects in the network are changed at discrete times in response to events on an event list”. The other simulators work with fixed time steps (typically 1-second intervals). Given the type of analysis we perform in this paper, such coarse-grained analysis with fixed time steps is not appropriate. We need to deduce the exact time at which an accident occurs. Of the three simulators that were event-based, and thus potentially useful for our study, the FLEXSYT-II system makes use of stochastic movement patterns, making it difficult to precisely control the movements of individual vehicles. The SIGSIM system is focused on signal-controlled junctions for the evaluation of signal control policies. Hence, adapting this simulator to our scenario would not have been straightforward. Finally, SIMNET has the purpose of evaluating traffic control strategies in general, and not on analyzing specific accident scenarios. In sum, we believe that the ECAM system complements today’s existing traffic simulators, and will be a valuable tool for future analysis of complex accident scenarios.

8. Concluding remarks

We have investigated the feasibility of using vehicular communication for supporting the avoidance of intersection collisions involving older drivers. Our results indicated the communication to be an effective mean for supporting accident avoidance in many cases.

While the results are promising, it is important to note that our study is early work, and that a number of key steps need to be taken before safety systems based on vehicular communication can become a commercial reality. For example, the question of how a safety system should handle a warning message is crucial. Should the system take action and brake automatically, or should a warning message be displayed to the driver so that he or she remains in control? Still, researchers tend to agree that vehicular communication is the key to a future with safer traffic, where old people can maintain mobility.

References

[1] Andrisano O., Verdone R., Nakagawa M., "Intelligent transportation systems: the role of third generation mobile radio networks", IEEE Communication Magazine, pp. 144-151, Sept. 2000.
[2] Bernauer E., Breheret L., Algers S., Boero M., Taranto C. D., Dougherty M., Fox K., Gabard J-F., "SMARTEST – Review of Micro-Simulation Models", SMARTEST Project Deliverable D3, Institute for Transport Studies, University of Leeds, UK, 1998.
[3] Bishop R., "Intelligent vehicle applications world-wide", IEEE Intelligent Systems, vol. 15, pp. 78-83, Jan./Feb. 2000.
[4] Caird, Creaser, Edwards, Horrey: Contributing Factors to Accidents by Older Drivers R&D Plan and Empirical Studies, Cognitive Ergonomics Research Laboratory, University of Calgary, Canada, 2002.
[5] Chisalita I., "Traffic safety-oriented communication in mobile networks for vehicles" (tentative title), Licentiate Thesis, Linköping University, Sweden (forthcoming 2004).
[6] Chisalita I., Shahmehri N. "A context-based vehicular communication protocol" IEEE Personal, Indoor and Mobile Radio Communication Conference, Barcelona, 5-8 Sept. 2004, in press.
[7] Corben, Fildes, Oxley: Older Drivers Highway Design: The development of a handbook and training workshop to design safe road environments for older drivers, Accident Research Centre, Monash University, Melbourne.
[8] Gartner N., Messer C., Rathi A. (eds), "Traffic flow theory", U.S. Federal Highway Administration, Turner-Fairbank Highway Research Center, 2002.
[9] Hakamies-Blomqvist L., "Aging Europe: the challenges and opportunities for transport safety", European Transport Safety Council, Brussels, Jan. 2003.
[10] Hakamies-Blomqvist, Helmers, Henriksson, "Trafikmiljö för äldre bilförare – Analys och rekommendationer utifrån en litteraturstudie (Traffic environment for older drivers – analysis and recommendations from a literature study)", Väg- och transportforskningsinstitutet, VTI rapport 493, 2004.
[11] Jones W. D., "Building safer cars", IEEE Spectrum, vol. 38, pp. 82-85, Jan. 2002.
[12] Jones W. D., "Keeping cars from crashing", IEEE Spectrum, vol. 38, pp. 40-45, Sep. 2001.
[13] Kiefer R., LeBlanc D., Palmer M., Salinger J., Deering R., Shulman M., "Development and Validation of Functional Definitions and Evaluation Procedures for Collision Warning/Avoidance System", US National Highway Traffic Safety Administration Technical Report, USA, Washington, Aug 1999.
[14] Kowalski R., Sergot M., " A logic-based calculus of events", New Generation Computing No. 4, pp.67-95, Springer-Verlag, 1986.
[15] McCoy G.F., Johnson R.A., Duthie R.B., "Injury to the elderly in road traffic accidents", Journal of Trauma 29, pp. 494-497, 1989.
[16] McDowd, Shaw R., "Attention and Aging: A functional perspective", The Handbook of Aging and Cognition, Lawrence Erlbaum Publishers, 2000.
[17] Miller R., Huang Q., "An adaptive peer-to-peer collision warning system", IEEE Vehicular Technology Conference, Birmingham, USA, pp. 317-321, May 2002.
[18] Owsley, C., "Driving Mobility, Older Adults, and Quality of Life", Gerontechnology 1(4), pp. 220-230, 2002.
[19] Pierowicz J., Jocoy E., Lloyd M., Bittner A., Pirson B., "Intersection Collision Avoidance Using ITS Countermeasures", U.S. Department of Transportation, National Highway Traffic Safety Administration, Office of Advanced Safety Research, Sept. 2000.
[20] Preusser D., Williams A., Ferguson S., Ulmer R., Weinstein H., "Fatal crash risk for older drivers at Intersections", Journal of Accident Analysis & Prevention, Vol 30, pp. 151-160, Mar 1998.
[21] U.S. Bureau of the Census, "World population profile: 1998", Technical report WP/98, US Government Printing Office, Washington DC, 1998.
[22] Vägverket, "Older driver's problems in traffic", Publikation 63, 1998.

Sound processing for Health Smart Home

Dan ISTRATE*, Eric CASTELLI**, Michel VACHER*, Cong-Phuong NGUYEN**
**CLIPS-IMAG, BP 53, 38041 Grenoble Cedex 9, France*
***International Research Center MICA - 1 Dai Co Viet - Hai Ba Trung - Hanoi - Vietnam*
Eric.Castelli@mica.edu.vn

ABSTRACT. Sound in smart home are usually encountered for friendly man-machine interfaces, but sound information extraction is a complex task because of environmental noise and of multichannel processing need. A multichannel sound processing system capable to detect and identify sound events in noisy conditions is presented in this paper. The multichannel sound processing allows us to localize the sound in smart home and to select appropriate signal for identification procedure. This sensor is real time implemented on PC. The event detection module is carried out for each channel in real time. The classification module is launched in a parallel task on the channel chosen by data fusion process. The aim of this process is to select the channel with the biggest signal to noise ratio when a multiple detection occurs. The system validation is made on a test set and is presented with the proposed methodology of evaluation for a medical telemonitoring application. The obtained results are allowing us to develop smart home applications.

KEY WORDS: Acoustical Signal Processing, Noise, Multichannel Processing, Real Time, Sound Detection & Classification, Wavelet Transform

1 Introduction

Our days, sound became a preferred interface and information source for smart home. Sound contains low level information like class (silence/music/sound), speaker identity, sound type (impulsive/harmonic) and high level information such the lexical parts (words, sentences), sound class (door clapping, ringing phone, fall sound,...). Extraction of high level information is possible today in real time, thanks to many studies. The actual challenges are the multichannel processing, attenuation of environmental noise, multispeaker speech recognition.

In this paper we describe a multichannel sound processing system which detect and identify a sound between several predefined sound classes. The system input is composed, for instant, of data collected by 5 microphones and its output data is sent through a network (Ethernet). For a real time working purpose, the sound analysis is divided in three steps : sound event detection for each sound channel, fusion between simultaneously events and sound identification. The extracted information is sent through the network and if it is needed, the recorded sound can be transferred for latter analysis by network.

This system is a part of a medical telemonitoring project with the aim of detecting serious accidents. In these conditions we consider a *sound event*, an impulsive sound (door clapping, step sounds, dishes sounds, etc.) and a *noise*, a stationary signal (environmental noise, white noise, water flow noise, etc.).

The proposed sound processing system is implemented in real time with LabWindows/CVI software on a PC. Evaluation of the sensor has been carried out with real environmental noise on a generated test set. An evaluation methodology is proposed and discussed.

2 Sound database

In order to test and validate the smart sound sensor we have generated a *sound corpus*. It contains recordings made in the Clips laboratory (15% of the CD), the files of "Sound Scene Database in Real Acoustical Environments" [6] (70% of the CD) and files from a commercial CD (film effects, 15 % of the CD). Entire corpus is composed of 3354 files; every sound is sampled at 16 KHz and 44 KHz.

We have carried out *7 sound classes* from the sound corpus, for training the classification algorithm. The 7 sound classes are presented in the Table 1.

The *test set* used for smart sound sensor validation is a mix between the 7 sound classes and noise at different SNR. The noise is recorded in an experimental apartment named HIS. There are 7 files corresponding to the 7 sound classes. Each file is constituted by all sounds of the corresponding class inserted with silence periods of random time length (1577 events to detect and identify). For each sound, SNR can have a random value either between 10dB and 20dB or between 0dB and 40dB. For the first case, the SNR repartition is uniform and for the second one, the SNR repartition corresponds to real measures in the HIS apartment. Silence between consecutive sounds varies randomly between 5 and 60 seconds. Total number of useful sounds to be detected is 1577.

Table 1 - Sound class description

Sound class	N°. files	N° frames	Total length	Alarm
Door clapping	523	47398	379 s	NO
Glass breaking	88	9338	75 s	YES
Ringing phone	517	59188	474 s	NO
Step sounds	13	36480	292 s	NO
Screams	73	17509	140 s	YES
Dishes sounds	163	7943	64 s	YES
Door lock	200	6050	49	NO

3 Sound Processing Hardware

The proposed system is composed of 5 omni-directional microphones and an acquisition card (National Instruments PCI-6034E) plugged in the PC which is in charge with the sound analysis software (Figure 1). Each microphone is equipped with a HF transmitter. Acquisition card has 8 differential inputs and a maximal sampling rate of 200 ksamples/s. The sampling frequency was fixed at 16 kHz, a value usual in speech recognition. Before acquisition card a HF receiver is needed in order to receipt and demodulate sound information.

The sound sample acquisition use low-level functions in order to drive the card in real time. The detected events are saved on PC hard-disk and sent through the network. An history of detected events (detection time, detection type) is recorded in a text file. The abnormal detected signal is recorded in a standard Wave format (without compression) and could be sent in the same format through Ethernet network, if requested.

4 Sound Processing Algorithms

The sound processing system has been divided in three modules as shown in Figure 2. The first and second modules are making up the first parallel task. The third module is the second parallel task.

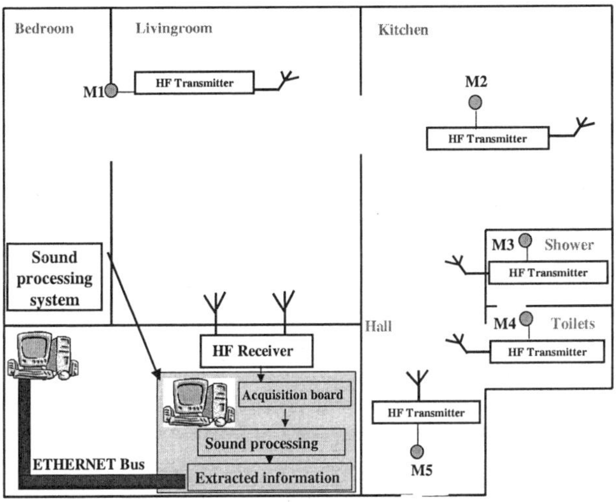

Figure 1 - System hardware

The first module is processed on each channel in order to detect a sound event and to extract it from signal flow. The fusion module selects the best channel in the case of a simultaneously event detection on several channels. The channel with the best Signal to Noise Ratio is chosen from estimation of SNR made for each channel. These two modules make up the first parallel task.

The last step is the sound classification or second parallel task. This module is receiving the sound event extracted (output of first task) and it estimates the most probable sound class. The proposed sensor classifies the sound in one of the seven sound classes.

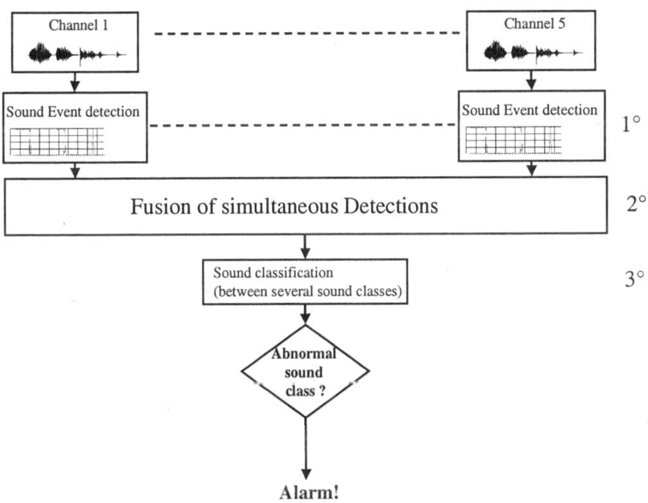

Figure 2 - Sound processing schema

4.1 Sound Event Detection and Capture

The event detection aim is to find impulsive signals in the noise and to extract them from the signal flow. The system must be capable to identify impulsive signals like door clapping, dishes sounds, fall sounds but also speech presence too, in a noisy environment. The performances of the first module are very important for the entire system because if an event is lost, it is lost forever.

There are many techniques for sound detection: energy threshold, statistical model, energy processing or wavelet processing [1]. We have validated three detection algorithms proposed by Dufaux [2] on our test set but the obtained performances for environmental noise are not suitable. We have proposed two other algorithms [4] with better performances either for environmental noise or for water flow noise but not for the two cases.

A wavelet based event detection algorithm is proposed in the following. Unlike Fast Fourier Transform, Wavelet Transform is well adapted to signals that have very localized features in the time-frequency space [3]. This transform is frequently used for signal detection and audio processing. We have chosen Daubechies wavelets with 6 vanishing moments to compute DWT. A complete orthonormal wavelet basis consists of scalings and translations of the mother wavelet function, a function with finite energy and fast decay.

Wavelet Transform on a 512 sample frame corresponding to a 32ms window allows good signal enhancement in noisy conditions. Analyzed sounds are impulsive and so, better enhanced by Wavelet Transform. Discrete Wavelet Transform is applied on the sampled data and its output forms a vector of the same length than the signal (512). This vector has a pyramidal structure and is composed of 10 *wavelet coefficients* (see Figure 3).

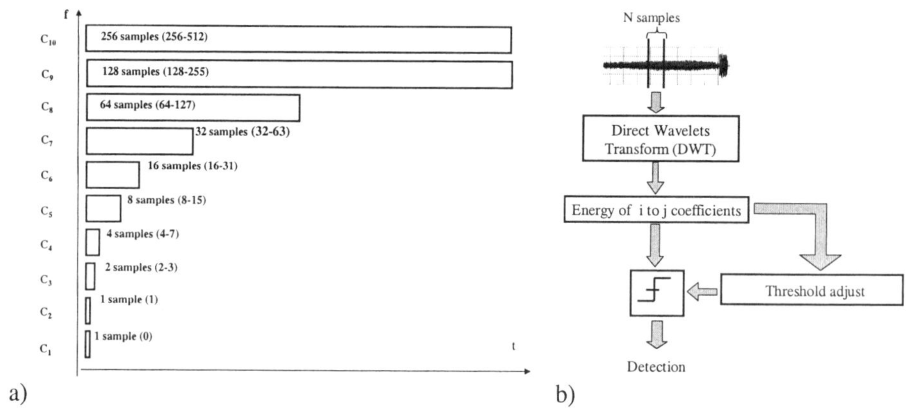

Figure 3 - a) Wavelet coefficients repartion; b) Flowchart of the wavelet based algorithm

The algorithm (flowchart in Figure 3) calculates the energy of the 8, 9 and 10 wavelet coefficients (the three higher order coefficients), because the significant wavelet coefficients of the sounds to be detected are rather high order.

The detection is achieved by applying a threshold on the sum of energies of the three highest order wavelet coefficients. The threshold is self-adjustable and depends on the average of the 10 last energy values. Overlap between two consecutive analysis windows is 50%.

An example of sound detection achieved by the presented algorithm is shown in the Figure 4. The amplitude of the sound signal that contains a mixture between a ringing phone at 3.2 second and a water flow noise at 0 dB of SNR can be seen in the first window, in the Figure 4, while the second window shows the wavelet energy outlined in black and the self-adjustable threshold in grey. The detection signal presented in the third window shows clearly that the algorithm detects the signal from noise despite their close amplitudes.

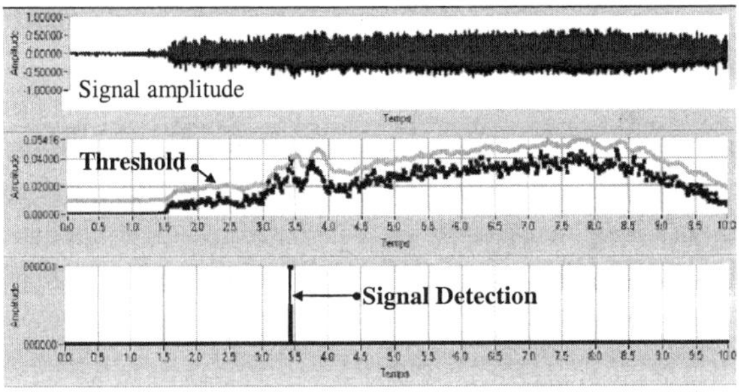

Figure 4 - Detection of a ringing mixed with water flow noise at 0 dB of SNR with proposed algorithm

The presented algorithm detects only the signal beginning and not the end. A first approach is to consider a fix duration sound as detection output. However, the sound classification system is very sensitive to long silence parts. Therefore, we detect the end of the signal by applying the same algorithm on the time inverted signal.

The procedure used to realize an everyday life sound event detection and capture involves the following steps: the output signal starts simultaneously with the detection and lasts 7 seconds. Then, the signal is time inverted and the detection algorithm is applied once again. In the next step the detection of the end of the signal is used to extract the sound (the output signal has a variable length). This procedure is allowing classification algorithm to analyze only the typical part of the detected signal.

4.2 *Fusion between Channels*

Event detection is continuously operating on each of five audio inputs. According to Figure 2, a fusion is necessary between these 5 inputs in the aim of choosing the best channel and implicitly, to localize the sound source, when multiple detections occur simultaneously. We consider *simultaneous detections* two or more detections occurring at less than 0.5 seconds after the first detection (the propagation time and the algorithm structure determine this time).

In case of simultaneous detections, the best channel is considered the one with the biggest Signal to Noise Ratio (SNR). The SNR is estimated for each channel like the ratio between average sound power (1 second of signal after an event detection) and average noise power (1 second of signal before event detection). The average noise power is buffered continuously in memory. The output of fusion module gives the event signal.

4.3 *Classification*

The classification module looks to identify the event sound between predefined sound classes. This module uses a **G**aussian **M**ixture **M**odel (GMM) method [5]. This method evolves in two steps: a training step and an identification one. Identification module is the only module involved in real time constraints. Classification does not use directly signal samples, but a vector of acoustical parameters calculated on analysis windows. The acoustical parameters are determined for each analysis window of 16ms with an overlap of 8ms.

The training is initiated for each class of signals from sound corpus and gives a model containing the characteristics of each Gaussian of the class. The training is achieved after 20 iterations of an "EM" algorithm (Expectation Maximization) following a K-means algorithm.

Each extracted signal is a series of acoustical vectors. The membership likelihood of a class for each acoustical vector is calculated for all classes. The likelihood of the entire signal is obtained by geometrical average. The signal belongs to the class for which likelihood is maximum.

4.3.1 Acoustical parameters

There are many types of acoustical parameters but only few of them are appropriate to the sound classification. After a statistical study based on Fisher Discriminant Ratio (FDR) and a validation on a test set, a combination of 16 MFCC with ZCR, RF and Centroid has been chosen (error classification rate was 10% on a 1577 test set). MFCC are cepstral coefficients based on triangular filtered energy in different frequency bands (Fourier Transform with a Mel frequency scale followed by logarithm and Inverse Fourier Transform). The Zero Crossing Rate (ZCR) is the number of crossings on time-domain through zero-voltage. The Roll-off Point (RF) measures the frequency which delimits 95% of the power spectrum, while the Centroid is the frequency which divides the power spectrum in two equal parts.

5 System Validation

5.1 Implementation

The whole sound analysis flow-chart (Figure 2) is implemented by a software written with LabWindows/CVI on sound analysis PC. This software drives simultaneously the real time sound acquisition on 5 channels at 16 kHz sample rate. The acquisition is made by a double buffering of 2048 samples by channel. Between 2 acquisitions of 2048 samples, the event detection is made on each of 5 channels. In the same time the signal power is calculated and stored into memory (this value is necessary for SNR estimation).

In case of event detection the fusion module is launched in order to select the best channel. The signal of the selected channel is recorded on the hard disk (7 seconds after event detection). The number of selected channel is shown on the software front panel, like sound localization information.

Before launching a second event detection procedure, the detected signal is time inverted in order to estimate the signal end. After signal extraction at founded signal end, the classification algorithm is started up. The most probable sound class is shown on the front panel. All these modules are launched in a parallel task in relation to real time sound acquisition task.

When a sound event is detected, the system is emitting an information frame through the network. The frame contains: date and time detection (day, month, year, hour, minute, second, milliseconds) and a character field. This character field is composed by: the three most probable sound classes with their corresponding likelihoods and the localization of the sound event (the channel).

On the software front panel (Figure 5) are shown the signal of last detected event, the localization of last event (the room in our experimental apartment), a chronological account of detected events, and, on apartment plan, the event localization once again.

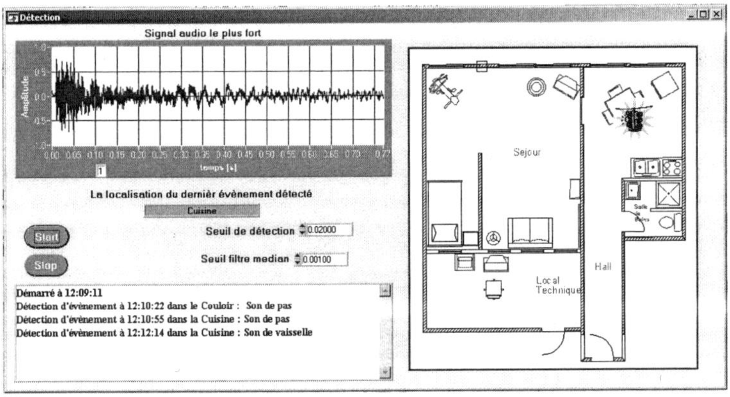

Figure 5 - Front panel of smart sensor. Detection of step and dish sounds

5.2 Proposed Methodology for Sound Processing Evaluation

The evaluation of the smart sound sensor for a telemedicine application must take into account the different characteristics of both detection and classification modules. For detection module we define a *good detection* (G) as an event detection occurring between 0.5 seconds before signal start and signal end. A *Missed Detection* (MD) is a lack of detection in the previously defined time interval and a *False Alarm* (FA) is a detection occurring outside of this time interval.

For classification module, the 7 sound classes are divided in two categories: class with alarm (A) and class without alarm ($\overline{A}$). Possible errors are :

- **Error without consequence (W)** = a sound of a class with alarm is classified in another class with alarm *or* a sound of a class without alarm is classified in another class without alarm
- **Missed detection (MD)** = a sound of a class with alarm is classified in a class without alarm
- **False alarm (FA)** = a sound of a class without alarm is classified in a class with alarm

All errors for the two tasks are illustrated in the Figure 6. The proposed Global Missed Detection Rate (GMDR) and the Global False Alarm Rate (GFAR) are defined in following equations in accordance with Figure 6.

$$GMDR = \frac{MD_{Detect} + MD_{Class}}{Total\ Number\ of\ event\ \text{detections}} \qquad GFAR = \frac{FA_{Class}}{Total\ number\ of\ event\ \text{detections} + FA_{Class}}$$

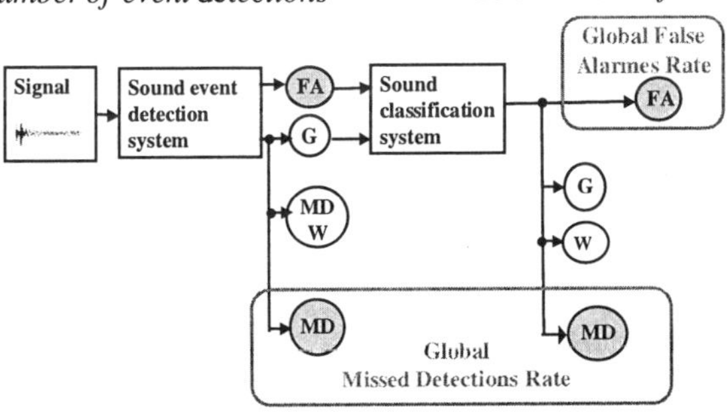

Figure 6 - Global False Alarm Rate and Global Missed Detection Rate representation

5.3 System Evaluation Results

The results of system evaluation on the test set are presented in the Table 2. Test set contains a mixture between real noise (recorded in the test apartment) and everyday life sounds. These results were obtained by using wavelet based algorithm for detection of the start and of the signal end. The classification module was achieved with 4 Gaussian models and 16 MFCC coupled with energy, zero crossing rate, roll-off point and centroid. For classification module a *leave one out* protocol has been used: the model of each class is trained on all the signals of the class, excepting one. Next, each model is tested on the remaining sounds of all classes. The whole process is iterated for all detected files.

There are not many missed detections, GMDR=3% for the two test sets. This value can be considered as acceptable for our application because the sound extraction system will be coupled with other sensors. False alarms remains below 15%, GFAR≈12% in the same conditions.

Table 2- Sound processing system performances on 1577 tests

	SNR∈[10,20] dB	SNR∈[0,40] dB
GMDR	3 %	3 %
GFAR	12.3 %	12.7 %

6 Conclusions and Perspectives

In this paper we have presented a multichannel sound processing system which detects sound events and identifies sounds among 7 predefined sound classes. It was designed to work in the framework of a medical telemonitoring application. We have proposed an evaluation methodology in relation with the application. The obtained results in real noisy environments are acceptable.

Actually, the system is composed of the data acquisition card plugged in a PC. To make it physically independent, we can implement the sensor system inside the digital signal processor card. We have chosen to test the sensor algorithms using a PC because of the facilities in terms of implementation and verification.

Acknowledgements

This work is a part of the DESDHIS-ACI ”Technologies for Health” project of the French Research Ministry and is a collaboration between the CLIPS (*Communication Langagière et Interaction Personne-Système*) laboratory, the TIMC (*Techniques de l'Imagerie, de la Modélisation et de la Cognition*) laboratory and the MICA Center *(Multimedia Information, Communication and Applications - Hanoi - Vietnam).*

References

[1] Takeshi Yamada and Narimasa Watanabe, “Voice activity detection using non-speech models and HMM composition,” in *Workshop on Hands-free Speech Communication, Tokyo, Japan*, 2001.

[2] A.Dufaux, *Detection and Recognition of Impulsive Sounds Signals*, Ph.D. thesis, Faculté des sciences de l'Université de Neuchatel, 2001.

[3] L. Daudet, *Représentations structurelles de signaux audiophoniques - Méthodes hybrides pour des applications à la compression*, Ph.D. thesis, Marseille, 2000.

[4] M.Vacher, D.Istrate, L.Besacier, E.Castelli, and J.F.Serignat, “Smart audio sensor for telemedicine,” in *Smart Objects Conference 2003, Grenoble, France*, 15-17 May 2003.

[5] D. Reynolds, “Speaker identification and verification using gaussian mixture speaker models,” in *Workshop on Automatic Speaker Recognition, Identification and Verification, Martigny, Switzerland*, April 1994, pp. 27–30.

[6] Real World Computing Partnership, “CD – Sound scene database in real acoustical environments, ”http://tosa.mri.co.jp/sounddb/indexe.htm, 1998-2001.

Toward a Human-Friendly Assistive Environment
D. Zhang and M. Mokhtari (Eds.)
IOS Press, 2004

Toward an evaluation methodology for computer accessibility

R. Kadouche[1], B. Abdulrazak[1], M. Mokhtari[1 2]

[1]Handicom Lab GET/INT,. Evry, France.
[2]INSERM-U483, Université Pierre & Marie Curie, Paris, France
Rachid.Kadouche@int-evry.fr

Abstract. Our research work focus on the accessibility of assistive technologies dedicated to people having severe disabilities, particularly providing quantitative and qualitative evaluations methodologies on human-machine interaction while getting access to a computer. We aim to design compensation strategies developed by people having sever motor disabilities in order to use physical input devices to control a computer. This paper discusses and presents our quantitative evaluation methodology on human-machine interaction while getting access to a computer. This method allows choosing among several input devices, the optimal one with respect to the effectiveness of using this input device for each population of users with disabilities. Preliminary results using three inputs devices (mouse, Trackballs, Joysticks) are presented. Moreover users mainly having spinal cord injuries and muscular dystrophies from the rehabilitation hospital of Garches and the French Muscular dystrophies Association (AFM) participated in the experimentations.

1 Introduction

Access to, and independent control of, a computer can be an important part of everyday life for people with disabilities[5]. For example, people whose impairments prevent communication through writing and/or speaking by using appropriate technology, perform these activities with computer assistance. Improved computer access has also been shown to give significant gains in educational success and employment opportunities for people with disabilities. However, in order to be of benefit, computer systems must be accessible [6].Most problems encountered by people with disabilities are related to the use of human machine interfaces (**Figure 1**). Their capabilities in acting on a system can be analyzed with various available peripherals (keyboard, joystick, mouse, etc.). The handling of these peripherals requires a number of degrees of freedom (ddl), a specific movement amplitude and/or a specific strength to control output signals, either continuous (e.g. mouse), or discontinuous (e.g. keyboard). These characteristics condition the various actions which could achievable by each end-user.

Many interfaces are designed using user behavior models that have been derived exclusively from able-bodied users [9], and several software like Virtual keyboard, Head Tracker, Visioboard ,..., have been developed in order to improve their computer accessibility.
The key to developing truly effective means of computer access lies in a user-centred approach [7]. It is especially important to understand how users with disabilities differ from able-bodied users in their interaction behavior. Several works highlight these differences, and show the incapacity of these users to handle the input devices[8], [6], [10]. The principal features of computer access using an input device are: the ability to move anywhere the cursor on the screen, the functions click, double click and the drag and drop.
Knowing explicitly how People with disabilities differ from their able-bodied counterparts may assist the design of genuinely more inclusive interfaces. It is necessary to define accurately the users needs, and in particular, their physical abilities. Thus it is important to describe as closely as possible their motor incapability and evaluate their behaviors while using human-machine input devices [1, 2].

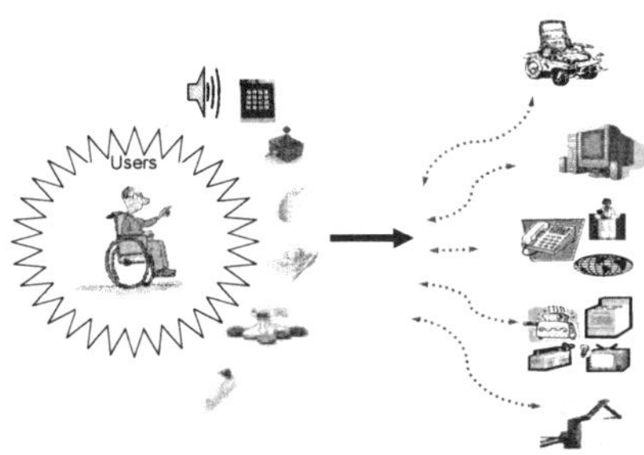

Figure 1: The environment access for people with disabilities

In this paper we will focus mainly on the analysis of users' strategies when using three computers input device which are : standard **mouse**, **Joysticks** (Penny and Giles) and **Trackballs** (Orbit) (**Figure 2**) by the development of an evaluation method based on software application who allow us to determine the most adapted interface for each population of users with disabilities.

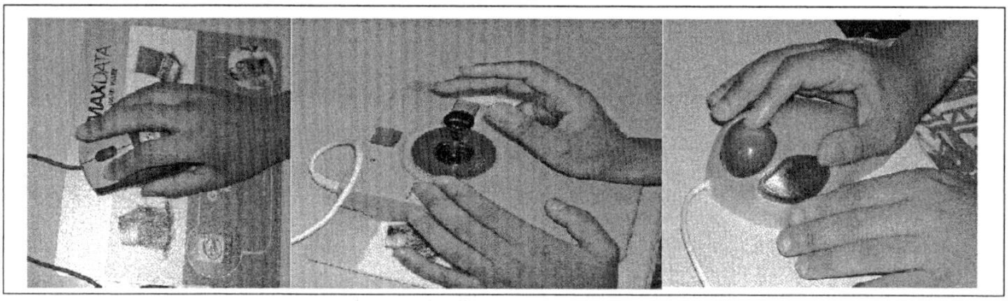

Figure 2: The input devices tested

2 Evaluation method

To evaluate users' behavior while using computer input device, we have designed a quantitative evaluation strategy based on the use of a newly developed software. Besides the qualitative approach, an ergonomist performed a qualitative evaluation method using a questionnaire [4].to report the mains information about the patient (identity, personal feedback); in addition input device apprehension phase was video recorded.

The quantitative evaluation method is based on innovative software development for online tracking of user commands performing a specific task. The main identified parameters recorded are:

- **Accuracy** of the cursor on the screen which consists on analyzing the trajectories deviations,
- **Ability** to carry out a simple click, a double click, and drag and drop,
- **Time** necessary to perform the task.

The evaluation method that we have developed is based on three tests which include all possible functions necessary for a computer interface access [3].

Two types of analyses were developed: the **user tests** and the calculation of the corresponding **errors** corresponding to each test. The duration and the cursor trajectory were recorded in a log file. The three tests evaluate all the operations which can be processed by the device (XY moving of the cursor, simple clicking, double clicking, drag and drop).

- Test 1: consists in connecting two graphical targets by clicking on the first target then, clicking on the second one. It compute the cursor speed according to the time to perform this task.
- Test 2: following a trajectory imposing angles and curves, without having to click. It compute the accuracy error done by the user to perform this task.
- Test 3 is a Drag and Drop test. It compute the number of clicks while carrying out the task.

As shown in the figure bellow, the error accuracy of test2 is quantified by a surface between the real layout and the ideal one. It is computed by recursive algorithm which counts the dots which do not belong to the surface and deduces the desired surface from the total surface.

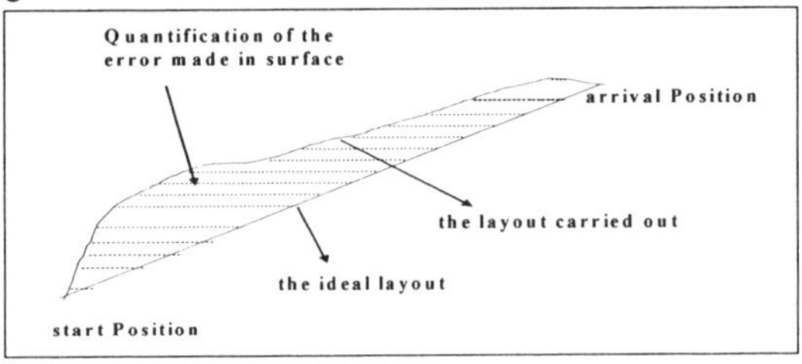

Figure 3: Error calculation based on a recursive graphical algorithm

3 Preliminary results

These preliminary results correspond to two months of evaluation, 13 adults users with no professional activities, took part in our experimentation. 8 of them having spinal cord injuries and 4 with muscular dystrophy and one person having cerebellar ataxia. Among this group there were 2 women. The age, type of disability and the computer skills(CS) of each user are presented in **table1**. Users from AFM are coded by AFMxx, form rehabilitation Hospital Garches by GCHxx (The different computer skills are: 4: daily use, 3: frequently use, 2: seldom use, 1: never use)

User Code	User Age	Type of disability	CS
AFM01	44	Cerebellar ataxia	4
AFM02	24	Becker muscular dystrophy	4
AFM03	28	Duchenne muscular dystrophy	4
AFM04	21	Duchenne muscular dystrophy	4
AFM05	48	Becker muscular dystrophy	4
GCH01	27	SCI-C6	1
GCH02	27	SCI-C6	4
GCH03	22	SCI-C5	1
GCH04	33	SCI-C6	4
GCH05	30	SCI-C5-C6	2
GCH06	18	SCI-C6	4
GCH07	25	SCI-C5-C6	1
GCH08	34	SCI C4-C5	1

Table 1: Users' diagnosis

The experimentation were preceded by learning phase to familiarize this interface with the user. Mainly the average duration of the task is one hour. Results for the three input devices (mouse, Trackballs, Joysticks) are presented as 3D color histograms (**Figure 4, Figure 5**), with the two axes, the test number and the used input devices. Duration task of test 1 (in tenth second unit), the surface errors of test 2 (number of pixels divided by 10^3) and the clicks number of test 3 (multiplied by 10), are presented with three different color bars. Each users' experimentation using the three input devices, was represented by 3D histogram. For example the histogram of AFM01 corresponds to the following table:

Input devices	Test1(tenth of second)	Test2(the number of pixels divided by 10^3)	Test3 (the number of clicks multiplied by 10)
JOY	159	51,391	30
MOUS	60	16,523	20
TB	102	20,922	30

Table 2: the results of AFM01

In the rest of the paper, all comments about the three input devices, correspond to the types of these interfaces, for example Joystick's remarks, correspond only to the Penny and Giles Joystick used in this experimentation, and the same for the mouse and trackball.

The following graph (**Figure 4**) correspond to the results of the muscular dystrophy users

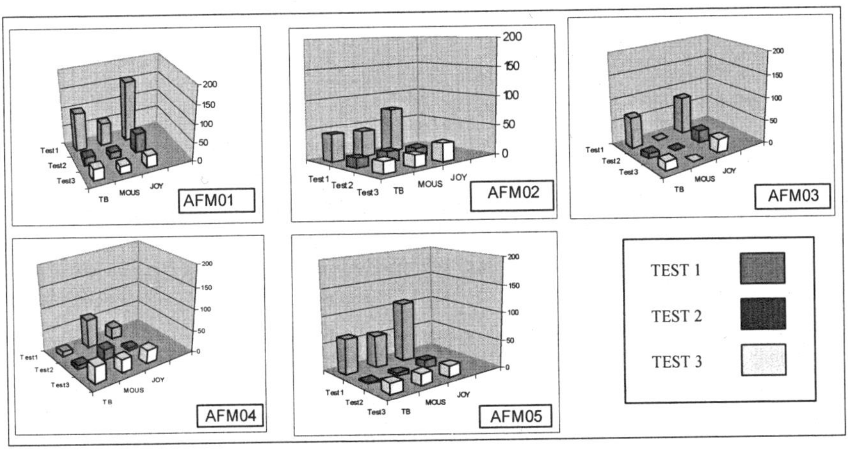

Figure 4: Experimentation results of users with muscular dystrophy

The CS of these users, which is daily use, allows them to have good scores in cursor speed, error accuracy and number of clicks except AFM01 which have cerebellar ataxia with spastic movements.

This figure indicate that people with muscular dystrophy had good results with TrackBall and the mouse compared to the Joystick results, due to the accuracy of their fingers movement.

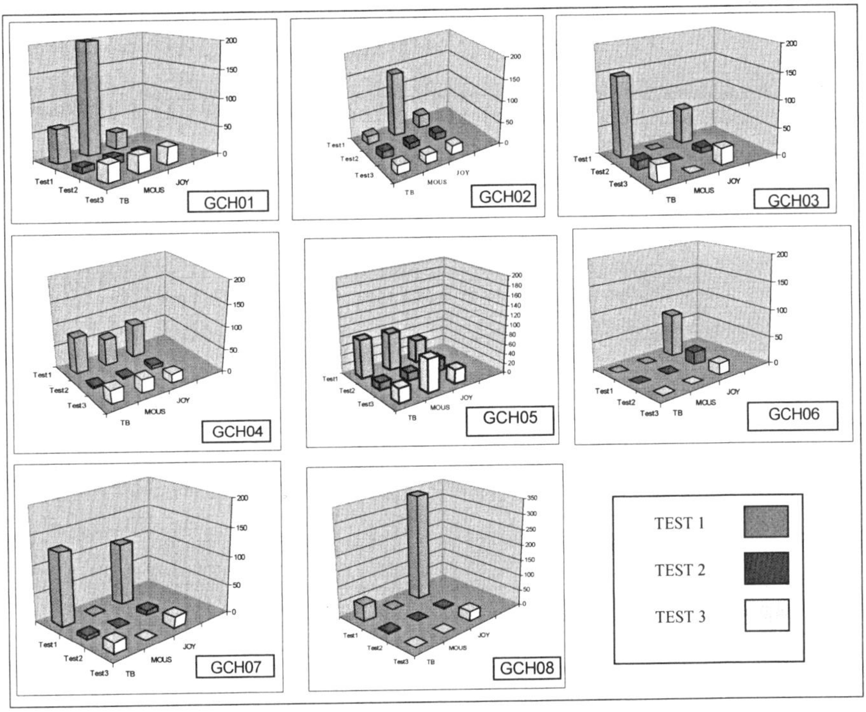

Figure 5: Experimentation results of quadriplegic users

We notice that (**figure 5**), as users with muscular dystrophy, CS of GCH02, GCH04, GCH06, which is daily use, allows them to have good scores in cursor speed, error accuracy and number of clicks using the three input devices.
GCH06 didn't use the mouse and the Trackball because he had been in hurry for his medical consultations appointments.
The quadriplegic people, either didn't use the mouse or made bad score with it. Except to GCH04, he hade good results using this input device, due to his recent accident and his daily computer use.
The absence of the results in the two graphs above (the mouse for AFM03, GCH03, GCH07 and GCH08) is due to the non possibility or the rejection to use this interface from the user.

We found that, even if the joystick seems not adapted for computer application, it provide a solution for people with shakiness and spastic movements(AFM01).
Most of people with muscular dystrophies have good results with Mouse and bad results with Joystick, due to the accuracy of their finger movements.
Quadriplegic people have good results with Joystick because of their ability to move their shoulder in the space dimension. Trackball gives overall good results for both populations.

Conclusion

This work allows us to know the reaction and the behaviors of both populations (people with muscular dystrophies and quadriplegics people) using the three different input devices (mouse, Trackballs, Joysticks) and to identify the adequate interface for each user. The evaluations highlighted the difficulties to use input devices and proved the ability of the users to compensate their handicap. General conclusions can be validated, so mouse provides the better scores rather than trackball and the joystick. Actually we are not able to explain this effect, due to the limited number of users. Therefore we are aiming at a more significant end-user group and several interfaces to complete this study. Even if the joystick is used to control their wheelchair, we observed that people with disabilities mainly don't believe that they can use this interface as computer input device.
In addition we are working on the modeling of the upper limb posture during the grasping phases to model the description of the residual motor capabilities and evaluate human behavior while using human-machine input devices. Coupling the modeling of residual motor capability with resulted actions on the cursor, should provide a better understanding of the user profile and consequently adapt the human-machine interfaces[11]according to the context [12]. The ability to re-calibrate these interfaces, or develop new ones, is essential for the successful design of assistive devices for people with disabilities. As hardware costs drop and computers become increasingly widely available, the population of users grows both in number and diversity. The user profile is the basis for adapting systems to cater for the varied needs, interests, preferences, background, and other characteristics of that diverse user population.

5 Acknowledgements

The authors would like to thank the users who have participated actively in this research work and the occupational therapists who assist the experimentations. This project is funded by the GET and by the industrial foundation Louis Leprince Ringuet.

References

1. Mokhtari, M, : Interaction Homme-Machine : Application aux aides technologiques pour la réduction du handicap moteur HDR, (Novembre 2002)
2. Kadouche.R : analyse de l'interaction Homme-Machine dans le cas d'un handicap moteur. Rapport DEA. (2003).
3. Martina Ziefle :Is the trackball a serious alternative to the mouse ? A comparison of trackball and mouse with regard to cursor movement performance in manipulation tacks. Proc HCI'2003, Vo 3. (2003) 158-162
4. Institute of physical deficiency rehabilitation : http://www.irdpq.qc.ca/index.html
5 .G. Busby, "Technology for the disabled and why it matters to you," IEE Colloquium Digest, Computers in the service of mankind: Helping the disabled, Digest No. 97/117, 1997, pp. 1/1-1/7.
6. Keates S, Clarkson PJ, Robinson P: Cursor measures for motion-impaired computer users. Proc ACM (2002) 135 - 142
7. Stephanidis, C. User interfaces for all: New perspectives into human-computer interaction, in Stephanidis, C., editor, *User Interfaces for All* (2001), Lawrence Erlbaum, 3-17.
8. Tomas A. Stapleford and Richard M. Mahony : Improvement in computer positioning performance for people with cerebral palsy. Proc RESNA 1997. 321-323
9. Keates S, Clarkson PJ, Robinson P. Investigating the applicability of user models for motion-impaired users, in Proceedings of ACM ASSETS 2000 (Arlington VA2000), ACM Press, 129-136.
10. William W. McMillan Computing for Users with Special Needs and Models of Computer-Human Interaction CHI 92 143-148
11. Abdulrazak B., Mokhtari M., Feki M.A., Grandjean B., Rodriguez R.; « Generic user interface for people with Disabilities: Application to smart home concept » Proc ICOST 2003, 1st International Conference On Smart homes and health Telematics, "Independent living for persons with disabilities and elderly people", Ed. IOS Press, pp.45-51, Paris, September 2003.
12. Feki M.A. , Abdulrazak B., Mokhtari M., « XML Modelisation of Smart home envirement », Proc ICOST 2003, 1st International Conference On Smart homes and health Telematics, "Independent living for persons with disabilities and elderly people", Ed. IOS Press, pp.55-60, Paris, September 2003

Toward a Human-Friendly Assistive Environment
D. Zhang and M. Mokhtari (Eds.)
IOS Press, 2004

Research into Telecommunications Options for People with Physical Disabilities

Toan NGUYEN [1,2], Rob GARRETT [1], Andrew DOWNING [2],
Lloyd WALKER [1], and David HOBBS [1]
[1] *NovitaTech, Adelaide, SA, Australia*
[2] *School of Informatics and Engineering, Flinders University, Adelaide, SA, Australia*

Abstract. People with a disability do not have equitable access to the modern telecommunication medium. Not only do they experience difficulty typing, handling the phone, or dialling and answering calls, but for those who are unable to speak, the only option is to type messages using whatever parts of their bodies that are functional. This research was aimed at providing practical ways for people with a disability to participate in the extensive community of home and mobile phone users.

Part of this research focussed on text messaging solutions for people who have physical disabilities, as this is expected to be a significant communication means for those who use an electronic communication device to speak. An important aspect of this project is the promotion of the principles of Universal Design (or Inclusive Design) to ensure that future products and services take into account the needs of people with disabilities. For further information, e-mail: rob.garrett@novita.org.au

1. Introduction

Accessing telecommunication technology and the broad range of services behind it has been an ongoing challenge for people with disabilities. With technology continually changing and mobile phones shrinking in size, the gap between people with disabilities and telecommunication technology has grown. This research trialed and evaluated new configurable 'off-the-shelf' technological options that can improve the lifestyle, independence, security and social interaction of people with physical disabilities. The trials involved ten participants, drawn from the 1300 children and adults for whom *Novita Children's Services Inc* (formerly The Crippled Children's Association of SA, Inc or CCA) provides a service. The trial group included people with mild, moderate and severe physical disabilities affecting movement and speech. The trials tested the ability of the participants to make and receive calls and, for those participants that can use the Short Message Service (SMS), to create and send text messages efficiently.

2. Project Background

The aim of this research was to trial and evaluate new technological options that can improve the lifestyle, independence, and social interaction of people with physical disabilities through the use of telecommunications. This work is the continuation of research conducted by NovitaTech (formerly Regency Park Rehabilitation Engineering), the technology division of Novita, performed in collaboration with the School of Informatics and Engineering, Flinders University, Adelaide.

Preliminary research through a focus group session [2] and the "*Mobile and Home Needs Analysis Survey*" questionnaires [1,3] carried out by NovitaTech and Flinders University, in May 2002, indicated that people with disabilities within the community are able to use, and want to have access to, mobile telecommunications. It has also highlighted that most people with a disability are not aware of the available technology and, if they are, do not use it to its fullest extent. Fewer respondents were actually using the available or add-on mobile phone technology available to them. Of the forty seven respondents, modest numbers expressed interest using available add-on technology or mobile phone features available on more advanced models such as a cordless headset (32%), personal hands-free (32%), speakerphone function (28%), speed dialling (27%) and voice recognition (23%).

This research looked at alternative solutions (such as using car kits, voice recognition and hands-free technology, and network features such as voice mail) to improve the awareness and the telecommunications experience of people with physical disabilities. The aim of the trial was to enable these members of the community to participate and experience telecommunications technology to the same extent as able-bodied people currently do. The research hypothesis was "*that through the use of wireless mobile phone technology, people with disabilities will become more active and participating members of the community, leading to an increased sense of social inclusion, independence, and security*".

3. Research Methods and Procedures

A broad range of participants representing a spectrum of age, disability, gender, and telecommunications experience with telecommunications equipment was sourced. Participants were chosen for the trial based on their needs and the available telecommunications equipment at the time of the trial. This was carried out through an initial assessment of "matching the participant with the available technology". This assessment identified the participants' communication needs and accessibility problems. A priority scale was implemented to measure the "Importance" and "Needs" of the participants, while a rating scale was used to measure the "Performance" and "Frustration" when accessing telecommunications equipment. All participants were subjected to the same questions to guide the researcher to match the participants' needs with the appropriate available solution.

Following the selection of ten participants from the initial assessment, each participant was able to trial the technology that was assessed as being most suitable for them for three weeks. Prior to the trial, each participant received training in the use of the provided technology, whereby all the features and associated applications of the technology were explained in detail. This was a standard protocol for all participants. Re-training was an ongoing process throughout the trial when required by the participants. Due to the nature of the participants involved and the possible problems that may occur due to the technology, some trials ran in parallel depending on the uniqueness of the individual's needs, while other trials ran in series for those where similar solutions were implemented.

An "ABA" style approach was implemented throughout the trial period:

A – Before intervention: without recommended equipment (prior to the trial);
B – During intervention: with recommended equipment (end of the trial);
A – After intervention: when equipment had been withdrawn for two weeks or more.

This process involved a measure of the participant's performance and satisfaction relating to the problem areas identified by the participant at the beginning of the trial. At each stage during the trial an assessment was carried out, through the use of a customised *Canadian Occupational Performance Measure* (COPM) questionnaire [4]. COPM is a standardised outcome measure tool designed to detect change in a participant's self-perception of occupational performance over time. It was used throughout the trial to measure the performance and satisfaction of the broader issues, concerns and problems that a participant had with phone technologies to evaluate the research aim and hypothesis.

Trial participants included those with a mild physical disability with limited mobility and restricted movement, reduced strength or muscular dystrophy, to those with severe Athetoid Cerebral Palsy. Their ages ranged from fourteen to eighty, with some participants having no previous exposure to telecommunication technology. Their details are shown in Table 1.

Table 1: The trial participants, their previous telecommunications experience, and the technology that was provided to them.

PARTICIPANT	AGE	DIAGNOSIS/CLINICAL CONDITION	PREVIOUS TELECOMMUNICATIONS EXPOSURE WITH MOBILE PHONES	TECHNOLOGY PROVIDED
1	17	Cerebral Palsy (CP), limited mobility (walking aid & wheelchair)	Nokia 5110	Panasonic GD95
2	80	Restricted to wheelchair (mobility), hearing aid user	Some exposure, from a family member's handset	Kyocera QCP 3035
3	18	Muscular Dystrophy (Duchenne's)	Panasonic GD75	O_2XDA
4	53	CP mild	Ericsson A2618	Panasonic GD95
5	23	Restricted to wheelchairs (limited movement) and reduced strength	None	Bluetooth Car Kit
6	39	Limited mobility and restricted movement	None	Advanced Car kit
7	18	Muscular Dystrophy	Motorola Talkabout	Kyocera QCP 3035
8	14	CP – cognitively more than physically	Philips Savvy	Panasonic GD95
9	16	Athetoid CP (severe)	None	RehaPhone
10	50	CP (severe)	Nokia 3310	Advanced Car kit

The performance indicators (where applicable) for the trial involved the use and/or access to the following features:

- Voice calls (through various methods such as speed dialling, voice dialling or other methods);
- Text messaging (SMS) and/or email (open, create & send);

- Voicemail (retrieve as well as use);
- Access to the information services (weather, news, sports, lotto numbers etc...) via WAP (Wireless Application Protocol);
- Browsing the Internet (website specified); and
- Other features on the phone (Extras – voice memo or commands plus any other features, depending on the product).

A review of the initial assessment results concluded that the ten participants could be classified into three distinct groups:

GROUP 1 (Grp 1): Participants with mild physical disabilities that prevent them from using standard telecommunications equipment effectively and efficiently. Typical problems were associated with small keys, displays and difficulties relating to lifting or holding the phone for the duration of the call. Three participants belonged to this group.

GROUP 2 (Grp 2): Participants with moderate physical disabilities (eg. Cerebral Palsy) that typically restrict them to the use of one mode of communication such as text or voice and/or limited use of both. Four participants belonged to this group, and one of them is shown in Figure 1 below.

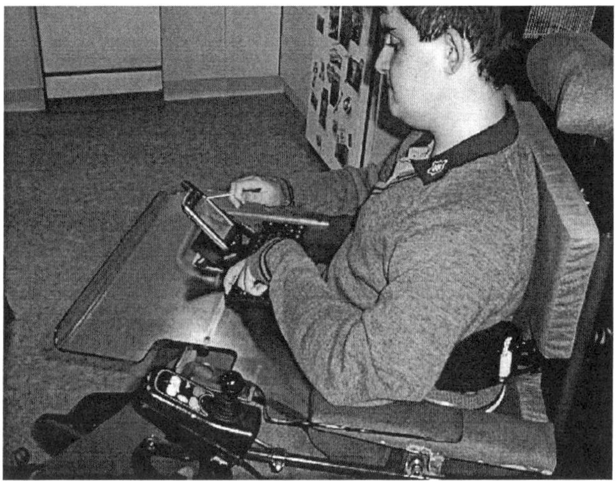

Figure 1: A Group 2 participant trials a new piece of equipment (an O_2XDA personal digital assistant (PDA) and mobile phone) that was matched to his particular needs.

GROUP 3 (Grp 3): Participants with severe physical disabilities (eg. severe Cerebral Palsy). Two individuals used switches to operate an Augmentative and Alternative Communication (AAC) device. A carer normally operates the phone on behalf of these participants. Three participants belonged to this group. Finding an off-the-shelf solution for these participants proved difficult. It required a combination of technologies, innovative thinking and various trials to find the right technologies to operate a mobile phone. Significant time and effort was spent on recommending a solution for participants in this group.

4. Results

Initial interviews with the ten participants revealed that voice calls and text messaging were the **most** important communication needs. Mobile communication solutions that the majority of participants identified to be essential and/or important include:

- Speakerphone capability;
- Voice dialling and speed dialling;
- Predictive text (word prediction) for faster text messaging;
- Voicemail; and
- Larger display.

Other mobile phone solutions that were considered useful by participants included the control of a mobile phone via a computer and an attachable computer keyboard for the phone. Those mobile phone technologies that were considered "not required" by many participants included headsets (cord and cordless) and attachable keypads for a mobile phone.

Nine of the ten participants showed high to very high outcomes. One participant from Group 3 showed only slight improvement in performance and experienced reduced satisfaction with the solution provided. This was due to a technical problem experienced with the telecommunications equipment during the trial period. The voice control system for the mobile phone behaved erratically and did not function as technically specified. Efforts were made to correct this malfunction through software upgrades and hardware replacement, to no avail. Although the trial was not as successful as anticipated, the participant indicated that had the total hands-free solution worked as specified, the solution would have been significant for them.

Figures 2 and 3 show the overall satisfaction and performance results of all of the participants that took part in the trial. It should be noted that during each interview, "1" was the minimum score and "10" was the maximum score. Participants could not score a particular performance or level of satisfaction as being below "1" (i.e. zero) or above "10". The average score for each participant is presented in the figures, and follows on from the "ABA" approach that was described in section 3. The horizontal axis labels in figures 2 and 3 follow the convention "Grp Y (X)", where 'Y' represents the group that the participant was identified as belonging to (i.e. Group 1, 2 or 3 as outlined in section 3) and 'X' represents the particular participant. Using this notation, "Grp 1 (8)" refers to participant 8 who was identified as belonging to Group 1.

The use of car kits that incorporated speakerphone, with voice and speed dialling such as that from *SonyEricsson* and *Nokia*, when installed on wheelchairs proved successful for three participants of the trial. For these participants, the privacy of a conversation was not an issue and the concept of installing a car kit onto a wheelchair was unknown to them. For two of these participants, the increase in performance and satisfaction was significant. Therefore, having speakerphone capability and reduced effort to control the phone through voice and/or speed dialling with the car kit was a very effective solution. The provision of the car kit and elimination of any effort required to control the phone benefited one participant from Group 3 immensely, since prior to the trial the participant had **no** form of independent access to the mobile telecommunications network. The car kit system also has great potential for improving the telecommunications needs of people with disabilities that fit into Group 2 and 3 categories of the trial, and requires promotion by telecommunications providers to further publicise these options.

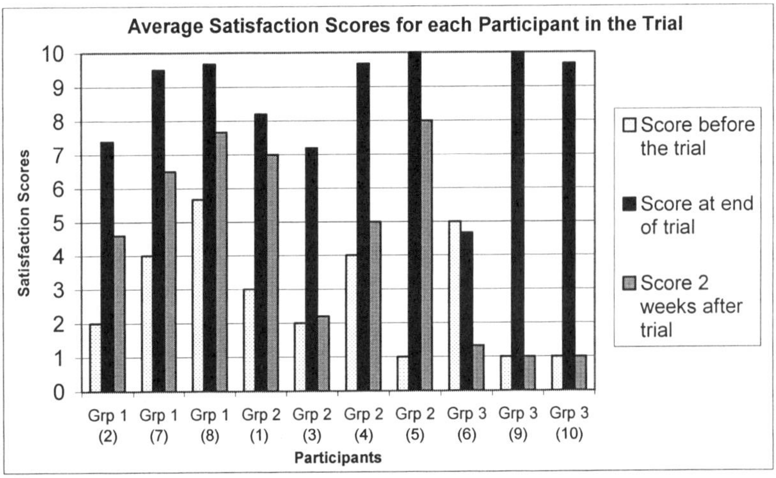

Figure 2: Average satisfaction scores of the 10 participants throughout the trial.

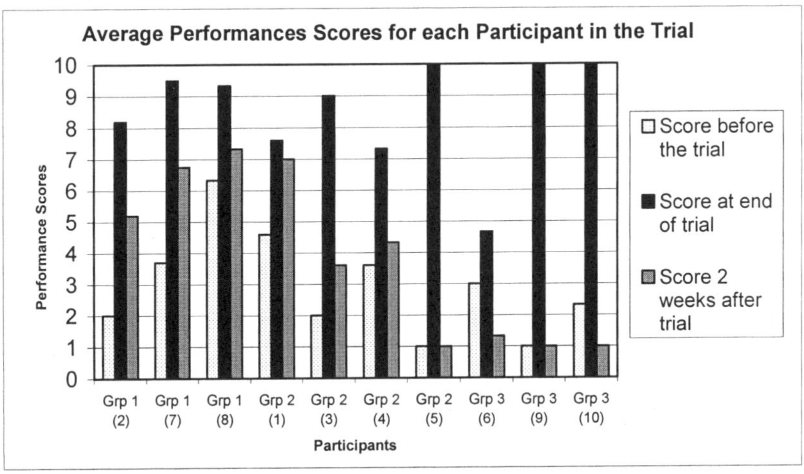

Figure 3: Average performance scores of the 10 participants throughout the trial.

5. Discussion

This research and clinical trial was able to demonstrate that current, off-the-shelf telecommunications equipment can enable people with disabilities, even severe physical disabilities, to access the telecommunications network. Prior to the trial, the researchers were confident that solutions did exist for people with mild to moderate physical disabilities, and were satisfied with the results in these areas.

However, even the researchers involved in this work, who have extensive experience in the disability sector, were surprised when off-the-shelf solutions were found for the participants with severe physical limitations. It was expected that it would be very difficult to find a satisfactory match for these clients, yet a solution was found, and these trial participants can now access the telecommunications network. This was a profound outcome of the trial.

Pivotal to the success of these trials was an in-depth knowledge of existing mobile phone technology options and features, a clear understanding of the client's telecommunication needs and abilities, and the matching of appropriate technology to an individual. This matching process led to 4 of the 10 participants purchasing the solution that was tailored and recommended for them.

Another important outcome from this research was the discovery that most trial participants were not aware of the full capabilities of their current mobile phone (if they had one), and hence **education** played a big factor in improving the way they now use their phone.

6. Conclusions

With the right policies, processes and support (appropriate user skill and equipment matching, education, training and delivery) in place, solutions can be found. This research and trial was able to demonstrate that current off-the-shelf solutions can help alleviate problems and improve the lifestyle, social interaction, security and independence of many people with physical disabilities in terms of telecommunications access.

The trial results showed that:

- There is no insurmountable barrier to the use of phone technology by people with a disability. Features of existing technologies offer affordable solutions to problems of accessibility previously considered unsolvable;
- Mobile telephone technologies can provide improved access, functionality, social interaction, independence, safety and security. These are all areas of high priority for people with a disability;
- Nine out of ten participants showed high to very high results in terms of their overall performance and satisfaction with the use of the telecommunication equipment provided (a technical difficulty prevented an effective evaluation of the 10th participant);
- Participants that had an inadequate solution are now aware of an adequate solution (or alternative solution) to access telecommunication equipment and services. The provision of hands-free features such as speakerphone and voice and speed dialling on phones proved to be essential. Mobile phone car kits also proved to be a practical solution for participants restricted to wheelchairs. Voicemail and text messaging was also important;
- Participants that had no independent access to telecommunication equipment can now access the phone network successfully.

The provision of an effective telecommunications solution for a person with a disability can be achieved within an overall total of half a working day, even for the more challenging situations. Even more substantial is the increased independence each participant gained through an appropriate equipment match, and hence a decreased reliance on a third party to perform a previously impossible task.

Through this research it was concluded that people with a range of physical disabilities **can** use and **should** have equal access to telecommunications equipment and services. With the right policies, processes and support (equipment matching, education, training and delivery) in place, current off-the-shelf solutions can help alleviate problems and improve the lifestyle, social interaction, security and independence of many people with physical disabilities.

7. Acknowledgments

This project, "*New technological options for people with physical disabilities, through the use of telecommunications equipment*", was supported by the Australian Commonwealth through the Telecommunications Research Grant Program of the Department of Communications, Information Technology and the Arts. Telstra's Disability Services also provided additional funding for the purchase of telecommunications equipment and access to their network.

References

[1] Nguyen, T. (2002), Mobile and Home Phone Needs Analysis Questionnaire, Unpublished master's thesis, Flinders University, Adelaide, Australia.

[2] Nguyen, T. (2002), Focus Group: Accessible Mobile Phones, Unpublished master's thesis, Flinders University, Adelaide, Australia.

[3] Nguyen, T. (2002), Accessible Mobile Phone Project, published in the ARATA News, No. 28, Summer 2002, pgs 1-2.

[4] Law, M., et al. (1999). Canadian Occupational Performance Measure, (3rd ed.), CAOT Publications ACE, Ottawa, Canada.

Chapter 2

Smart Home and Healthcare

Toward a Human-Friendly Assistive Environment
D. Zhang and M. Mokhtari (Eds.)
IOS Press, 2004

Potential of Smart Home Technology at Homes of European Elderly

Mervi HIMANEN, PhD
Senior research scientist, VTT Building and Transport; Docent, Helsinki University of Technology
P.O. Box 1800, FIN-02044 VTT, Finland, +358 9 4564570,(fax) +358 9 463251,
mervi.himanen@vtt.fi

1. Abstract

Smart home and information and communication technology (ICT) is expected to assist growing groups of senior citizens if help is needed for independent living at home. The feasibility of technology is dependent on skilled R&D work and feedback of end-users. The paper will summarise results from a few pre-occupancy type studies carried out in some European countries: Denmark, Finland, France, the Netherlands, United Kingdom and Spain. The end-user feedback and attitudes towards smart home and ICT at home among the senior citizens has been in focus.

The seniors are by no means onlookers when ICT is in concern, in spite of the fact that a certain portion of them, who already have reached relatively high age, most probably may at all make acquaintance with it. Although the Finnish senior citizens have not purchased all ICT tools available for use at homes, they wish to have and to learn how to use smart home and ICT applications. Although Finns in particular are considered to have positive attitudes towards technology in general, this positivism is not rare in the other European countries either. The use of ICT at homes follow from the advance of information society and the cap between leading information societies and the followers is closing up - especially, after information has spread of how new technology can assist independent living of elderly.

2. Background

The operating systems of the houses are becoming as essential as other building services – water piping and plumping, heating and cooling, etc. In old building stock where elderly people currently live, planning and refurbishment of new routes, networks and equipment presume special know-how of the methods and costs. New ideas and pioneering experiments concern also intelligent construction materials and products as well as the technical systems. The latest housing production already incorporates many products with electronic intelligence.

It can be taken as given that a large numbers of elderly people wish to be able to live independently as long as possible at their homes, and according to the social policies of European countries the governments wish the same while coping with the growing numbers of elderly. Among other things, technology is expected to aid in solving the problems of growing population of senior citizens in need of assistance. The elderly has been considered to be a special group with special needs. Many solutions for smart housing, independent living and gerontechnology have been tailored to fulfil these expectations.

Attempts to develop a turnkey smart home "product" for world wide markets have pop up every now and then. TRON -house in Japan in 1980's was among the very first ones. However, no ready made smart homes are available. If one wants to have a smart home, lot of design and contracts are needed to build it up from components, which are not necessarily easily accessible, compatible and affordable. In the first place, smart home has been a media home with ICT tools, automated home appliances, advanced home electronics and home control systems connected to building automation. More sophisticated applications - making the house smart in a more wise sense - such as active structures have developed quite slowly.

In the beginning of this millennium, a Finnish housing and facilities management corporation introduced a housing product called the media home. The period of home automation with cabling for ICT networking adapted to mainstream housing stock had started in Finland. To call it a media home demonstrated good knowledge of building concepts, not mixing the house with ICT facilities with a smart house, it is, an intelligent building which covers also the other forms of building intelligence than building logic, in other words electronic intelligence (cf. Section Definitions).

The years after the first media homes were built, were not very successful for the ICT business while the stock exchange value of it collapsed and the hype of it blew up. However, ICT continued to be applied in everyday products and used also in housing. In spite of booming housing markets, for example in Finland, markets of smart home applications have not succeeded. In the Netherlands Smart Home Foundation has not been a great success story either. The business of implementing wireless technology, which is feasible especially in the current housing stock, has not flourished yet. It seems that a certain point have been reached, where a new direction for the R&D of smart home technology has to be taken.

A mean to solve the problem of unsaturated markets is to turn to the residents and ask their needs and wishes in order to get to know about future demand. The construction sector has put efforts on development of design and methods that can satisfy the needs of different customers now and in the future cf. e.g. [11], [12]. Finland is a mini laboratory for studying feasibility of new technology such as ICT and smart home features; it is one of the advanced information societies and small enough (~ 5 million inhabitants). In addition to the surveys to be discussed in this paper in detail, Tampere University of Technology has just recently finished a study on the popularity of smart home features among residents of all ages (http://www.tut.fi/dmi/projects/tatu/semma.htm). A finding was that the residents did not know of the possibilities which new technology can offer. Often potential customers do not know what smart home is. Undergoing work on the ´Book on Smart Homes Evaluation´ by Greger Sandström and Ulf Keijer at Royal Institute of Technology in Sweden will offer further information of end-user feedback.

Students of facilities management at Helsinki University of Technology have made research on the housing providers' and developers' visions of the future smart homes; their market prognoses, as well as reasons for retardation and means of winning new markets [1], [5], [7], [13] and [29]. Similarly to other radical technologies[1], in evitable, new smart home and IC technology is here to stay but it takes time before it becomes a part of standard home building routines. Unexpectedly, the professionals – not the home builders and consumer and housing associations – retard the implementing new products in housing

[1] Radical innovations are products which are meant for market, which does not yet exist [18].

sector and several reasons for that can be found from the building design tradition of conservative building sector [17], cf. e.g. [26].

Although the communication networks will constitute the backbone of our lives now on, the good standard of e-services is essential to the spread of the use of ICT. ICT can be employed even more effectively if systems and practices can be simplified by the means of systems design - even the target should be that some system will disappear after to be recognised unnecessary by systems design. Thus the service load can be decreased or service power moved there where it is best in use in society, or in companies and families. The user-friendliness or good usability and the high quality of information content are needed because human ability to comprehend the information is essential before the ICT can keep its position as a useful tool. Comprehension turns information into knowledge. It is the human skill of selecting valid or relevant information from the vast variety of piles of information available in the new media without any useless negative emotions towards areas still unknown, and put it in use.

3. Definitions

Smart homes are related to the phenomena of automated and intelligent buildings, which sometimes are mixed. There is no universal definition of intelligent buildings. However, certain consensus of the intelligent building concepts exists and efforts for agreement on the definition are available cf. [4] and [29]. The latest of them is available of the automated buildings [30]. The end-user feedback represented in this article is rather on media than smart homes. That is because the residents have experience of the use of ICT at home. However, the use of scenarios in data gathering has made it possible to look at the end-user feedback of the ideas of smart homes too.

To differentiate intelligent buildings from other building concepts the forms of Building Intelligence (BI)[2] have been studied [9] which are derived from the forms of human intelligence[3]. Automated or integrated buildings are intelligent buildings, where logic is the key attribute of the design, and the human ability of mathematical and logic intelligence is the motor for the R&D of solutions and implementation of them. Building automation and ICT services are the leading applications for this form of building intelligence, in the case of housing, the form of BI of media homes. The other forms of building intelligence assist in making the building logic work for the benefit of older residents and housing facilities management, as well as companies working in social housing management and welfare services.

4. Objectives and method

Next will be summarised results of a few previous pre-occupancy studies carried out in some European countries. These studies have used end-user feedback as a measure for the feasibility of technology. A study made in Central Finland already in 1995 among elderly, aged of 55 to 70 years, has worked as a preliminary study for the two others: the

---

[2] *Building-connectivity* (speaking and speech recognition including music and linguistics; user-connectivity and control: either personal or automatic or defined by the organisation in concern); *Building self-recognition* (building knows the state it is in; a kind of consciousness); *Spatiality* (a more conscious understanding of the spatial expression of the architecture, structures, interior design); *Building kinaesthetic* (a sense of change, active structures, moveable structures, furniture and equipment, adjustable technology or building services), and *Building logic* (embedded sensors to monitor the occupants' daily activities, combinativity).

[3] The seven forms of human intelligence by Gardner are (1983): *Logical-mathematical, musical, linguistic, interpersonal, intrapersonal, visual-spatial and bodily-kinaesthetic.*

Elderathome project (QLK6-CT-200-00405) carried out in addition to Finland, in Denmark, in the Netherlands and in Spain. The Demulog project with target groups of all-aged applicants of social housing in Finland, in France and in United Kingdom is used for comparison.

The Finnish survey has been carried out from the viewpoint of the building developers who were improving the quality of housing products, facilities management and welfare service provision. The Demulog project looked the feedback from the energy suppliers' perspective heading to prevent peak hours in electricity consumption, and still serving their tenants with acceptable housing and technology. The Elderathome project promoted independent living and housing conditions of elderly in their present homes.

This paper covers the use of ICT at home for safety, home appliances, home control, communications, as well as, the need of home office and the purpose of using computers and Internet. It is possible on the basis of some European experience of senior citizens to draw a quite clear picture of the difficulties and possibilities faced in smart home market but means of winning the future markets will most probably be dependent on new ideas of applying smart housing in a broad sense - lively debate wanted.

The data gathering has taken place by face to face interview in other case studies except the Finnish one which was carried out by posted questionnaires. The demography of the respondents of the selected cases was quite similar to the average national demography of elderly. Some times there were more men in the sample than in average and also the educational and income levels of the respondents were by no means the best of the elderly. More detail descriptions of the cases in research reports [10], [2] and [20].

The questionnaire of the Elderathome interview was divided into four parts as follows: (1) present situation, the future needs and wishes of dwelling, surroundings, services for independent living, (2) testing feasibility of current standards (Table 1), (3) scenarios of daily activities and services of food or nutrition, eating, cooking and shopping, cleaning and personal business and mobility, and (4) demographic data (age, gender, education, household type, income) including also health condition, activity level and willingness to pay possible extra costs due to needs of getting older.

5. Results

The attitudes of elderly towards the use of automation and smart house solutions are quite positive among the respondents of the Finnish survey of needs and wishes of elderly [20]. Just retired - those in the so called third age - are most interested in activities, hobbies and services. Those still working and the eldest age group are more in need of getting help at home. Then it could be time for adopting technology which promotes good health and function, and keeps up active social life and mobility preventing impairments of old ages [10], cf. [11]. The result corresponds to the heath condition of the respondents. Time for the aid of independent living and gerontechnology is after the health condition starts to demand for it, making helping technology natural and acceptable – even in some cases the video monitoring is desired. This does not mean that old ages is time for suffering from diseases, which can and should be cured.

Housing needs of elderly are quite similar to those of younger generations. If the households of elderly have not as many items as the younger families they are planning to pay some in the future. Already in 1995 14 per cent of respondents aged from 55 to 70 had a home computer and 24 per cent wanted to have a one [21][20], while in average 25 per cent of all Finns had a home computer at that time. On the other hand, 47 per cent of the elderly respondents didn't have any type of ICT at home, not even a mobile phone and only 25 per cent wanted to keep it that way in the future.

Table 1. Topics of the smart home applications of the Elderathome interview.

PERSONAL HYGIENE
A temperature limiter (thermo-regulator) in the faucet.
A hydro-massage system in a bath or a shower.
SAFETY
The floor material (looking normal and stylist out) that prevents slipping.
The colour choices, which are not only beautiful, but help to see things easily.
The stylist handrails in a dwelling in other parts too than bathroom and stairs,
An alarm system which can easily be installed in the future.
Residents are informed about safe behaviour and receive instructions for the use of installed facilities.
HOME APPLIANCES
Domestic appliances that prevent the incorrect use of them.
The appliances can be maintained by users themselves.
Use of fixed resetting and control for safety reasons, e.g. one button to turn all electric appliances off.
HOME CONTROL
Remote control possibility of home appliances and home electronics, e.g. lightning or opening the door.
Alarm buttons, safety bracelet, motion censor and other such equipment to facilitate connections to other people in emergency situation.
Lamps that turn on automatically, when entering a room and which turns off, when no-one is present.
FOR ONE'S CONVENIENCE
Kitchen fitment that can easily be moved either manually or automatically by pushing the button.
Flexible thresholds that will fall down when you step on them.
Using Internet for looking for medical advice or making booking for the appointment to the doctor.

Roughly a quarter of elderly respondents to the Finnish survey, wants to use new technology at home unquestioningly. More than a third of them take it if the solution is good enough and 16 per cent of them will use it if there is no other help available. Men more often than women looked after the quality of technology if it is good enough, and women rather than men decided between technology and manual help. Finally, a share of 16 per cent does not want to use home automation. Contradictorily to the willingness to use home automation a third of elderly told, when asked, how much they are willing to pay for home control system, that they are not ready to take it although they will get it free [22]. Need and wish is not the same thing as the final activity which is a compromise. Most of the respondents to the Finnish survey of needs and wishes of elderly in 1995 said that they either will learn how to use computers if needed or had those skills already [23].

5.1. Connections

In the Mediterranean countries personal social contacts are numerous compared to the Central and Northern European countries (Statistics Finland 1997). Accordingly the response to the Elderathome interview from Finland and Spain give clear proof to the fact; in Spain most of the elderly meet friends or relatives regularly or often while only one fifth of Finnish respondents visit others that often. They had however a chance to talk with some-one daily about worries or when something nice has happened or some had good neighbours whom to visit but not everyday. Relatives and friends of the Finnish respondents live far away or it is otherwise difficult to meet them on regular basis a quarter of Finnish respondents keep contact frequently with them by phone, by mail or via email.

Almost all Finnish elderly respondents of the Elderathome interview had or wanted to have both wired and mobile phone, while younger generation has started to use only mobile phones and the number of fixed phone lines is declining; it was in 2002 52.4 per 100 inhabitants and the number of mobile phones 86.7 per 100 inhabitants (Statistics Finland 2004). The shift from the majority of fixed phone lines to mobile phones took place in 1998 (Statistics Finland 2001). The corresponding figures in Spain were in 2002 quite the same; 50.6 and 82.4. However, in Spain the number of fixed lines is still increasing. Also all Spanish elderly respondents had or wanted to have wired phones but the number present or future holders of mobile phones was some more than half of all corresponding the national situation in average.

The elderly in Helsinki, the capital of Finland have information and communication tools at home in 2003 to same extent as the results of the wishes of the elderly of the previous survey in Central Finland in 1995 prognosticated.

More than a half of the Finnish respondents had or wanted to have a connection to information networks while every tenth within respondents of Spanish cases had or wish to get access to information networks. Signals towards increased use of services of information society are seen also in Spain where the progress of it is not yet as advanced as in Finland; the level of Internet accesses has risen from 9.6 per cent of households in 1999 up to 25.2 per cent of households in 2003 in Spain (Eurostat 2004). The level of Internet accesses was 47.4 per cent of households in Finland in 2003.

The most important reason for having ICT at home in Spain is to keep in contact with relatives and friends and for safety reasons (Table 2.). In Finland multiple purposes are reported about how to use ICT.

Table 2. Most important reason for information and communication channels (the Elderathome interview).

Percentages of the respondents	FIN[1]	E[1]	DK[1]
Safety	47	43	33
Working	11	11	13
Hobbies	41	14	40
Keeping contact to relatives	66	84	33
Keeping contact to friends	64	40	20
Running errands (e.g. telebanking)	77	2	13
Getting services	65	1	27[2]
Other	3	1	13
n	98	96	15

[1] FIN ≡ Finland, E ≡ Spain, [2] Modified question: asked of information access

Table 3. Internet access of households in 2001 (Eurostat).

Netherlands	Sweden	Denmark	Finland	United Kingdom	Ireland	Austria	Luxembourg	Germany	Belgium	Italy	France	Portugal	Spain	Greece
NL	S	DK	FIN	UK	IRL	A	L	D	B	I	F	P	E	EL
64	61	**59**	**50**	**49**	48	47	43	38	36	34	**30**	26	**25**	10

Bold text ≡ within this study

Table 4. The number of home computers in 2001 in some EU countries per inhabitants (Eurostat).

FIN	NL	UK	F	E
36	36	30	22	12

[1] FIN ≡ Finland, E ≡ Spain, NL ≡ the Netherlands, UK ≡ United Kingdom, F≡ France

Table 5. The possession and preference to have a computer (the Demulog project).

Percentages of the respondents	FIN[1]	UK[1]	F[1]
Possession	63	44	19
Wish to have	91	64	48
n	103	100	100

[1] FIN ≡ Finland, UK ≡ United Kingdom, F≡ France

Table 6. Acceptance of restrictions on timing of the use of equipment (the Demulog project

Percentages of the respondents who accept	FIN[1]	F[1]	UK[1]
Electric cooking stove	11	53	46
Washing machine	21	38	49
Other, excluding TV	27	50	35
Other, including TV	18	21	8

[1] FIN ≡ Finland, UK ≡ United Kingdom, F≡ France

Connections to relatives and friends seemed important to the elderly also according to the results from the experiment of the Net corners and telecommunication for home help services in the town of Joensuu in Eastern Finland [27]. Email, writing letters and reading newspapers as well as tele-banking were the most popular purposes to use the Net corners. Pollanen [28] points out that elderly start up using computers, because they want to keep up their memory functions, to learn new and to integrate thereby to the society better, or the computer skills are more valuable in daily life than for example the skills in languages which cannot be used on daily basis.

Similarities and differences were found from the result of the Elderathome interview in contacting various target groups: children, relatives, friends, neighbours, health care, social workers and home help. Health care and social workers were contacted hardly at all. The Spanish respondents kept touch with children, relatives and friends by phoning and meeting while Finnish respondents in addition to that used also mail and email. Mail was never used in Spain but a few uses of email were found also in Spain to keep in contact with close by.

According to Finnish and Spanish case studies the phase of the information society influences the use of communication tools (Table 3 and Table 4). In advanced information society they are used frequently and for multiple purposes. The elder are not the leaders in the use of ICT, but they are by no means against to use new technology, as it was found already in 1995 among elderly in Central Finland [20].

Video phones are not at all popular, although experiments of the use of them in senior service homes in the town of Tampere have given proof of its usefulness for example in preventing loneliness, because the contact by video is more personal than by voice phone. The low quality of the video image transfer has been recognised as a reason for the inconvenience of using video phones. The elderly in Central Finland in 1995 thought that the most important purpose for using video phone could be to get help in emergence situations – women thought so more often than men did [25]. Secondly, the possibility to know, how relatives are doing was a good reason to have video phone.

5.2. Energy and lighting control

The survey of the needs and wishes of the elderly in Central Finland revealed that end-users in the age of 55 to 70 stick to the traditional control devices [20], [24], [19], [16]. Of new lighting control devices (dimmer, timing and pre-settings for various occasions) a natural light control was more often accepted by elderly than by other age groups.

Such home control which is related to safety (alarm buttons, safety bracelet, motion censor and equipment facilitating connections in emergency situation) is very well accepted according to the response of the Elderathome interview. For example, most of answerers had already a temperature limiter in the faucet. Most of the respondents in Finland and in Spain were fond of home control facilitating easy living and energy efficiency such as lamps that turn on automatically, when entering a room and which turn off, when no-one is present. But there were also quite many who did not want to have such luxury.

The Demulog project studied the possibility with thc smart home technology save energy by reduced room temperatures and limited use of electricity for home appliances among adult respondents. The possibility to save water was also checked. The results of the referable room temperature are as follows [3]: (1) a large majority (> 80 per cent) accepts lower temperature when nobody is at home or during the night, (2) a small majority (50 to 57 per cent) accepts lower temperature in bedrooms than in other living spaces, but one third (a share of 35 to 45 per cent) wants to have same temperature all over the dwelling, and (3) a large majority (95 per cent in Finland, 93 per cent in France, 72 per cent in UK) wants as high or higher temperatures in the bathroom and toilet than in the living areas. It is expected that elderly want to have warm housing without draft even more than others. Often their housing is aged too and needs repair and better indoor air [10].

In Finland a share of 71 per cent of the responses and in France a share 55 per cent are against an energy saving system after the result of the Demulog interview [2]. Only in UK was found a share 58 per cent of the respondents who is in favour of savings by restrictive technology. However, in Finland 80 per cent of the respondents wish to have a modern safety equipment (not asked elsewhere). Acceptance of proposed energy-saving measures based on the time limitations of the electricity supply was not very well welcomed (Table 6). But the acceptance of low energy consuming home appliances was very good in Finland (in most cases 99 per cent), good in UK (in most cases from 91 to 96 per cent or more) and although not as good in France (in most cases from 64 to 70 per cent) not at all bad in there either. The acceptance of water saving measures was good (Finland 69 per cent, France 70 per cent, UK 87 per cent), but the acceptance of a composting latrine was not that good (Finland 19 per cent, France 18 per cent, UK 29 per cent).

The lesson of the result of the Demulog interview teaches that although residents seem flexible in timing during daytime - maybe without any compulsory ties - the daily routines of society are still usually followed and changing the timing of domestic work in not necessary possible. It is unstudied if this is true also among elderly having free time.

5.3. Safety and home appliances

The answers to the questions about safety aspects were all accepted by the respondents from Spanish and Finnish cases (Table 1). They were more in use in Spanish than in Finnish cases. The only exception was an alarm system which can be installed easily in the future. A quite good number of Spanish respondents don't want to have it.

As younger families also the Finnish elderly interviewed in 1995 liked the safety facilities such as safety stove, movement monitoring, water leakage or fire alarm, etc. [20]. The equipment helping in reaching objects such as dishes and china, or aid for moving around are popular, as well as, the HVAC equipment for good indoor climate are important for elderly – more important than smart control [10], [16] and [19]. Kitchen fitment that can easily be moved either manually or automatically by pushing the button seems to a favourite of "European elderly". Only Danish and Dutch (relatively small samples) were not interested in to have adaptable kitchen cabinets or sanitary facilities.

The security of surroundings was not in favour among respondents from the Finnish and the Spanish cases of the Elderathome interview although the question was testing the Dutch design recommendation, the "Woon Keur Certificate" about paths behind housing to be social secure, conveniently arranged and not inviting for unauthorised people. This unpopularity of the Dutch recommendation within Finnish and Spanish cases might have something to do with the population density which in the Netherlands is the highest in Europe and the lowest in Finland [8]. The possibility to come across with someone violent or with other bad intentions is not that high in the last mentioned countries.

Response to questions of home appliances varies (Table 1). The Finnish respondents want to have safety home appliances when needed, but not equipment which has to be maintained by them selves. The Spanish favour domestic appliance which prevents incorrect use of it and which can be maintained by the end-users.

The Finnish elderly respondents (three quarters willing) were far more willing to use new housing technology in general than Spanish (two thirds not willing). This is contradictory to the fact that quite many of the new solutions were in use in the Spanish dwellings. The similar difference is found when looking the response of the willingness to learn how to use new technology; four fifths of the Finnish respondents are willing to learn after there will be a need for it and half of the Spanish respondents are not at all interested in learning new any more. This confirms the earlier opinions of use of ICT of Finnish elderly [20].

The scenarios of the lifestyles revealed that if copying with independent living turned out difficult, the Finnish elderly respondents favoured solutions which allow to be served at home while the Spanish respondents looked help from their own neighbourhood. A good share of Finnish respondents was trusting also on ICT; services via Internet and emails. They were also otherwise technology fans; if help was needed for cooking they like to solve it either with getting meals-on-wheels or using modern technique for easier cooking.

Questions of home appliances and of course the questions of home control were on very new solutions. In addition to the previous mentioned, such as flexible thresholds that will fall down when you step on them were asked. On one hand ignorance and on the other clear opinions of the respondents can have influenced on some contradictory response and in some cases missing answers on new technology. Also the questions about the knowledge of renovations revealed that senior citizens do not necessarily know that new technology can help them live longer in their present homes.

6. Conclusions

The information society in terms of use of communication technology is here already, and the elderly are by no means onlookers when ICT is in concern, despite the fact that a portion of them most probably may at all make acquaintance with it. More sophisticated applications such as active structures have developed quite slowly. The senior citizens are ready to use technology at home and wish to have smart home and ICT applications quite as willingly as the younger generations. The use of ICT at homes follow from the advance of information society and the cap between leading information societies and the followers is closing up

It seems obvious that in the e-Europe senior citizens are not a special group which is not interested in the latest ICT helping their every-day life and rather the problems appear because they do not necessarily know that new technology can help them live longer in their present homes. Some solutions elderly want to have after grown old enough to need them – not necessarily earlier. Flexible spaces and adaptable technology is able to serve residents when needed.

The end-user feedback is a good tool when determined which implication takes place first. Those who think they are eager to adapt new are not all ready to act right away and on the other hand some of those who say that they are not interested, in fact, are the first to use new technology if it becomes available.

7. Acknowledgements

The results from the EU 5FP project Demulog was carried out in co-operation with Mr. Pascal Girault EDF in France, Dr. Dragana Avramov, Population and Social Policy Consultants (PSPC) in Belgium and Dr. Helen Mulligan Cambridge Architectural Research Ltd (CAR) in United Kingdom, and Elderathome with Dr. Pirkko Kasanen from TTS Institute in Finland.

References

[1] Aaltonen, J., (2004). *Älykoti – asukkaiden toiveet ja tarpeet.* Espoo: Helsinki University of Technology. Institute of Real Estates Studies. 15 p. (in Finnish, to be published)

[2] Avramov, D., (2001). *Living Conditions and Preferences of Families in Housing Need. Results from the Demulog Survey.* Brussels: Population and Social Policy Consultants (PSPC). 19 p. (unpublished working paper)

[3] Avramov, D., (2001)., pp. 16-17

[4] Clements-Croome, D. (ed.). (2004). *Book on Intelligent Buildings.* London: Thomas Telford Books. (to be published Sep 2004)

[5] Estama, E. (2004). *Tuotevalmistajien ja -suunnittelijoiden odotukset älytalosta.* Espoo: Helsinki University of Technology. Institute of Real Estates Studies. 18 p. (in Finnish, to be published)

[6] Eurostat., (2001). *Telecommunication Indicators in the Eurostat Area.* Brussels: European Commission. Statistical office of the European Communities. Directorate D: Business statistics. Unit D-3: Production. & ITU, International Telecommunication Union. Short term business statistics. 17 p.

[7] Granvik, S., (2004). *Sosiaalinen isännöinti ja näkökulmia älytalon mahdollisuuksista sen tukemiseksi.* Espoo: Helsinki University of Technology. Institute of Real Estates Studies. 12 p. (in Finnish, to be published)

[8] Haffner, M. E. A., Dol, C. P., (2000). *Housing stattistics in the European Union 2000.* Delft: Delft University of Technology. OTB Research Institute for Housing, Urban and Mobility Studies. 82 p. , p. 6

[9] Himanen, M., (2003). *The Intelligence of Intelligent Buildings. The Feasibility of the Intelligent Building Concept in Office Buildings.* Espoo: VTT. VTT Publications 492 (ISSN 1235-0621). 497 p. ISBN 951-38-6038-8, pp. 284-342

[10] Himanen, M., Rauhala, R., Sjögren, A.-M., Masides, A., Codina, J., Hoogendoorn, F., Gottschalk, G., (2004). *Universal Housing Styles and Cultural Differences. Some European Cases of Elderly - Needs and Wishes of Dwelling, Surroundings and Services.* Brussels: European Commission. Deliverable 3 of Elderathome (The Prerequisites of the Elderly for living at home: Criteria for Dwellings, Surroundings and Facilities (QLK6-CT-2000-00405). 85 p. (to be published), pp. 6-10

[11] Himanen, V., Himanen, M., (2003). *Connecting Homes of Senior Citizens to Services and Recreation.* In: The proceedings of the ICADI, International Conference on Aging, Disability and Independence Advancing Technology and Services to Promote Quality of Life. Track of Transportation. Dec 4-6. 2003. Washington, DC: University of Florida, American Society on Aging, European Commission. (to be published)

[12] Himanen, M., Himanen, V., (2003). *Human Engineering in Studying Residents and Housing.* In: Methodologies in Housing Research, Theme 4. How do we identify the structural relations between cultural, social and psychological factors related to the design, meaning and use of housing. Stockholm 22-24 Sep 2003. Available at: http://www.infra.kth.se/BBA/?lang=sv.

[13] Jokinen, S., (2004). *Älytalojen kysyntä ja tarjonta.* Espoo: Helsinki University of Technology. Institute of Real Estates Studies. 23 p. (in Finnish, to be published)

[14] Kärnä, S. (1992). *Keski-ikäisten tulevaisuuden näkemykset ja toiveet omasta vanhuuden palveluista. 45-64-vuotiaisiin varkautelaisiin kohdistunut kyselytutkimus.* Kuopio: University of Kuopio, City of Varkaus. 90 p. (in Finnish)

[15] Lehto, M., Jantunen J., (1991). *Älykäs rakennus. Markkinatutkimus. Otto Wuorio Oy.* Espoo: VTT Yhdyskunta ja rakennustekniikka. 16 p. Appendix 56 p. (in Finnish, confidential)

[16] Lehto, M., (1999) *Applicability of Smart House Features for Homes of Elderly. Intelligent and Responsive Buildings.* In: G.Klepfisch (ed.), Proceedings of 1st International Conference on Intelligent and Responsive Buildings in Brugge, Belgium. March 29th - 30th 1999. Antwerpen: Technologisch Institut vzw, Belgium Centre for Domotics and Immotics (BCDI), CIB Working Commission WO98. pp. 195 - 203. ISBN 90-76019-09-6

[17] Lehto, M., (2001). *Commercialisation of the technologies developed in the RAKET research programme.* Helsinki. (The LINKKI 2 Research Programme on energy Conservation Decisions and Behaviour. Publication

25/2001, ISSN 1456-5013). 160 p. ISBN 951-788-338-2. Available also at: http://www.tts.fi/linkrap.htm. (in Finnish, with an abstracts in English), pp. 9, 108-109, 142-146
[18] Kivisaari & al. in: Lehto, M., (2001), pp. 24-25
[19] Lehto, M. (1998a). *Smart House Features in the Homes of Elderly - An End User Oriented Approach.* In: Alistair D.N. Edwards, András Arato, Wolfgang L. Zagler (eds.), Computers and Assistive Technology proceedings of ICCHP '98, 6th International Conference on Computers Helping People with Special Needs, Vienna Austria - Budapest Hungary. 31th Aug.- 4th Sep. 1998, vol. 118 and CD-ROM edition. Vienna: Österreichische Computer Gesellschaft on behalf of the International Federation for Information Processing (IFIP). pp. 198-202 ISBN 3-85403-118-1.
[20] Lehto, M., (1998). *Tekniikkaa ikä kaikki – käyttäjän käsitys asumisen automaatiosta.* Helsinki: Ministry of Environment. Housing and Building. (Finnish Environment 244. ISSN 1238-7312), 180 p. ISBN 952-11-0339-6 (in Finnish with English and Swedish summary), pp. 128,160
[21] Lehto, M., (1998)., p. 153
[22] Ibid., p. 140
[23] Ibid., p. 131
[24] Ibid., p. 149
[25] Lehto, M., Karjalainen, S., (1996). *Uuden tekniikan käyttö ikääntyvien asumisessa. Käyttäjäkyselyn tulokset erityisesti TPO:n käyttöön.* Espoo: VTT. 24 p. (in Finnish, confidential), p. 19
[26] Mikkola, K., Riihimäki, M. (2002). *Omakotirakentajien valmius ympäristöystävällisiin rakennustapoihin.* Espoo: VTT Research Notes 2170. (ISSN 1235-0605) 53 p. ISBN 951-38-6095-7 (in Finnish with English abstract) Available at: http://www.inf.vtt.fi/pdf/tiedotteet/2002/T2170.pdf, ISBN 951-38-6096-5, ISSN 1455-0865
[27] Pollanen in: Piirainen, T., Tedre, S., (year unknown). *Telematic services for the elderly. TSE project 1999-2001 in the Health Care and Social Services. Evaluation.* 58 p. (Orders: mailto tuula.piirainen@jns.fi), pp. 17, 19
[28] Pollanen in: Piirainen, T., Tedre, S., (year unknown)., pp. 18-19
[29] So, A., Ting-pat. (2001). *The Intelligent Building Index (IBI) Manual.* Hon Kong: Asian Institute of Intelligent Buildings. May. 2001. 84 p. ISBN 962-86268-1-7
[30] *Technology Roadmap for Intelligent Buildings.* (2002). Ottawa: National Research Council. 60 p. ISBN 0-662-33203-2, available also at: www.caba.org, referred 8.4.2004.
[31] Viranko, N., (2004). *Älykoti – rakennuttajien brandit ja kokemukset.* Espoo: Helsinki University of Technology. Institute of Real Estates Studies. 15 p. (in Finnish, to be published)

Toward a Human-Friendly Assistive Environment
D. Zhang and M. Mokhtari (Eds.)
IOS Press, 2004

Exploring New Ways of Enabling e-Government Services for the Smart Home with Speech Interaction

Christian A. **Schiller**, *IBM, Germany*
Yi Min **Gan**, *IBM, China*
Charles **Kemper**, *Voice Insight, Belgium*
Borivoj **Tydlitat**, *IBM, Czech Republic*

This paper discusses how in the future e-Government services can be enabled with easy Speech Interaction and are made ready for a dynamic service delivery environment. The European Union 6th Framework project "SAFIR" (Speech Automated Friendly Interface Research) is creating an innovative paradigm in the area of Human-Machine interface, combining Voice & Graphics. The outcome of the SAFIR project will give each citizen and special user groups an equal opportunity to access and modify at any time interactively existing up to date e-government information through easy-to-use devices as a television (TV), wired and wireless devices (cell phones or Personal Digital Assistants [PDAs]) from anywhere by usage of own voice in his daily language. Imagine the citizen at anytime everywhere simply speaking to his TV or PDA to request and fill E-Government forms and transactions. This paper focuses on the "Smart Home" aspect of delivering E-Government services, through the use of Residential Service Gateways and Set-top boxes.

1. Overview of SAFIR project goals

1.1. The Societal Problem

Modern democracies are facing the growing challenge of the information of the citizens:

- How to inform the citizen?
- How to give access to existing data?
- How to maintain this data, so that the information is properly up to date?
- How to collect information from the citizens in an efficient and easy way?
- How to give a positive feeling that the administration is really servicing the population?

As a result, a key societal problem is the communication between governmental sources and all citizens with no discrimination; more precisely it can be described now as the challenge on how to give an equal opportunity to both Internet literate and Internet illiterate citizens to access reliable governmental data sources.

At the same time special (mobile) governmental users (national, regional, municipal employees, police, fire brigades, civil protection...) are facing a similar problem while being in the field. The problem is enlarged by the fact that in some circumstances they should also update the governmental data repositories with new facts to maintain the reliability of those data sources.

1.2. The Goals

Consequently, the first goal of SAFIR is to **give an equal opportunity** to individual citizens and groups of European citizens, public bodies or private companies (e.g. Fire Brigade, Municipal field employees, police and security officers, Doctors, ...) to access, through easily usable devices, existing authorized content without having to be PC literate using the simplest human interfaces: voice + graphics (eye). For the PC literate users it will increase efficiency when accessing data being mobile.

The second objective of SAFIR is to create the tools, techniques and methods to build and maintain reliable content up to date, by sending people in the field with voice activated mobile devices: This addresses the second goal of the project - the governmental services to the population and the way of working of the administrations could be effectively improved by speeding up the creation of reliable and up to date repositories.

2. State of the Art Technology

This chapter outlines the technologies and concepts which are to be used in the SAFIR project for the "citizen" user group, using so-called Set-Top Boxes (STB) to access e-government services. An STB is a small computing unit which usually connects to a television set, or is already built into a television set. Common uses for STBs *today* are the reception of digitally broadcasted TV programs (DVB) and, using a Smart Card as authentication, the decryption of Pay TV programs. Additional features such as Electronic Program Guides, Video Recording functionality and even internet browsing capabilities are increasingly offered by STB manufacturers.

This is, however, not enough to provide multimodal access to e-government services. Today's STBs are closed systems designed specifically to serve the defined purposes. Also, the only human-machine interface usually is an infrared remote control. In SAFIR, we are extending this concept of STBs with the open-standard application platform approach of the OSGi Alliance.

2.1. Speech Recognition and Synthesis

Recent progress in human speech and language processing technologies has made it practically feasible to use human speech as a means of human-machine interaction. While the state of the art is still far from offering a real "talk" with a computer, there already are speech technologies efficient and robust enough for successful business deployment. At the same time, advances both in computer technology and in speech processing have made it possible and practical to use speech interaction not only with servers and desktop computers, but also with various portable and embedded devices.

There are several technologies related to speech and language that are already practically useable. The principal ones are speech recognition and synthesis, speaker validation and identification, natural language generation, translation and understanding and various text search and information retrieval techniques. The technologies most relevant to speech-based user interfaces are speech recognition, synthesis and simpler forms of language understanding.

Most examples of existing speech and dialog-based user interfaces can be found in telephony, where automation of call centres using server-based speech recognition, understanding and synthesis is becoming common. Speech on desktop has found only a limited number of customers so far, but there is an important group of users with visual and other disabilities, who greatly benefit from technologies like screen readers or dictation.

With nowadays' tremendous growth of portable and embedded devices and their ever increasing capabilities, the time has come to utilize speech-based user interfaces on portable computers, PDAs, cell phones, multimedia devices, smart appliances and other equipment for home, office and industry. An example of success of embedded speech is the automobile – numerous manufacturers already integrate speech control in their cars. Such systems provide for example cell phone name dialling, integrated messaging, navigation, diagnostics or voice control of those car functions where it is acceptable from safety point of view.

2.2. *"Smart Home" Device Middleware*

As illustrated in Figure [F1], Home Gateway is the central controller in an home to support Smart Home solution, it bridges community broadband data networks to internal home networks, enabling customer to receive a whole new class of services. Home Gateway provides Internet access, facilitates networking in home and brings value-added services including digital Audio/Visual entertainment, control, security, management and more that will be offered to improve the home life experience. Home Gateway can be implemented as Set Top Box (STB) or Residential Service Gateway, or a device combined both functions.

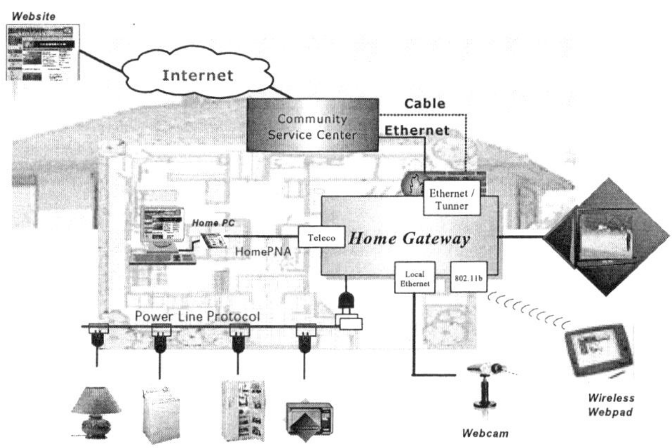

[F1] Home Gateway Network Connectivities

2.2.1 *Smart Home Device Software Architecture*

Figure [F2] shows the common software architecture of smart home devices, Home Gateway is one kind of such devices. This architecture is targeted at supporting economically viable device deployments by device manufacturers while simultaneously supporting the scalability needs and protecting the investment of service providers, content authors and application programmers as new device classes emerge.

Network connectivity to support the delivery of both data and application services brings in a range of additional requirements. These include security, device management, user management, content formatting and software distribution requirements. End to end runtime solutions defined to meet these requirements create additional requirements associated with managing user subscription, application and device life cycles and the potential mismatches between them. The increase in overall system complexity has created the need for appliance middleware. This middleware is intended to address the broad range of network appliance platform requirements, while simultaneously maximizing reuse among the components that are used to instantiate it.

To respond to the widely heterogeneous collection of devices and requirements, IBM's device architecture is a composable collection of subsystems. There are five categories of subsystems that make the architecture. These subsystems are Operating System, User Interface, Communications, Security and Application subsystem. These subsystem services work together in a cohesive manner to enable the construction of different device reference platforms to address the different classes of device capability. Components from each subsystem may require other components, potentially from other subsystems, to operate (i.e. many of these components cannot stand alone).

Each of these subsystems contains a number of components. These components represent a collection of both native and Java based implementations. Reference platforms for different device classes are built from appropriate collections of these subsystems and, more accurately, collections of components from each of these subsystems integrated into a single reference platform. In some cases, both a Java and a native implementation are available for inclusion in a reference platform.

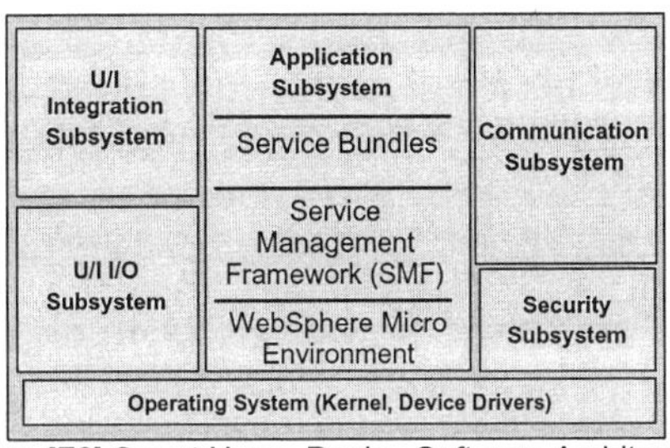

Figure [F2] Smart Home Device Software Architecture

Linux, originally developed for the desktop and adapted for servers, has done well in these markets and is making in-roads into the highly fragmented embedded market, offering developers and users the promise of a common operating system across these platforms. Availability of source code, royalty-free, and reputation are key criteria for selecting Linux. The open source community represents a powerful movement and open development model driving innovation.

2.3. "Smart Home" Services and Business Context

This chapter is an excerpt from the IBM White Paper "Smart Home In-house and Backend Architecture" [R1], which discusses in more detail how Smart Home services can be delivered to consumers by a Service Aggregator. The excerpt in here is used to enable the basic understanding of the Smart Home context.

It is important to realize that the consumers of Smart Home Services are predominantly ordinary non-technical people. They will be happy to "outsource" the management and delivery of Smart Home Services based upon the appliances they have in their homes to someone, instead of taking care of that for themselves by dealing with a possibly large number of service providers. This creates a new and fascinating business opportunity for a company taking the role of a *Smart Home Service Operator (SHSO)*. Ideally, a Smart Home Service Operator has already a business relation to potential Smart

Home Consumers and offers some simple IP connectivity to them. It leverages its communication channels into the home, to the consumer premises equipment and establishes financial relations to the consumer and the level of trust a SHSO has in the consumer's mind. This is, because the SHSO has already been serving the consumer successfully for some time, compared to Service Providers acting directly over the Internet.

The SHSO manages the RSGs and all software running on them. He provides a service delivery environment to which Home Service Providers may connect to. The SHSO makes it easy for consumers to subscribe and unsubscribe to a variety of Smart Home Services and to pay on a per-usage model. The SHSO operates a backend platform which Service Providers may utilize to offer and deliver Smart Home Services to the consumer, thus making Smart Home Services an *on demand business.*

The Smart Home Service Operators hold the key to manage and deliver Smart Home Services to their consumers. From our point of view, Smart Home Services, such as Security, Entertainment, Health / Elderly Care, Home Office and Meter Reading will soon achieve a good market acceptance. The business model for a SHSO is challenging but viable. IBM executed studies where this viability could be proven for specific customers. These studies showed that there is no one and only business model, but a specific one dependent on the customer, its locale and its clientele.

As depicted in figure [F3], the Smart Home Service Operator (SHSO) acts as a mediator between the Service Providers (which provide a set of services as described in the previous chapters) and the homes. It is aggregating the Smart Home Services and may act as a single "face" to the consumer for all Smart Home Services offered by Service Providers through the SHSO. Delivering Smart Home Service is complex from a technical perspective. This includes the management of the Residential Service Gateway and the applications that are running it. Smart Appliances have to be integrated and connected to the Service Providers and have to be made accessible for the consumer at home and out of the home. The SHSO hides this complexity from the consumer.

The SHSO supports the consumer in the home providing a local interface to the Smart Home Services running on the RSG. It supports the consumers out of the home by giving them access to the Smart Home Services via a Family Portal from different types of devices. A Family Portal is the portal which consumers use to register and manage user IDs and Smart Home Services as well as to access their home over the Internet. The SHSO supports the Home Service Providers by leveraging the RSG infrastructure in the home and by providing the connectivity. In addition, the Service and Device Management functions are shared. Home Service Providers may get access to the appliances they run at the consumer's premises, if the consumer agrees to.

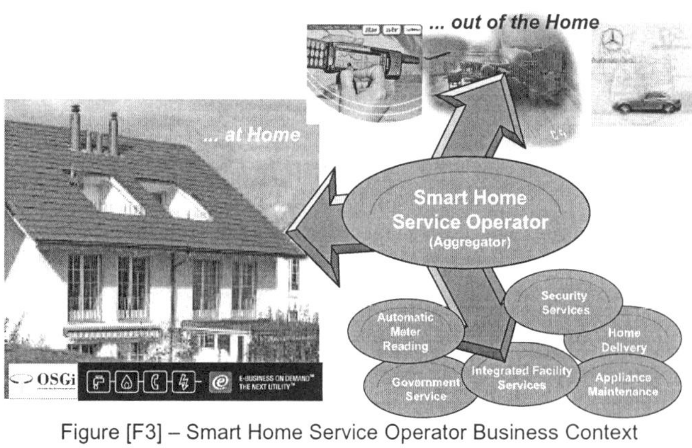

Figure [F3] – Smart Home Service Operator Business Context

2.4. *Voice Query Language*

2.4.1. *Introduction: The problem*

Despite the enormous advances made in the core voice technologies (recognition, synthesis and authentication) on which they are based, to be able to deploy voice applications in such a manner that they attain a high degree of acceptance and, at the same time, operate economically, is still today a challenging task.
The user really wants voice applications that are comfortable and easy to use.
However, most of the voice applications today are specifically developed using more or less proprietary tools or still emerging standards like VoiceXML and SALT.

But specially developed, custom-built systems, even using object technologies and emerging standards, require an enormous configuration and programming effort. Because of the high degree of complexity in these proprietary voice applications, economical operation is nearly impossible on a large scale.

To be really deployable voice technology should be in a position to take any existing repository or application and allow the user to start to interact without having to program all the possible interaction scenarios: An almost impossible dream when you add the additional problems of ontology, and phonetic ambiguities – especially in a multilingual and multicultural space like Europe.

2.4.2. *A conceptual solution: The Voice Query Language from Voice-Insight*

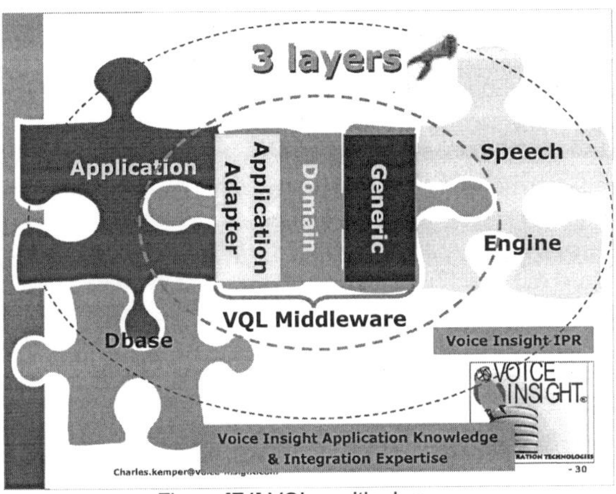

Figure [F4] VQL positioning

Speech Engines are of 3 basic types :

- Voice Synthesis or Text To Speech (TTS)
- Voice Recognition or Speech To Text (STT)
- Voice Authentication

Voice recognition software, or software that converts a human speech recorded by the sound card of a PC into a text document, is becoming a commodity item. Companies like IBM, Scansoft, Nuance, Panasonic and Microsoft are developing those packages for instance. The so called *Speech Recognition Engines* need various information elements in order to function among others :

- ☞ A list of words or dictionary
- ☞ A list of phonetic representations
- ☞ A list of rules about how to use those words to create sentences

Statistical data to document the probability for a word to occur in a particular context (words preceding or following the word under consideration).
Speech Recognition Engines are by now common off-the-shelve (COTS) products.

Information systems, like GIS (Geographical Information Systems), ERP (Enterprise Resource Planning), DM (Document Management) and PDM (Product Data Management) manage business data that are vital for companies. The data managed by those systems is very often stored in a database management system. Although the software is commonly available, most companies have invested enormous amounts of money in both the customisation of the systems and in the creation of the data managed by the systems. Therefore, the information systems and their data represent a considerable asset to these companies.

The Voice Query Language invented, developed and implemented by Voice Insight is addressing the following mission:

VQL makes it possible for users to use COTS speech technology (both speech recognition and speech synthesis) to interact with existing Information Systems.

The main features of VQL™ that make this possible are:

1. A Natural Language syntax based voice command interface.
2. A domain concept that contains generic elements common to a particular class of applications (typically linking application topological relations with generic linguistic forms).
3. Automatic dictionary and grammar creation based on information from the domain model, from the information system (system commands, usually actions) and from the managed data set (objects to which actions are applied).
   The dictionary is created at runtime and can be dynamically adapted to the application context, allowing to create the voice interface automatically on the fly.
4. Seamless vocal access to multiple applications through multiple active dictionaries and grammars. This feature makes VQL a Vocal Application Browser.
5. Integration of speech technology through industry standard interfaces and possible proprietary interfaces
6. Dictionary swapping management system.

2.4.3. Dialogs, Syntaxes, Natural language and Domains and Ontologies

User interfaces can be either syntax or dialog based. Graphical user interfaces are dialogs because at each selected menu level, the system responds with next available menu choices. Dialog interfaces can be very awkward, especially when many successive choices have to be made. Natural language is syntax based. People understand a sentence because the language syntax is wired in their heads. Sentences can carry a whole lot of information at a cost of being very complex to analyse.

Vocal interfaces using natural language are best suited to a syntactical approach, especially when a graphical feedback exists. Dialog based systems could be acceptable when voice is the only interface. VQL uses a domain based natural language syntax approach and supports dialogs. The purpose of the VQL™ solution is to allow a user to query or command **existing** information systems through spoken language. Commands involve the activation of information system functions. Those functions can in most cases be described as actions on items managed by the information system.

The richness of natural language vocabulary and syntax allow actions to be requested in a multitude of different ways. The task of understanding natural language is a considerable one. Even if there would be no technical limitations in the speech recognition engines, it still would be very elaborate to describe the syntax and vocabulary people uses effortless while composing daily requests for action. Complex natural language analysis would be needed to extract the meaning from the stream of words understood by the speech recognition engine. Only then the intention of the speaker could be translated into actions in the information system.

The core VQL uses the opposite approach. If one knows the set of objects and related functions that an information system makes available to a user (in a given context), commands that apply to these objects can be phrased in a "generic" way. Only those VQL phrases applicable to the particular user, the particular context, the set of objects available to the user in the information system need to be made available at that particular time.
This principle reduces both the complexity of the grammar of allowable commands and the size of the dictionary of words that need to be understood. VQL application adapter does implement the actions related to the understood phrases. This adapter program maps the recognized request for action on information system supplied logic.

The EC funded SAFIR project will use the current VQL technology and push it a step further by adding domains (e-Government / e-Payment), translations, ontologies, modes and user adaptiveness.

3. SAFIR Set-Top-Box System Development Kit

3.1. *Solution Overview*

In the introduction it is outlined that the SAFIR project will create a new paradigm in combining Voice, Natural language and Graphics user interface.

The project will first integrate in one SAFIR Software Development Kit (SDK) different innovative layers:

- Device and User Adaptative Voice Engine
- On the Fly user voice natural interface for existing e-Government content
- Bi-directional communication between an in-home Intelligent Remote Control (IRC) and a service gateway-based Set-Top Box
- Spatial Ontology Mediator

With more traditional layers innovative by their combination with the above:

- Cross-language term substitution and Routing translation engines
- E-Government smart card mask for voice interaction

And other needed components:

- Voice Synthesis and Authentication techniques
- Mobile Devices such as an Intelligent Remote Control for the Home
- STBs and Residential gateways

Those elements are represented in this functional representation in the following figure:

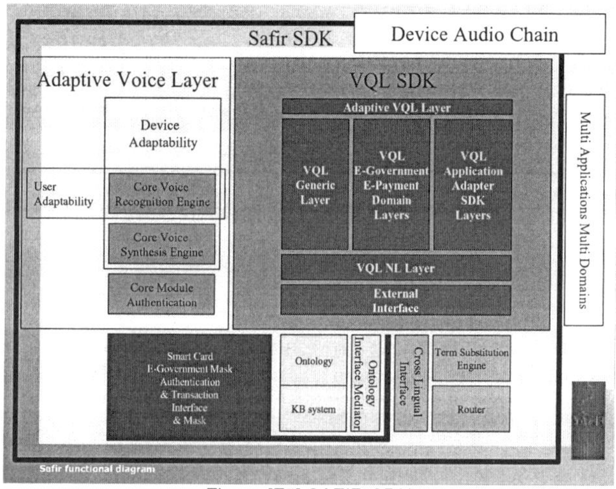

Figure [F5] SAFIR SDK

The SAFIR exploitable SDK will within the SAFIR project be used to create application oriented software development kits selected to be innovation with high exploitation potential and societal impact for more targeted user populations.

In the previous chapters, the state of the art technologies of the Speech HMI and Smart Home service delivery domains were outlined. In the course of the SAFIR project, those two worlds are "married" for the first time, enabling service aggregators and governments to deploy Smart Home and e-government platforms over the same basic technology platform. The following chapter outlines how the advantages of this solution.

3.2. *Benefits of the Solution*

3.2.1. *For Citizens*

For Citizens, the benefit of the SAFIR STB SDK will become tangible as soon as the SAFIR project enters the pilot phase with actual citizen users in late 2005. For the first time, citizens will have the chance to interact with the e-government services in a wholly new way – with three selected pilot regions in Europe, citizens will be able to interact with the services their local government can provide to them via their TV set and in natural spoken conversation.

The aim of the SAFIR project is define a viable solution for handling voice interaction for e-government services. Due to the modular and flexible architecture as outlined in the previous chapter, device manufacturers of mobile devices, Set-Top Boxes and Residential Services Gateways who base their software stack on open standards will be able to reuse the SAFIR components and thus make their devices SAFIR compliant. That way, those devices will be able to serve as clients for the SAFIR e-government applications provided by the administrations. Citizen users are then provided with a STB either through the government or through third parties. Most likely, telecommunications companies will take that role, but in some cases also governmental institutions could go that way. One example for the latter is the Naestved Kommune in Denmark, which is taking an innovative approach in providing healthcare and security solutions for their citizens by providing them with a Residential Service Gateway.

The main benefit of the SAFIR approach for the citizens is that a new group of people will be able to gain access to e-government solutions, the group of internet-illiterate people. By making the interaction with government processes as easy as turning on the TV and leading a natural language conversation instead of having to cope with the typical maladies of PCs, the reach and benefit of those e-government applications will be greatly increased. Another benefit is that citizens can access multiple services through a single piece of hardware (the STB) installed in their home. Knowing the short device life cycles especially in the consumer goods market, an open standard approach for the software middleware ensures that applications will still run on new devices with new capabilities and new services.

Thus, the decision for the citizen to buy a device incorporating the SAFIR technology is eased. At the same time, viewed from another angle, this fact encourages STB manufacturers to incorporate the SAFIR approach into their devices.

3.2.2. For Service Providers and Aggregators

The home and office networking market needs converging towards open standards based connectivity to enable interoperability. With emerging technologies like Universal Plug and Play and the dynamic service delivery platform defined by the OSGi Alliance, this trend is visible, but still in early stages of market penetration.

In a networked world without open standards and interoperability, the complexity of heterogeneous home networks can be managed neither by the end user (the consumer of services), nor by any kind of management instance like a service provider or aggregator. This, in the end, does not benefit the end user, who will be getting more and more frustrated by complex, non-cooperating technology bits and pieces. For a specific service provider this means that the quality of service they can promise to their customers will deteriorate, as many kinds of yet unknown incompatibilities or interferences of other networked home equipment with the service provider's equipment make it increasingly impossible for them to determine the root cause of a problem with the service.

The SAFIR approach, combining the manageability of an OSGi platform with an innovative way for realising a speech user interface, allows service providers and aggregators to leverage SAFIR compliant STBs and RSGs for the integration in their services portfolio and thus enable a better quality of service for their customers.

As governments can be seen both as a service provider (of e-government services) and as a Service Aggregator (maintaining a platform communicating with STB/RSGs deployed to their citizens).

For governments, the SAFIR approach in general allows them to improve the image of government processes by providing an easier to use and more reactive service to their citizens based on their needs. Going to the administrations to fill out forms, sit in waiting lines at the government offices is a chore to every citizen. Especially in times where the government image is not the best one and bureaucracy has reached and all-time high, the SAFIR solution can help greatly to improve the citizen-government relationship.

When cooperating with a third party service provider, governments can rely on existing, open standards based infrastructure to design their service offerings and connect them with the service provider platform. When acting as a service aggregator themselves initially, they can think of extending or leasing this platform to 3rd party providers in order to share infrastructure costs with them.

The following figure [F6] outlines the envisioned architecture and usage of the SAFIR solution. Citizen users will be able to use a multimodal interface to interact with services provided either by their government (regional, municipal) or Third Party service providers such as Multimedia Content Providers, Healthcare Providers or Safety&Security Providers.

The SAFIR solution is not restricted to being used on Set-Top Boxes only. With clearly defined interfaces and a modular architecture concept, it will be possible to transfer the benefits of adding a domain-specific speech user interface to other kinds of devices, like Residential or Office service gateways as well. Also, there are several possibilities of how to realise the so-called Intelligent Remote Control. It can range from high-end devices such as Tablet PCs or PDAs down to simple audio-capturing equipment like Bluetooth-enabled microphones.

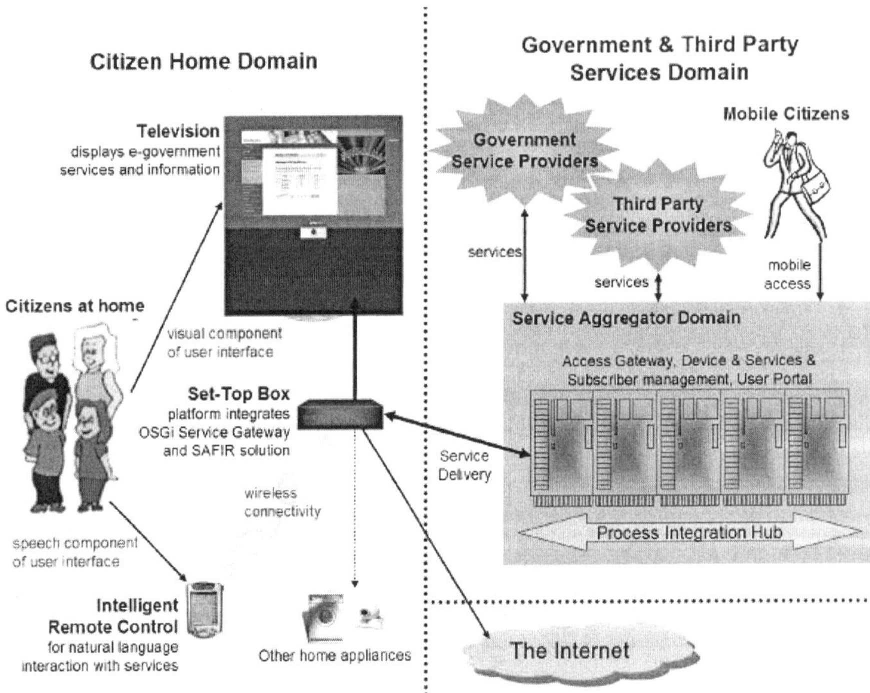

Figure [F6] SAFIR Architecture Overview

References

[1] White Paper "Smart Home In-house and Backend Architecture", IBM 2003

Trademarks

About the authors

Christian A. **Schiller**, *IT Architect, IBM, Germany*
(christian.schiller@de.ibm.com)

Christian Schiller, Dipl.-Ing. (BA) and BSc, studied Information Technology Management and graduated from the University of Cooperative Education Mannheim in 2001. Since then, he is working in the business development team of IBM Global Services Strategy & Marketing department. There, he is working on new offerings and solutions in the area of Mobile and Pervasive Computing as an IT Architect, focusing on the emerging market of broadband service delivery to heterogeneous home networks ("Smart Home").

Yi Min **Gan**, *Manager, IBM, China*
(ganyimin@cn.ibm.com)

Yi Min Gan is managing the Pervasive Computing and WebSphere Portal software product development teams in IBM China Development Lab. He has been involved into the development of embedded software and pervasive middleware since 2001. Prior to that, he has led a team for eCommerce product development and customer services for 2 years. Yi Min Gan joined IBM as a Research Member at China Research Lab in 1996, focused on the research of Internet multimedia technologies. Yi Min Gan received his Master degree of Automatic Control Theory and Application from Tsinghua University in 1995.

Charles **Kemper**, *CEO, Voice Insight, Belgium*
(charles.kemper@voice-insight.com)

Charles Kemper has extensive executive and managerial experience in the GIS, Document Management, CAD/CAM, and Consumer Electronics industries. Previously, Kemper served as executive vice president in Sales and Marketing with Brics/Brics Net. He also was managing director for Intergraph, a Benelux company with BEF 300 million revenue. Kemper also held the position of CAD support group manager for Philips Consumer Electronics, where he managed the organization responsible for the evaluation of the technical automation needs (CAD/CAM PDM...) of the worldwide C.E. product division. His early career positions also included Engineering, IT and CAD consulting positions with GE Calma, ComputerVision and Gerber Systems Technologies. Kemper holds an engineering degree from the Polytechnical School of the University of Brussel, where he started his career as assistant professor in fluid mechanics and thermodynamics (acoustical research on fluid mechanics). A frequent industry speaker, Kemper was the keynote speaker at the USGS GIS conference in May 2001 & 2003, and the Oracle/Compaq Ebusiness conference in the Hagues NL in February 2001. Kemper has also spoken at the last four International ESRI UC conferences in San Diego and at the European GIS conferences in Greece (2000, 2001,2003) , Turkey (2000), Portugal (2002), Nederlands (2000), Belgium (2003) and France (2001, 2003) , at the last ITS seminar in Paris (2003) as well as at the SpeechTek exhibition in New York (2003).

Borivoj **Tydlitat**, *Software Engineer, IBM, Czech Republic*
(borivoj_tydlitat@cz.ibm.com)

Ing. Borivoj Tydlitat studied Computer Science at Faculty of Electrical Engineering of Czech Technical University in Prague. He worked in several companies as a software developer and architect. He joined IBM Research in 1997 and has been working on the technologies of speech recognition, natural language understanding, multimodal user interfaces and their applications. Today he works at IBM Voice Technologies and Systems on embedded speech recognition.

Toward a Human-Friendly Assistive Environment
D. Zhang and M. Mokhtari (Eds.)
IOS Press, 2004

A Proposal for a Software Architecture of the Intelligent Health Home

ROY Jean-François, PIGOT Hélène, FRAPPIER Marc
{jean-francois.roy3, helene.pigot, marc.frappier}@usherbrooke.ca
Département d'Informatique
Université de Sherbrooke
Sherbrooke (Québec)
Canada

Abstract. Problems associated with aging include Alzheimer's disease. Cognitive deficits are important parts of the disease. Many elders want to continue their normal lives even when sick. An Activity of Daily Living (ADL) sometimes requires external help since the elder may not have all the resources (physical and cognitive) to complete an activity. The Intelligent Health Home (IHH) assists the elderly in their ADL through its residence and apparatuses. This paper describes the services that we plan to offer through the IHH. These services are the core of the software architecture that will give the framework of the IHH system. The system is used by the resident and other actors, such as a medical staff, proxies and technicians. Additional services must be added to the framework to support these actors. The description of the services through a software architecture is then schematised.

1 Introduction

1.1 Context

Elders are living longer through a better healthcare infrastructure and a better lifestyle. Living longer means a higher risk of diseases and infections. The risks of developing cognitive degeneration (like Alzheimer's disease) are thus directly correlated to the age factor. Nowadays, the elders are institutionalised when they reach a health risk for themselves and their family. While institutionalisation is the main solution of the cognitively deficient, it is not the solution of choice for many reasons. First of all, the costs of a hospital-style health home are prohibitive and require specialised personnel and equipment. Also, many elders prefer to stay in their residence [1]. It's important for an elder to live in an enjoyable environment. We must define another way of helping the resident at home with restricted costs. The Intelligent Health Home is a new solution to meet the elder's needs.

The Health Home (HH) has existed for many years. The earlier health homes focussed exclusively on remote monitoring. The main issues associated with remote monitoring are the lack of direct interventions to the elder when dangerous situations arise. This is where

Intelligent Health Home (IHH) expands on the original Health Home definition. The IHH is a Health Home with a cognitive approach to its resident's Activity of Daily Living (ADL) together with a detection and prevention of dangerous situations. The problem solving part of the ADL is a responsibility of the IHH itself; hence, the IHH must be a self-contained computer system to help the elderly. This definition of the IHH has been accepted by many researchers. Remote monitoring has long been perceived as a way to save money and add services at home. The IHH is meant to give a better quality of life to the elder in a secure and autonomous environment [2]. This departs from the actual elder homes and their services that cut the links between generation, thus reducing the independence and the quality of life while giving an archaic aid [3]. The IHH are meant to be supported by many actors.

Defining the software architecture itself needs answers to this simple question: How the IHH helps the resident through his ADL without requiring external actors? The information of the resident is first captured by sensors located in the home. By analysing data provided by sensors, the IHH should be able to discover the resident's ongoing ADL, identify difficulties experienced by the resident, and identify a solution to the resident's handicap and apply this solution to the resident's surrounding environment. The solution is delivered through intelligent appliances and/or actuators. If a dangerous situation can not be safely managed by the IHH systems, the IHH must contact external actors to come to the rescue of the resident. With the problem in mind, the construction of the framework must be modifiable easily and rapidly if changes occurs to the definitions of the services. Moreover, the system must preserve the confidentiality of the resident. Additionally, the security of the resident must prevail over everything else.

The objective of this paper is to provide an overview of a software architecture that we have defined for the IHH. This architecture contains a service model, class diagrams, a framework, and a software prototype that illustrates the connections between the different modules. The service model contains four main services: task assistance, remote monitoring, intervention to the resident, and home adjustments. This architecture has been defined through the following steps: i) define the needs of the resident in his daily life activities, in order to preserve his autonomy and security; ii) define the roles of each actor; iii) model the needs and roles of each actor through software engineering; iv) build a framework of the IHH; v) construct a prototype proving the initial concept of the IHH.

To intervene in a resident's ADL, the system must have a way of detecting what is the ADL itself. This is by far the main problem of the DOMUS' IHH. Since human intelligence is used when achieving an ADL, a comparative cognitive architecture must be used to analyse the resident's actions. The IHH is modelled with that architecture in mind. The IHH reacting to the resident's actions is, by itself, a service offered to the resident. The system must support other functionalities to be usable. These extra services are defined, along with the actors that use them. Services are the basis of any software; they must be precisely defined and be complete.

The results of the research are based on the formalisation of the services of the system and its characteristics. Parts of the results include a prototype. It is currently in development and will be briefly introduced in the paper. There are many ways to describe a system. Here, a top-down approach is used for the DOMUS' IHH.

2 Related Work

Technological improvements over the years in health care brought medical sensors at reasonable prices. Researchers at the MIT Media Lab developed portable sensors that are able to study the vital signs of the resident in a constant manner [4]. The extracted data gives a personalised tracking of each resident which may be used in a Health Home. Thus began the Health Home: remote monitoring at home with medical tools. Early HH architectures were principally meant to do data acquisitions from the resident, removing the need of a specialised nurse. All of these sensors sound good in practice, but the fact is that when an emergency happens, the medical tool can't help the resident directly: someone must come to the rescue of the resident.

The HH slowly evolved and became more "intelligent". The apparatuses added functionalities to the home and could respond positively to the resident's medical needs. Technological tools are available but it is important for the resident that his private life must be kept that, private [5]. Quantitative data can be gathered by sensors, and by analysing it, a solution may be found and an action taken by the apparatuses. This is not an IHH by the DOMUS definition, an IHH must resolve both physical and cognitive problems, and offer an intervention to the resident.

Physical monitoring is widely available for a good reason: it's much easier to analyse quantitative information than qualitative. It's also much cheaper. This is why IHH are just the tip of the iceberg technology wise: there's much work to be done on the ADL analysis and intervention.

Many IHHs are in the prototyping phase. The CHU Grenoble's IHH and the University of Washington's IHH are meant to be intelligent describers of the resident's ADL through various monitoring. The monitoring is akin to the previous Health Home's remote monitoring. What distinguish the DOMUS' IHH from others is clear: the IHH is not only meant to monitor the resident in his ADL, but also intervene when he encounters a handicap situation.

The IHH of CHU Grenoble, is meant to detect physical deficiencies, specially fall detection, and respond to that [6]. The SIMBAD (Smart Inactivity Monitor using Array-Based Detectors) is another major tool in fall prevention, which is a major cause of institutionalisation [7]. At the University of Washington, the researchers are interested in high level activity detection from low level captors [8]. It's interesting for the DOMUS' architecture since they have a similar approach for the resident's ADL detection. The University of Rochester's IHH is again meant to help a person with cognitive disorders. The Smart Medical Home offers a memory enhancing technology for tracking objects using cognition [9]. They focus more on the visual behaviour of the resident, which poses an additional problem for the confidentiality of the resident. The Georgia Institute Home Aware IHH concentrates on living in security despite of autonomy losses and is constructed on the importance of having a laboratory to prove the partnerships between the human and the machine [10].

DOMUS' IHH (DIHH) distinguishes itself by using an elaborate cognitive model. Instead of building small systems for the analysis of each task, the system will analyse the resident's problem as a whole. To do so, the Rousseau model is used in DIHH because it links the various elements of the system components [11]. The model enables an intervention based on these principles: the person, the activity and the environment. A diagnosis is made through an analysis of these concepts [12].

3 Services Model

3.1 Actors

When an elder is institutionalised, many persons take part in his everyday life: nurses, doctors, and the elder's family. These bonds still exists in the DIHH. Thus the resident is not the only actor who uses the system. The actors using the system have specific needs and preferences. These needs must be defined in addition to the needs of the resident. The actors may be human individuals as well as electronic devices. We consider the following actors. The resident is the person who receives the help from the IHH. The medical staff consists of doctors, nurses, and anyone who provides formal medical help. A caregiver is a person who formally assists the resident in his daily activities. The family includes the persons who have a formal relationship with the resident. A technician has the responsibility of the IHH software and equipments. Sensors are apparatuses that receive data only. Actuators are apparatuses that dispatch information through the environment. Intelligent apparatuses receive and send data and can process higher level information. The actors interact with the system in two possible ways: they could activate a process of the system, or, receive information from a process.

3.2 Services

The services are the functionalities provided by the system to satisfy the user needs. Our architecture consists of four main services: task assistance, remote monitoring, intervention to the resident, and home adjustments. These services were included for the resident only. Since many actors were defined, in addition to the resident, additional services are required. They are: i) protecting the access to sensitive data, ii) securing the physical equipment of the IHH, iii) modifying the files describing the resident's profile and other actors, iv) setting up the IHH.

A representation of the diverse services includes the relationships between the system modules. Since task assistance and remote monitoring are provided directly to the resident, they form the Resident Supervision module. The environment services include the intervention to the resident and the set up of the IHH; they form the Environment Management module. The Files Management module contains the services needed for the modification of the files in the system and the protection of sensitive data. The last module, System Failure Management, includes the securing of physical equipments.

Since the main objective is to create the architecture for supervising the resident in his ADL, the Resident Supervision module is described thoroughly. The Figure 1 describes how the main modules interact among themselves. To secure the life of cognitively impaired people, immediate dangers like a stove fire must be prevented quickly. These dangers could be prevented in the task assistance or the remote monitoring services. In order to respond very quickly, immediate dangers are addressed by a specific module, the danger monitoring service, which takes immediate action when necessary.

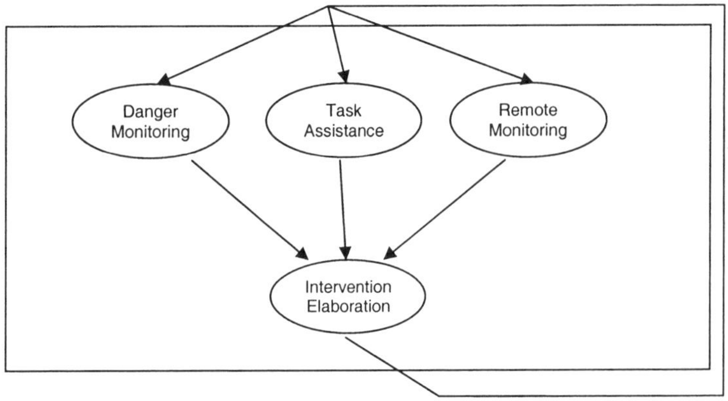

Figure 1 : Cyclic Resident Support

3.2.1 *Danger Monitoring*

Some apparatuses can be dangerous if they are left without monitoring. Intelligent apparatuses can detect dangerous situations and notify the IHH. When a zone of danger is reached, an alert is given. The unessential services are temporarily disabled. In all cases, there's a management of priority that takes place. Scenarios of cognitive assistance are defined to recognize these zones of danger, along with the vital stats of the resident.

3.2.2 *Task Assistance*

Thanks to the various intelligent apparatuses and sensors, data is collected constantly upon the environment and the resident. With the data, the system checks its files for an existing activity that is being done. Activities may not be properly recognized, due to the uncertainty of the information gathered and the high variability of ADL patterns. When a task is achieved, the system tries to determine to which activity this task belongs, and will try to envisage the evolution of the activity. The resident can carry out, in parallel, several activities; the system must hold account of it. The IHH analyzes changes in the environment, the resident or the activity. Various situations of handicap can occur in the current ADL. They correspond to an inadequacy between the resident, the activity to be realized and the environment. A task can be too demanding for the physical or cognitive capacities of the resident. In the same vein, the environment may not be suitable for the task, or tools needed for the ADL's completion may not be available. The goal of the IHH is to mitigate through the environment the handicap situation.

3.2.3 *Remote Monitoring*

Remote monitoring makes it possible to gather information on the resident. Contrary to the danger monitoring module, this treatment is carried out on a longer term. Collected information relates to the IHH, the physical problems of the resident and the evolution in the realisation of his ADL. This remote monitoring makes it possible to detect and extrapolate on future failures of the resident or the IHH.

3.2.4 Environmental Intervention

The environmental intervention module knows the preferences of the resident and the degree of importance of the problem. When a situation requires an intervention, priorities management is done in order to offer the best intervention available. In a situation of a handicap, an intervention is not always carried out; time must be given to the resident to complete his tasks. Any intervention is personalized according to the resident's preferences. This intervention is made through the IHH's intelligent apparatuses and actuators.

3.2.5 Other services

The other services needed for the use of the IHH are properly defined. While these services are important to the system and its actors, they can be overlooked since they are not meant to complete the objectives directly. They consist of file management, user privileges and other non life-threatening services.

4 Framework

4.1 Framework

There are two primary ways to construct a large computerised system: a top-down approach where the foundations of the system are given and additional pieces start from there, or a bottom-up vision, where the system is built from the combination of many independent components. The basic idea behind the software architecture of the DOMUS' IHH is simple: an open framework that can be filled later in a top-down approach.

Many researchers working on an IHH are opting for the bottom-up vision. For example, the Georgia Institute uses this approach and they came up with many different teams working on various aspects of the IHH. One potential difficulty with this approach is that the integration of these individually developed components may be difficult to realise since their connections may not have been carefully planned from the beginning.

4.2 Software architecture

Our software architecture has been defined using UML. Since teamwork is an important issue in the software's construction, UML has been selected to streamline communication between team members. DOMUS' IHH includes pervasive computing, distributed systems, cognitive modeling and plan recognition. The architecture must support them all; hence, we must plan in advance how they will be integrated.

UML use-case diagrams have been defined; they are omitted here for the sake of concision. These diagrams define connections between the four services and the actors of the system. They are hierarchically decomposed, in order to define more precisely the expected behaviour of each module and to facilitate their understanding.

A static model has been defined using class diagrams, in order to provide a common data structure framework that can be used by all team members, when they develop their components. We hope that it will ease the integration of these components, by avoiding names clashed, data redundancy, and structure clashes. These issues are particularly difficult to handle when several team members work independently on various pieces of the software.

4.3 Prototype

Work on the DIHH was started a year ago and many pieces are coming up together to be added to the prototype. Its first version was really basic: it was a user interface with XML support and predefined classes following the Rousseau model. It was then refined to include a prototype of the Resident Supervision module. The recognition of ADL is simulated through scripting. There is currently no communication link between the various apparatuses and this prototype; we have a graphical user interface that allows a simple simulation of the apparatuses. We are continuously improving this prototype in order to add new functionalities as defined in the services model. As the software prototype evolves, we will be able to distribute it in the real size DIHH, which will be available by the end of this year. The real-life testing will then be the ultimate test.

5 Conclusion

Our main objective was to build the Intelligent Health Home software architecture, capable of handling the deficiencies of an elder with physical and cognitive problems by using the IHH's environment. This will be part of the solution of building the DIHH.

Through the diverse services offered and functionalities implemented while building the IHH architecture, the framework offers a powerful yet simple development environment. The DIHH objectives are of course not yet completely achieved. It is a long term project attacking very difficult issues. Furthermore, we still need to validate if our services are correct, consistent and complete with respect to the needs of the resident and various other actors interacting with the DIHH. Since there are few studies in the field reporting on the effectiveness of an IHH and the level of acceptance by elder's when interacting with an IHH to conduct their ADL, validation remains an important issue.

From a software engineering perspective, we have adopted a gradual, top-down approach. Looking at the preliminary results of the prototype, it seems to be an efficient way of handling development. The DIHH is a complex distributed systems, that will contain large databases of tracking and analysis data, web applications, ubiquitous computing, real-time components, and wireless communications. Integrating all these aspects requires a careful planning. We hope that our architecture is a right step in supporting this integration.

While completing the framework, the next big step remains the transfer of the prototype to the real-size IHH lab. There's no better proof of a system's architecture than having the system functioning with real human beings.

References

[1] Martin M, *Étude de la perception de qualité d'un programme d'adaptation domiciliaire selon la perspective des usagers aînés*. Direction de la Santé publique de Montréal-Centre, 2000.

[2] Tang P., Venables T., *Smart Homes and Telecare for Indepedant Living*, J. Telemedcine and Telecare Vol.6 No.1, 2000.

[3] Fisk M., *Our Future Home: Housing and the inclusion of Older People*, Help the Aged, 1999.

[4] Pentland A., *Healthwear: Medical Technology Becomes Wearable*, Computer Vol.37 No.5, 2004.

[5] Rialle V. *La santé par des capteurs au domicile : entre « meilleur des mondes » et opportunités de solidarités nouvelles*, Publication du groupe STP (Sujet, Théorie et Praxis), Maison des Sciences de l'Homme, 2002.

[6] Rialle V., Duchêne F., Noury N., Bajolle L. et J. Demongeot, *Health 'smart' home: Information technology for patients at home*, Telemedicine Journal and E-Health, 2002.

[7] Sixsmith A., Johnson N., *A Smart Sensor to Detect the Falls of the Elderly*, IEEE Pervasive Computing Vol.3 No.2, 2004.

[8] Patterson D., Liao L. Fox D., Kautz H., *Inferring High Level Behavior from Low Level Sensors*, Fifth Annual Conference on Ubiquitous Computing (UBICOMP 2003), October 2003, United States.

[9] Randal Nelson and Isaac Green, *Tracking Objects Using Recognition*, International Conference on Pattern Recognition, August 2002, Canada.

[10] Abowd G., Atkeson C., Bobick A., Essa I., MacIntyre B., Mynatt E., Starner T., *Living Laboratories:The Future Computing Environments Group at the Georgia Institute of Technology,* ACM Conference on Human Factors in Computing System, April 2000, Netherlands.

[11] Rousseau, J. et al., *Model of Competence: A Conceptual Framework for understanding the Person-Environment Interaction for Persons with motor disabilities*, Journal of Occupational Therapy in health Care, in press.

[12] Pigot H., Mayers A., Giroux S., *The intelligent habitat and everyday life activity support*, 5th international conference on Simulations in Biomedicine, April 2003, Slovenia.

Toward a Human-Friendly Assistive Environment
D. Zhang and M. Mokhtari (Eds.)
IOS Press, 2004

A Pervasive Reminder System for Smart Homes

Sylvain GIROUX and Simon GUERTIN

Département d'informatique,
Université de Sherbrooke
2500 boul. Université, Sherbrooke, Canada J1K 2R1
{Sylvain.Giroux, Simon.Guertin,}@USherbrooke.ca
http://www.dmi.usherb.ca/~sgiroux/domus/

Abstract: One of the research projects at the DOMUS laboratory aims at the realization of smart homes and cognitive assistance for cognitively impaired people. The aimed system is a pervasive information system able to detect failure and anomalies in the behaviour of the habitants, and then to help them and notify other systems or people about potential danger. In this paper, we address the issue of finding the user and choosing the most appropriate device to transmit a message. As a prototype, a pervasive reminder system for message management explores the possibilities of dynamic cooperation between different kinds of devices, hardware, and software communicating through different networks. This pervasive system tries to locate, identify and notify the resident of upcoming appointments. The issues addressed are 1) localization and identification of the resident; 2) finding devices for communication and delivering messages according to the position of devices and the position of the user 3) spontaneous networking, discovery services, and service composition, and 4) migration of a running application. The latest allows a user working on a device to switch to another device more adapted to her task, making the application really pervasive.

1. Introduction

As Weiser said about pervasive computing, « The most profound technologies are those that disappear. They weave themselves into the fabric of everyday life until they are indistinguishable from it. » [1]. The DOMUS laboratory of the University of Sherbrooke studies pervasive computing and mobile computing. One of the research projects aims at the realization of smart homes and cognitive assistance for cognitively impaired people [2] [3]. People suffering from cognitive impairments —Alzheimer disease, schizophrenia, brain injuries...— often have no choice other than living in medical institutions. Smart houses [4] and mobile applications, e.g. activity compass [5], can play a central role in keeping them at home in their community. The aimed smart home would be a pervasive information system able to detect failure and anomalies in the behaviour of the habitants, and then to help them or to notify other systems or people about potential danger.

In this paper, we address the issue of finding the user and using the most appropriate device to transmit a message. As a prototype, a pervasive reminder system for message management explores the possibilities of dynamic cooperation between different kinds of devices, hardware, and software communicating through different networks. This pervasive system tries to locate, reach the user with the nearest or most convenient device and notify her of upcoming appointments. To do that, we need at the implementation level to address spontaneous networking, discovery services, service composition, and migration of a running application

First we sketch the general issues raised by smart homes for cognitive assistance (§2). Then we describe the prototype: the physical set up (§3) and the functional requirements (§4). Once the goal and setting are clear, we detail the distributed implementation of the various components (§5).

2. General Issues

Let suppose Mrs Smith is suffering from the Alzheimer disease. She is cooking a stew and preparing coffee when somebody rings at the front door. She goes to answer, chats a bit, and forgets something is cooking. And she listens TV in the lounge. The smart home detects the situation is hazardous: nobody is in the kitchen and the stove is on for a long time. The system decides to send a reminder to her. So the issue to solve is first to find where she is, then find what devices in the lounge can be used to present the reminder — TV, telephone, her PDA...—, and finally package the message and send it to the chosen device. Hence to finally provide Mrs Smith with the appropriate feedback, a pervasive system must face many issues. In this paper, we explore the combination of the following ones:

- *Identification and localization of the appropriate user*: there may be many people simultaneously in the house; they can move from room to room.
- *Heterogeneity of devices, hardware, software and networks' protocols*: in a house, there is a great variety of coexisting devices (electrical appliances, computers, TVs, PDAs...), software (server and client components, different operating systems and programming languages...), and networks (Ethernet, WiFi, Bluetooth, X10 [6]). They all have to collaborate.
- *Spontaneous networking and device and service discovery*: it is not possible to configure and to know beforehand all the devices and systems that will be present in the house; devices may join or leave the house dynamically; some are mobile, other are stationary.
- *Transitory coalition of devices*: devices and systems may offer complementary services that must collaborate for a moment to perform a task, for instance to deliver the message to a given user.
- *Pervasiveness*: interactions between components must be invisible and transparent to the user, furthermore a computation may have to migrate from one device to another. For instance, if the telephone is first used to reach Mrs Smith and she asks to see the state of the stove on TV, using the camera in the kitchen.
- *Zero-configuration*: obviously Mrs Smith cannot be asked to configure the system.

3. Prototype: A Pervasive Agenda System

The physical and software setup of the prototype incorporates multiple technologies that are not directly designed to work together (Fig. 1). In particular, the standard electrical hardware will bc interconnecting with the computer hardware and software systems through the X10 protocol. A system may use different electrical devices to enhance the user's level of comfort or to extract information about different physical aspects of the house. X10 devices are affordable and are already made for home automation. The X10 devices used in the project are:

- one X10-computer interface device connects to the serial port of a computer on one end and into an electrical outlet on the other end. The device enables to read and write X10 codes on the electrical wires. Model: X10 TW523 Two-Way Interface Module.
- two wireless motion detectors. Model: Version II Wireless X10 Motion Sensor.
- one RF base to convert the signals from the wireless motion detectors into the electrical system. Model : X10 16 Device RF Base.

To read and write X10 codes from and to the computer interface, we use standard serial port programming in Java. Other devices used are

- a PC running Linux Red Hat 9 mostly used to run different services of the Domus infrastructure.
- the user's PC running windows XP in the main room.
- a standard wired LAN setup
- a wireless transmitter base to allow WiFi connections to the network.
- a standard home router with DHCP capabilities is used to interconnect the networked hardware and allow connections to the Internet. Model: Lynksys Cable/DSL 4-Port Router.
- a printer enhanced with a Bluetooth antenna to allow printing from diverse devices.
- a HP iPAQ Pocket PC h5550 with Bluetooth and WiFi capabilities.

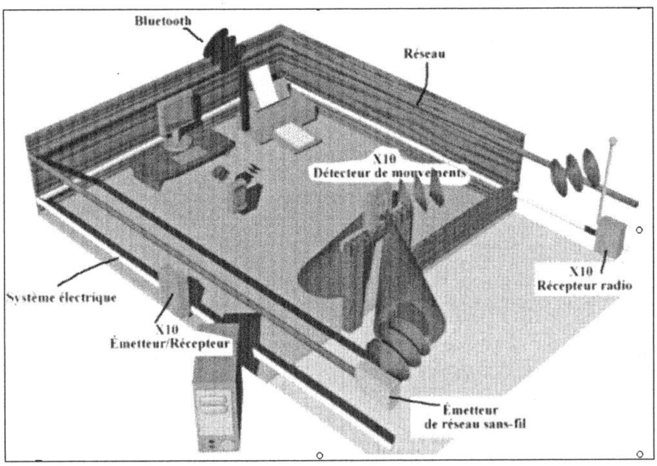

Figure 1. Current prototype implementation of the pervasive agenda system.

4. An Active and Pervasive Agenda System

The prototype built implements an appointment manager or agenda that keeps track of a user's appointments like any other agenda would do. Where the system distinguishes itself is that it is a distributed application that uses other distributed applications offering different services throughout the house. The agenda operates in conjunction with a messaging system to try to inform the user of an upcoming appointment. The system also uses other features from the house to better accommodate the user's needs.

To perform its duties, the system first must search for a device to notify the user (§4.1), then localize the user and prepare the delivery of the message to the user (§4.2), and finally support the migration of a user session from device to device to follow a user from room to room (§4.3). The next sections will present how these issues were addressed in the prototype.

4.1 Search of Devices for Message Delivery

When an appointment is approaching, the system has to notify the user. To do this, the system attempts to use any service implementing the messaging service. The system might or might not know where the user is in the house, so it disseminates the message to any resources that may communicate the information to the user. When the user reads the message, the system gets a confirmation the user got the message. The system then stops trying to reach the user and notifies other messaging services in the house so they can remove the read message.

4.2 Preparing Message Delivery to a Nearby User

When the system knows a certain user is nearby, it prepares to log the user in. Due to limited means of user identification in the current setup, we consider only one user. In this scenario, motion detectors work in collaboration with other software services running in the Domus infrastructure. The agenda is usually in standby mode in the main room. When the user enters the room as detected by motion detectors, the agenda login screen is filled with user name. If the user wants to use the application, she just needs to type in her password and start using the tool. The agenda program can do this because it uses a service that informs any client about the presence of a user in the room. When the user leaves the room, the agenda is also informed and reacts accordingly by removing the pre-filled login.

4.3 Migrating User Session from Device to Device

A user may need to migrate from one device to another when working with an application (in our case in the agenda). She may need better display capabilities. She may prefer to work in another room. She may need to work on a wireless device. When the user switches device, she wants to pick up the session where she left it. There are three cases when this happens:

- the user directly switches to the other device if it is available;
- the user stores her session on the server if no available device meets her needs;
- the user session is retrieved from the server when the device becomes available.

In the first two cases, the agenda system will log off the user from the current device when the transfer is successful. A login screen with the user name already filled in will be displayed to the user on the other device. The session will then be restored to where it was left on the previous device. In the second case, the user is logged off from the current device when the session is transferred to the server successfully. The user will then have to log on the appropriate device when it becomes available (third case). The session can then be restored from the server from the agenda's menu commands (or it could be automatically restored on a successful login).

5. Implementation

In this section we present implementation details of the prototype. First we explained the choices underlying the general infrastructure (§5.1). Next we present general services that must run in any cases (§5.2). Then we present specific services: services related to X10 components (§5.3) and services related to message delivery (§5.4). Finally the agenda system as a whole is described (§5.5).

5.1 Jini and Java as Backbone for the General Infrastructure

Indeed we want to build dynamic distributed system on heterogeneous components and supporting code migration. Hence we choose Java[1] and Jini. Java provided the compulsory multi-platform support and code migration through RMI. Jini provided

- *spontaneous networking*: services offered to the users or to other services may join and leave anytime.
- *service registration and discovery*: Jini discovery services enable to find the needed services in the DOMUS federation.

Reggie[2] is running on the Linux PC in a persistent and activable mode to save CPU resources. An http server is running also on this computer to make the necessary Jini jar files available for download on the house's LAN.

There is no centralized system but many different kinds of services that can have different physical or logical location. Services are grouped in the main federation: DOMUS. In fact, many sub-federations are used to realize the whole system (Fig. 2). A federation could either represent a room, a floor, the whole house or any logical boundary. With a good use of federations, a service or client can better choose a specific service depending where the desired service is registered, giving hints on its location.

5.2 General Services

For the Domus infrastructure, we developed a Domus server. This server is a service that provides basic information about this infrastructure. It also provide another HTTP server that allows to upload files that other services might need to store and make available to other programs that will use the system. Those files contain the code to distributed for a Jini service to work. These files need to be available through an HTTP server. This feature simplifies the development of new services.

The security server is a service that is used by any other servers or client program that needs to authenticate a user. This service also runs on the Linux PC. It is a small database that stores usernames and passwords.

5.3 Services Related to X10 Components

The X10 server allows the X10 technology to be incorporated in the Domus infrastructure. This server uses serial port programming in Java to interact with the X10 Computer Interface (§3). This computer interface monitors X10 codes travelling on the electrical

---

[1] We used JDK1.4 with the latest release of Jini. We needed to downgrade the version of Java we used when we incorporate the iPAQ because J2ME is only compatible with the JDK1.3.

[2] Reggie is the lookup service used in Jini to allow services to register themselves and lookup other services.

wires and stores them in the device's memory. With the X10 server, other services can read or write those codes to know the state of devices or to control them. To use it, a client or service of the Domus federation registers to the X10 server and specifies which codes it is interested in (Fig. 3.).

The room's motion detector and darkness detector service allows other services to show a more adapted behaviour in the presence of a user. This service is available to any other client or service interested in the state of occupation of the room or in the state of lighting. This service is composed of

- the two motion detectors that are placed back to back above the room's entrance;
- the wireless base that transmit the signals of the two wireless detector's X10 into the electric circuit of the house;
- the X10 server;
- the motion detector program that will handle the X10 signals.

The motion detector program registers to the X10 server and specifies X10 codes it needs from the motion detectors. It will then analyze the X10 codes received from the X10 server to determine either the room is empty or not, in full darkness or not. The algorithm can detect leaving or entering the room by analyzing the time elapsed between the X10 codes thrown by each motion detectors. Other services can then register themselves to the motion detector service to be informed of the room's occupation status.

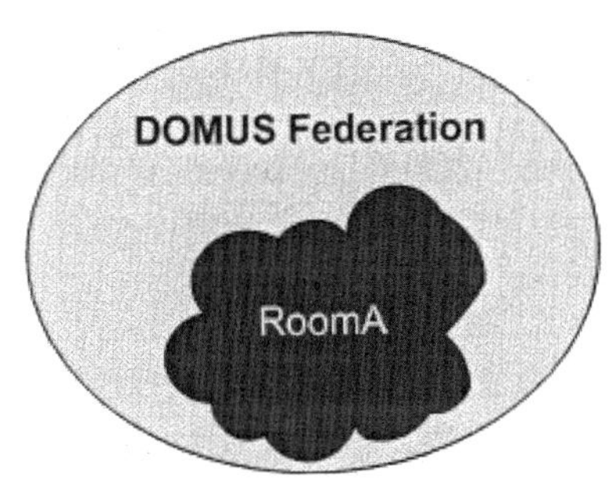

Figure 2. Organizing Domus into sub-federations.

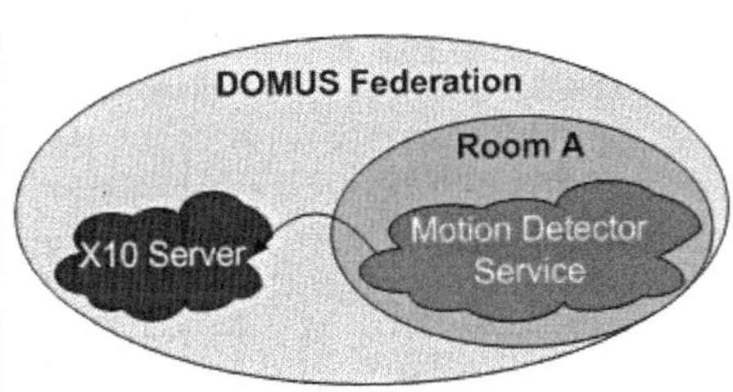

Figure 3. Detecting presence with X10 components.

5.4 Messaging System Server

To deliver messages to users in the house, we implemented a message server. This message server accepts request from clients that wants to deliver a message to a specific recipient. The message server processes the requests and looks up all the message clients in the Domus federation to deliver the message. The server can handle new message clients joining the federation. When a message has been read and confirmed by the recipient, the message client informs the message server of the successful delivery. The message server then proceeds to inform the originator of that message of the successful delivery. The message server also has to inform all the other message clients to remove this specific message from their queue.

Tasks of message clients are simpler. They have to display the message any way they want but they must keep a certain degree of confidentiality and integrity. The message client receives message request from the message server and then waits for a user interaction. For a user to read a message, she normally enters her password for confirmation. The message client confirms the user's identity with the security server. After successful user authentication, the message client then contacts the message server to acknowledge a successful delivery. Message clients must have the basic functions of adding a message and removing a message when requested by the server.

5.5 The Agenda System

The agenda server is a service that handles appointments for the users and tries to notify them of an upcoming appointment. The server has all the basic functionality an agenda server would have. That is to create, store, retrieve, and delete appointments. It uses the security server to authenticate users upon connection of clients. What makes the agenda server unusual is when time comes to notify a user. It searches the Domus federation for messaging services able to send out the notification to the right recipient (Fig. 4). Once the server has received a confirmation of reception by the messenger service it stops and marks the appointment as acknowledged by the user. The server also takes care of overdue appointments that were not acknowledged and the server removes them from the messenger service.

The server also supports the storage and retrieval of a user's session if she wishes to switch device. At the beginning of a session, the user gives a user name and password. She then uses the agenda like a normal agenda to browse, add and delete appointments. If she wants to switch from one computer to another that better suits her needs, she can browse the available computers and directly migrate her session to the new computer if it is available. If no computer is available, the user can store her session to the agenda server to retrieve it later from any other computer when available. When switching directly to another computer, a login screen with the user name is automatically pre-filled. The user enters her password and the session is restored as it was left on the previous computer. (Fig. 5.). There is no need to reopen windows or retype the information, even if not saved.

In the project we assume that it is always the same person that enters or leaves the room. When the client is started, it is looking for the motion detector service to be informed of the presence of a user in the room. There might be multiple motion detector services in the whole system, but the client will only be interested in a motion detection service that belongs to the same Jini federation as the agenda service. This permits the agenda to start the login process when someone enters the room. If there is no motion detector service for the room, the agenda client just behaves normally without inferring somebody is in the room. The client is also informed of the lighting of the room through the motion detector service. It could then open up a light or any other service that would enhance the environment for the user if she chooses to use the agenda (this is not yet implemented).

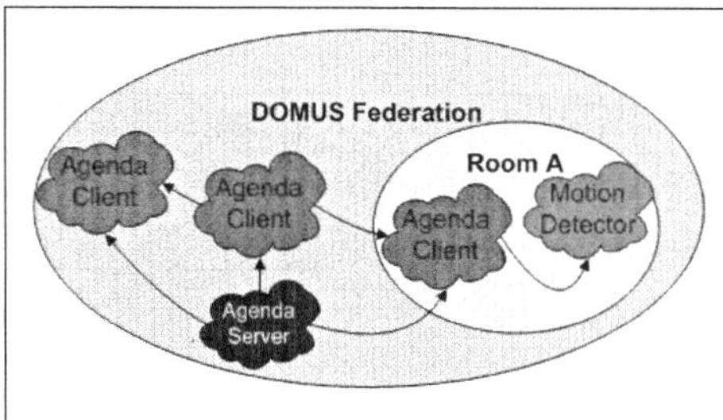

Figure 4. Agenda clients and server.

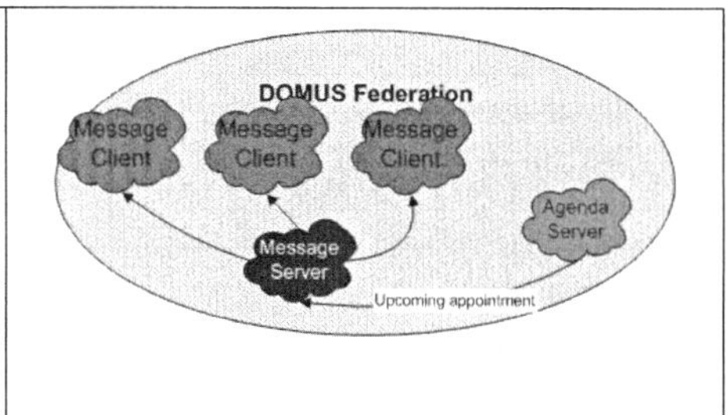

Figure 5. Request from the server to notify a user.

6. Conclusion

Smart homes providing cognitive assistance for cognitive impaired people raise many difficult issues. In the long-term, the DOMUS laboratory wants to implement such a smart home as a pervasive information system able to first detect failure and anomalies in the behaviour of the patients, and then to help them on-site and to perform some sort of tele-monitoring. Because it is a very complex task, we decided to address a simplified version of this problem.

In this paper we thus described the implementation of a pervasive distributed agenda system. This system has been used to explore how sensing and information devices can be integrated using a variety of communications services on the one hand and how information can be delivered to the user in a pervasive environment on the other hand. The emphasis was put on locating and communicating information to residents. The prototype enabled to explore the possibilities of dynamic cooperation between heterogeneous devices, hardware, and software communicating through different networks. This resulting pervasive system tries to locate, identify and notify the resident of upcoming appointments. Among the issues that have been addressed, let stress: 1) localization and identification of the resident; 2) finding devices for communication and delivering messages according to the position of devices and the position of the user 3) spontaneous networking, discovery services, and service composition, and 4) migration of a running application. The latest allows a user working on a device to switch to another device more adapted to her task. The user can then go on with the application without losing her work, making the system really pervasive. This distributed system is adaptive to changes of availability of services, devices and computers.

We intend to use the agenda system as a reminder system in an Agenda Home [7]. Robustness will then be a key issue to address. With respect to monitoring in a smart home, we need a way to store the vital information in case the network or a service is down. When the service or the network would become available again, the services would then report back the information that was saved locally.

Finally we intend to exploit the limited range of Bluetooth to build local coalition of devices based on physical proximity.

References

[1] Mark Weiser, *The Computer for the 21st Century*, Scientific American, 1991.

[2] H. Pigot, et al., *The intelligent habitat and everyday life activity support. 5th international conference on Simulations in Biomedicine*, Slovenia, April 2003.

[3] Pigot H., et al., *The role of intelligent habitats in upholding elders in residence. 5th Intl Conf. on Simulations in Biomedicine*, 2003, Slovenia. WIT Press

[4] Rialle .V, et al. *An experimental Health Smart Home and its distributed Internet-based Information and Communication System. MEDINFO 2001,* IOPress. pp. 1479-1483.

[5] Kautz, H. et al. *An Overview of the Assisted Cognition Project*, AAAI 2002, workshop.

[6] Boone, K, *Using X10 for Home Automation*, http://www.kevinboone.com/x10.html

[7] Pigot, H., and S. Giroux, *Keeping in Touch with Cognitively Impaired People: How Mobile Devices Can Improve Medical and Cognitive Supervision*, 2nd International Conference on Smart Homes and Health Telematics ICOST 2004, Sept 15-17, 2004, Singapore.

Toward a Human-Friendly Assistive Environment
D. Zhang and M. Mokhtari (Eds.)
IOS Press, 2004

A New Architecture for Smart Homes Based on ADB and Temporal Reasoning

Juan C. Augusto   Chris D. Nugent
School of Computing and Mathematics,
University of Ulster at Jordanstown, UK
[jc.augusto, cd.nugent]@ulster.ac.uk

Abstract. Smart home technology offers a viable solution to the increasing needs of the elderly, special needs and home based-healthcare populations. The research to date has largely focused on the development of communication technologies and intelligent user interfaces. The trend should now focus on the computational analysis to provide a means of user-profiled support to promote intelligent independent living.

We present an overview of a system that provides intelligent data analysis for smart homes. A key element of this system is the capability to handle time-related concepts. Our proposal exploits the mutual benefits of Active Databases and Temporal Reasoning to accommodate prevention of hazardous situations via processing of complex event detection. To maximize the reliability of the system behaviour we use tools to verify the set of ECA rules. We believe that this mix of technologies offers an innovative solution to both the research and the application domains.

1 Introduction

As people grow older their need for support in the home environment increases. Eventually, their comes a stage where people can no longer live independently with the only solution being relocation to a nursing home. It is common, following such a relocation, for a person to become depressed due to their lack of independence. Over the past decade there has been a surge of technological solutions being made available for use in the home. These aim to provide a means of independent living and extend the period of time a person can remain in their own home. Such environments maybe referred to as 'Smart Homes', whereby the home environment can proactively change to provide services that promote independent living. The underlying technology comprises three main components: communications, computing and user interfaces [12]. A variety of successful studies have been reported which employ each of these ranging from social alarms to healthcare monitoring to interaction with various home appliances. The majority of the effort has been directed towards engineering solutions as opposed to computational ones.

A key element in the implementation of computer based systems for Smart Homes is the ability to handle time-related concepts. Here we have addressed these through a combination of Active Databases (ADB) and Temporal Reasoning (TR). The resultant system is an ADB manager which, through the Event-Condition-Action (ECA) rules, can detect 'complex' events generated by a person. According to the context in which these events occur the system will produce warnings when potentially unusual or hazardous situations develop. In comparison with previous studies for ADB the language proposed for the ECA rules supports both instantaneous and durative events and is based on a formal framework that can account for a rich composition of events and states, which suits the description of the intended scenarios and their dynamic.

We believe reliability of the system's behaviour is paramount. This is an aspect of ADB systems that has not been explored as extensively as its importance suggests it should. Hence we consider providing means to ensure correctness at various levels. The most relevant being the verification that the set of ECA rules fulfill some desirable requirements and properties.

2 Our Case Study, a Smart Home

We have based our Smart Home model on a care institution in the United Kingdom. This institution is one of shared community care, where approximately 30 individual apartments are contained within the same building. Each apartment provides a means of independent living, through inclusion of a number of technology solutions. All of the apartments are linked to a central monitoring facility (CMF) to which alarms can be relayed when additional assistance is required. A typical layout of an apartment is shown in Figure 1.

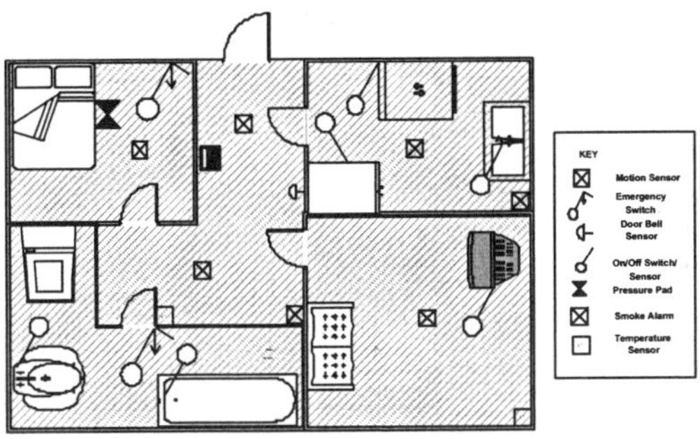

Figure 1: Layout of apartment with embedded technology to support independent living.

Motion sensors in each room have the ability to monitor the movement of a person through the home environment. Emergency switches (in the bathroom and bedroom) and smoke or temperature sensors can relay an alarm to the CMF when activated. Detection of a person getting out of bed is monitored by a large pressure pad placed at the side of the bed. Taps in the kitchen and bathroom are fitted with sensors to detect when they have been turned on/off. Additionally, sensors detect if the fridge has been opened/closed or if the cooker has been turned on/off. Given the vast amount of information which may be generated from these sensors, it is necessary to discriminate between normal and abnormal situations. The key issue is to primarily ascertain the current location of the person in the home, after which the sequence of their events can be assessed to determine normal or abnormal situations.

3 General Overview of the System

Our system is based on an ADB [11] framework. We focus in this study on the role of the ECA rules: `ON` *event* `IF`*condition* `DO` *action*. Our ECA rule specification language (see [2] for BNF definition) has been formally defined [6] and its interpreter has been implemented and tested (see [8] and [7]). Galton's proposal considers a set of operators that is mainly focused on events, states and their interaction. We use this as the basis for the specification of ON and IF clauses. Events in our framework can be primitive (sensors in the smart home being activated) or non-primitive (complex or composite), which are defined from other events by using some of Galton's operators. Also, they can be instantaneous or durative. To establish a link between the ON and IF clauses we use different calendar-related functions and qualitative temporal reasoning algebras. Calendar-related functions provide different utilities like `longerThan([T1,T2], 2hs)`, a function that determines whether the interval `[T1,T2]` lasts for more than two hours or not. Temporal references are dates which have the format `(YY, MM, DD, hh, mm, ss)`. We also use well known qualitative relationships providing temporal algebra operators considered in the literature of temporal reasoning for instant-instant, instant-interval, interval-instant [10] and interval-interval relationships [1]. For example, `during([T1,T2], [D1,D2])` to specify that $[T1, T2]$ is an interval that is comprehended by $[D1, D2]$. More details about the temporal reasoning layer can be found in [2].

A general depiction of the system is given in figure 2. Generic details of how the ECA rules are used in the ADB manager are given in the next section. More specific examples of their use are given in section 5 when we explain how the design of the ECA rules is supported by a verification framework. Rules with more complex events and states definitions are provided in [2].

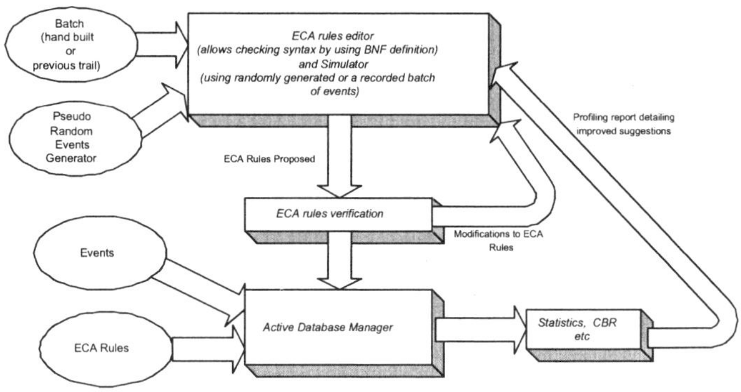

Figure 2: A general overview of the ADBM.

4 Expected Behaviour

The information generated from the sensors within the house and the interfaces embedded into common domestic appliances can be processed by the ADB manager to provide assistance to the person in a number of different ways; prevention of dangerous situations, comfort, security and health.

Prevention of dangerous situations: In these situations the information gathered from the person's environment can be assessed and also take into consideration previous actions of the person. The purpose is to provide an alarm when a person's actions may lead to potentially hazardous situations. For example, a person may leave a room within the house to go to another, but leave an appliance switched on in that room. If this is a light or a television this is not an issue, but leaving the cooker on and then running a bath can result in a hazardous situation and hence requires a form of intervention from the system. This can be represented with the following ECA rule schema:

ON "leaving a room"
IF "monitored appliance/device on"
DO "trigger close monitoring"

Comfort: This addresses the issues of the surrounding environment and changes this by taking into consideration the person's whereabouts in the house and their actions. For example, if a person gets out of bed in the middle of the night and moves into the reception area, switching the light on in the bathroom can be considered to be helpful, especially in the case of dementia sufferers. Another example may be if the ambient temperature rises or falls above the normal; these situations can be accommodated for by the following ECA rule schema:

ON "room temperature lower than NormalValue"
IF "house is inhabited"
DO "trigger heater"

Security: Our system can also be used as a means of security. The elderly are vulnerable to attack from intruders in their home environment. As such, our system can accommodate such instances and provide alarms when necessary. This can be exemplified by the following ECA rule schema:

ON "alarm has been issued of an intruder detected"
IF "no personnel expected at referred location"
DO "apply security emergency procedure"

Health: Here information can be accessed from self-operated healthcare devices, e.g. blood pressure or glucose monitors. It is often necessary to monitor vital signs over a period of time. For example, it is possible to represent with the following ECA rules the monitoring of a person's blood pressure. If this indicates a sustained increase for more than two successive recordings, following perhaps a medication change, then medical staff should be alerted of the condition:

ON "blood pressure higher than 200/175 for more than two successive samples"
IF "medication regimen to control blood pressure has been altered recently"
DO "notify clinical staff"

5 ECA Rules Verification

Why? Our system deals with a wide range of situations of interest including safety and health related issues. That is an extra motivation to ensure correctness of the ECA rules as a whole. There have been some reports on similar attempts in the literature, see for example [5], by using planning systems. While we address some of the properties considered in [5], here we offer an alternative solution to the problem that is closer to our framework and the methods and tools used in Software Engineering for verification and validation of software [3].

What? We are mainly focused on checking semantic correctness of the set of ECA rules as a whole. We consider here a list of properties whose verification can be automised in our framework and are important to obtain a more reliable set of ECA rules: a) *Consistency:* the actions triggered at each step should not be inconsistent. A separate check is performed to consider consistency of the incoming actions compared with the existing DB (but this second consistency check is undertaken at run time) (see [2]). b) *Triggerability:* this checks if each ON clause specification is such that it is always/sometimes potentially triggerable. c) *Joint applicability:* this checks if triggerability is possible for any subset. Due to the computational complexity of this goal N-Joint applicability can be explored meaning that only possible combinations of up to N rules are explored for joint applicability. d) *Rule coverage:* this checks if there are pairs (R1, R2) of rules such that the triggering conditions of R1 is a subset of the triggering conditions of R2. e) *Rule cascading:* this checks if there are any forced sequences of rule activations imposed by design. f) *Postcondition satisfaction:* this checks if a given postcondition is achieved after activation of a rule.

EXAMPLE **1.** Consider we wish to distinguish between those periods during the day where it is consistent with the person's habits to stay in bed and those when they are not in bed. We differentiate inactive periods (00AM-8AM) from active periods (the remaining hours). Suppose we have several rules in our ADB and some changes and additions have been introduced, by different people contributing to the design of the ECA rule base. Lets suppose that initially we have two rules stating that staying inbed for two hours is consistent with the persons' habits within (00AM-8AM).

```
Rule 1: ON occurs(po(inbed), [T1,T2])
        IF holds(inactive_period, [D1,D2]) ∧ during([T1,T2], [D1,D2])
           ∧ longerThan([T1,T2], 2hs)
        DO report_context_normal

Rule 2: ON occurs(po(inbed), [T1,T2])
        IF holds(active_period, [D1,D2]) ∧ during([T1,T2], [D1,D2])
           ∧ longerThan([T1,T2], 2hs)
        DO change_to_context_unusual
```

The intention of introducing rules 3 and 4 is to consider that some transition periods are hard to be labelled as unusual or not for being in bed. Unfortunately when rule 3 is entered the editor forgets to add the restriction nextDate([(Y1, M1, D1),(Y2, M2, D2)]) to make the two dates consecutive and hence to capture that the intended period elapses from 10PM until 1AM:

```
Rule 3: ON occurs(po(inbed), [T1,T2])
        IF during([T1,T2],[(Y1,M1,D1,22,00,00), (Y2,M2,D2,01,00,00)])
           ∧ longerThan([T1,T2], 2hs)
        DO change_to_context_intermediate
```

Another mistake when entering the dates to define the interval 7AM-10AM in rule 4 turns the '10' into '01' for the second date:

```
Rule 4: ON occurs(po(inbed), [T1,T2])
        IF during([T1,T2],[(YY,MM,DD,07,00,01), (YY,MM,DD,01,00,00)])
           ∧ longerThan([T1,T2], 2hs)
        DO change_to_context_intermediate
```

Finally a rule to capture the course of action when the system detected a potential hazardous situation:

```
Rule 5: ON occurs(failed_contact, T)
        IF holds(prog(context_unusual)),[D1,D2]) ∧ divides(T, [D1,D2])
        DO start_emergency_procedure
```

By using the rules provided in this example we can exercise the properties as follows:
Actions inconsistency: rules 2 and 3 will trigger conflicting diagnosis if change_to_context_intermediate is considered not compatible with report_context_normal.
Triggerability: because of the incorrect interval specification (the second date is earlier than the first one) in rule 4, it will never be instantiated.
Joint applicability: rule 2 can be activated together with rule 3 if the period during which the person is in bed is part of 10PM-01AM. Rule 2 cannot be activated together with rule 4 as this later one is not triggerable.
Rule coverage: because the omission of ensuring that the dates used to specify the interval in rule 3 are consecutive days the resulting period is any period that can be conceived between 10PM on one day and 01AM at any future day. Therefore, any state of the database allowing the triggering of rule 3 will also allow the triggering of either rule 2 or 1.
Rule cascading: it can be used for example to investigate if the triggering of rule 2 will be necessarily followed by the triggering of rule 5 and in case it does, if other rules can be applied in between (weak cascading) or not (strong cascading). Possibly the most important case of cascading to check is self-cascading, i.e. a sequence of rule activation leading to an infinite loop.
Postcondition satisfaction: we can use this for example to check if it is compatible with report_context_normal that some potentially hazardous devices can be on, e.g. the cooker. Because some rules can be only triggered after some others had been triggered and each one of these will have an effect on the database this property can be used to check if the conditions that allowed some previous rule to be triggered can persist when the last one is triggered, e.g. if the person has to be necessarily still in bed when the emergency procedure is started by the triggering of rule 5.

How? Our framework is conceived very much in the spirit of XTL (see [9]) however at present we use Metric Temporal Logic (MTL) as our framework for verification. We use an interpreter of the language proposed in [4] where a fragment of MTL, called *MTL-programs* is mapped to a constraint logic programming framework which admits efficient satisfiability checking of the constraints generated. Complexity is in the worse case linear in the number of variables involved. On the other hand, MTL offers a language which is expressive enough for us to map the language of our ECA rules into and to write the queries that allow us to check the properties described previously. We further restrict the expressiveness of *MTL-programs* by discarding the past fragment. We call this derived system *MTL-programs-F* because it is mainly focused on the use of operators referring to future computations: $\bigcirc$ ("next"), $\Diamond_c$ ("sometimes in the future subject to the constraint c: G is true"), $\Box_c$ (always in the future subject to the constraint c: D is true). A constraint can be for example the specification of an interval, so that $\Diamond_{[a,b]}A$ ($\Box_{[a,b]}A$) means that A is true sometimes (always) within the interval defined by a and b.

DEFINITION **1.** ([4], page 24, but without past operators) *MTL-programs-F* are made of *MTL-programs-F goals* and *MTL-programs-F clauses*. *MTL-programs-F goals* are defined as: $G ::= \epsilon | A | \bigcirc G | \Diamond_c G$ *MTL-programs-F clauses* are defined as: $D ::= A | \bigcirc D | \Box_c D | D \leftarrow G$ where ϵ denotes the empty goal, A denotes an atomic formula, and $c \in \mathbb{N}$.

This definition is complemented in [4] with some syntactical equivalences to make explicit that the metric operators can be used to define non-metric ones, so that in fact $\Diamond G$ ("sometimes in the future G") is also available as a body and $\Box D$ ("always in the future D") as a clause. For the list of properties considered above we do not require the capability of metric-based operators to write the goals or to encode the properties as at this stage we are focused on the order of the triggering and not on the duration of the triggered actions. However, we do require the capability to use metric-based operators to represent the duration based events and states that make the basis of our ECA representation language. Due to space restrictions we are not able to provide full details of this theoretical framework. Here we instantiate the general framework offered in [4] to a specific case study and temporal domain so formulas given below will refer to meaningful predicates used in the ECA rules and metrics will be refered to calendar dates. Although the initial framework considers an unbounded temporal structure we have natural initial and final times given by the time where the system started and the present, respectively. Also, before starting the verification process, the ECA rules have been translated and labelled so that a rule `ON E IF C DO A` will produce an *MTL-program-F*-based clause $do(\text{RuleID}, A) \leftarrow E \wedge C$. So that the rule will be identified by a unique RuleID.

Actions inconsistency, returns the IDs of rules which are conflicting in any sense that can be specified by using a predicate *conflictingActions*:

$$\Box(checkInconsistency(RuleID1, RuleID2) \leftarrow$$
$$do(RuleID1, A1) \wedge do(RuleID2, A2) \wedge conflictingActions(A1, A2))$$

Triggerability: $\Box(triggerable(RuleID) \leftarrow \Diamond(do(RuleID, A))$

Joint applicability, investigates triggerability for a pair of rules. By using conjunctions arbitrary sequences of rules can be tried manually or automatically, for example, all possible combinations of two or three rules:

$$\Box(jointApplicability(RuleID1, RuleID2) \leftarrow$$
$$\Diamond(do(RuleID1, A1) \wedge do(RuleID2, A2)))$$

Rule coverage:

$$\Box(coveredBy(RuleID1, RuleID2) \leftarrow do(RuleID1, A1) \leftarrow do(RuleID2, A2))$$

Rule cascading:

$$\Box(SBefore(RuleID1, RuleID2) \leftarrow do(RuleID1, A1) \wedge \bigcirc(do(RuleID2, A2))$$
$$\Box(WBefore(RuleID1, RuleID2) \leftarrow do(RuleID1, A1) \wedge \Diamond(do(RuleID2, A2))$$

Postcondition satisfaction, checks that after an action A has been applied a postcondition P is valid: $\Box(postconditionSat(RuleID, P) \leftarrow do(RuleID, A) \wedge \bigcirc(P))$

Hence the ECA rule editors can use the following *MTL-programs-F goals* to query the system about different properties: $checkInconsistency(Rid1, Rid2)$, $triggerable(Rid)$, $jointApplicability(Rid1, Rid2)$, $coveredBy(Rid1, Rid2)$, $SBefore(Rid1, Rid2)$, $WBefore(RD1, Rid2)$, or $postconditionSat(Rid, P)$.

One of the main reasons why we have choosen MTL is that it allow us to encode the language we considered in the ECA rules (see [2]). This translation can be automated, hence the ECA rule editors do not require knowledge of the underlying formalism. The only knowledge required is the ECA syntax and the list of predicates identifying the properties that can be checked.

6 Conclusions

Smart home technology at present offers a viable solution to the increasing needs of the elderly, special needs and remote home based-healthcare populations. The research to date has largely focused on the development of communication technologies and intelligent user interfaces. Here we focused on the computational analysis of user-centered data to provide a means of user-profiled support to promote intelligent independent living. We feel this addresses a new and challenging area in the overall concept of advances in technologies related to Smart Homes.

We presented an overview of a system that is based on an ADB framework with a formally defined language, providing representation for instantaneous and durative events, detection for non-primitive events throughout a rich set of operators that can relate events and states in a way that blends research between the DB and the AI communities. To maximize the reliability of the system behaviour we include as a part of the development process the use of tools that can be used to simulate, verify and validate the set of ECA rules. We believe that this mix of technologies offers an innovative solution to the research domain and also in promoting independent living in Smart Homes.

References

[1] J. F. Allen. Maintaining Knowledge about Temporal Intervals. *CACM*, 26(11):832 – 843, 1983.

[2] Juan Carlos Augusto and Chris Nugent. The use of temporal reasoning and management of complex events in smart homes. Technical report, School of Computing and Mathematics, University of Ulster at Jordanstown, United Kingdom, 2004. (`http://www.infj.ulst.ac.uk/~jcaug/TR-AugustoNugent2004a.pdf`).

[3] B. Berard, M. Bidoit, A. Finkel, F. Laroussinie, A. Petit, L. Petrucci, Ph. Schnoebelen, and P. McKenzie. *Systems and Software Verification (Model Checking Techniques and Tools)*. Springer Verlag, 1999.

[4] Christoph Brzoska. Temporal logic programming with metric and past operators. In *Executable and Temporal Logics, IJCAI'93 Satellite Workshop*, pages 21–39. Springer Verlag, 1993.

[5] P. Fraternali, E. Teniente, and T. Urpi. Validating Active Rules by Planning. In *Proceedings of the 3rd International Workshop on Rules in Database Systems*, volume 1312, pages 181–196. Springer, 1997.

[6] A. Galton. Eventualities. In Vila, van Beek, Boddy, Fisher, Gabbay, Galton, and Morris, editors, *The Handbook of Time and Temporal Reasoning in Artificial Intelligence*. MIT Press, 2004. (to be published).

[7] Rodolfo Gómez, Juan Carlos Augusto, and Antony Galton. Implementation and Testing for a Set of Event Detection Operators. Technical Report 398, School of Engineering and Computer Science, University of Exeter, United Kingdom, 2000. (`http://www.infj.ulst.ac.uk/~jcaug/rr398.pdf`).

[8] Rodolfo Gómez, Juan Carlos Augusto, and Antony Galton. Testing an Event Specification Language. In *Proceedings of the 13th. International Conference of Software Engineering and Knowledge Engineering (SEKE 2001)*, pages 341–346, Buenos Aires, Argentina, 2001.

[9] M. Leuschel and T. Massart. Infinite state model checking by abstract interpretation and program specialisation. In *Proceedings of Logic-Based Program Synthesis and Transformation (LOPSTR'99)*, pages 63–82. editor Annalisa Bossi, Venice, Italy, LNCS 1817, 1999.

[10] Itai Meiri. *Temporal Reasoning: A Constraint-Based Approach*. PhD thesis, Univ. of California, 1992.

[11] N.W. Paton and O. Diaz. Active Database Systems. *ACM Computing Surveys*, 31(1):63–103, 1999.

[12] J. Vanhala. A flood of intelligence. *ERCIM News*, (47):14–15, October 2001.

Toward a Human-Friendly Assistive Environment
D. Zhang and M. Mokhtari (Eds.)
IOS Press, 2004

Design of Health Care Life Support System based on Cybernectics

Tsutomu MATSUMOTO†, Yasuyuki SHIMADA†, Shigeyasu KAWAJI‡

† *Kumamoto National College of Technology,*
2659-2 Suya, Nishigoshi, Kikuchi, Kumamoto, Japan
{matumoto, shimada}@ec.knct.ac.jp
‡ *Graduate School of Science and Tecnology,*
Kumamoto University,
2-39-1 Kurokami, Kumamoto-city, Kumamoto, Japan
kawaji@cs.kumamoto-u.ac.jp

Abstract. This paper describes a concept and system implementation of health care support system. The medical consultation model is proposed based on analyzing task and information of medical consultation for creating a designing methodology to tele-health care system. The structure of proposed medical consultation model is created by idea of feed back control system. Clinician takes play of a controller and client is regarded with a controlled system in the model. How and Which parts of the model could be supported by computer and communication technology are discussed. The designing and implementation of collaboration among client, clinician and co-medical including family and establishment of communication channel are explained as one actual example based on proposed medical consultation model.

1 Introduction

The increasing population of senior citizens in the community requires the health care system to outreach to the people. However, it is not possible for the clinician and client's family to continuously monitor the client's everyday activities, over twenty-fours hours. There have been published papers related to this matters to improve this situation.

It is pointed out that the research to improve QOL (quality of life) of aged people has been a very important subject[1]. Ohta reported about the system which measures person's moving among rooms at home using infrared sensors[2]. He proposed the visualization of person's moving among rooms at home and total movement distance. It is considered that the non-contact type sensor is useful for measuring person's action, because it does not create additional burden on a subject. Monitoring system as similar as Ohta's way is also reported[3]. It is explained that finding method of the observed person's whereabouts can be obtained by a very simple statistics. Above mentioned reports focused on only the way of measuring vital signal or human behavior at home.

Papers related on Tele-medicine has been discussed on transferring medical image data to support diagnosis, medical counselling, sharing clinical information[4] [5].

Above reports have not cleared to support which parts of medical consultation, treatment or health care to client. This paper proposed a health care model with analyzing task and information of traditional medical consultation that clinician performs to clients. The designing and implementation based on the health care model are described in this paper.

2 Health Care and Life Support Model

Development of a health care and life support model including medical diagnosis by analyzing task and information is discussed in this section as a typical example of ill structure problem.

2.1 Task of Health Care and Life Support

In order to construct a medical consultation model, first we discuss the medical task of physician's diagnosis and giving therapy to patient. Physician interviews a new patient for acquiring various personal information, disease history of patient and family, life style, main complaint and so on. And physician does inquiry, inspection, auscultation to find abnormal states of patient. Physician orders blood check and/or bio-chemical medical check as occasion demands to clinical laboratory.

Physician estimates the state of patient using the data from patient and clinical laboratory data and inspection. Finally physician identifies the disease of client. Then physician makes a medical treatment plan after discussion on the subject with the client and/or family. After that, the physician makes a detail treatment plan. The treatment has two types. The one is to provide directly treatment to the client. The other is to provide indirectly to the client's treatment, for example through nursing staff. In this case physician gives an instruction to nursing staff then nurse staff carries out the instruction. There may be a case that physician gives a description to client and/or gives some advice to family. The family then cares for the client. Physician should confirm that treatment is given to the client.

In the case of health care and life support which include nursing elderly people, comedical who are family and nursing staff finds client's problem as client identification. For this decision making, Minimum Data Set is used. Then care plan is developed, is implemented.

Some time later physician and comedical evaluates the effect of treatment and/or care plan given to client and improves the plan. Above-mentioned tasks of physician and comedical are similar to an feedback control system configuration, a client as a controlled object, healthy as target and manipulated variables are medical treatment and care plan with cybernetics.

2.2 Information for Health Care and Life Support

Client information can be classified into two categories types of static and dynamic. The static information is not to change or even if change, time interval of changing is ignored, e.g. sex, age, etc. The dynamic information indicates variation with time and other causes, e.g. body temperature, auscultation sound, index of clinical laboratory data. In this paper client information is classified as follows. The zero order information is static information. And first - third order informations are dynamic.

1. Zero order information :
   Personal information(sex, age, disease history, career), disease history of family, life style (smoking, drinking, meal custom etc).

2. First order information : Obtaining directly or using simple detector
   Main compliant, inspection, auscultation, blood pressure, pulse count, body temperature etc.

3. Secondary information : Blood check and bio-chemical check up data
   Information from analyzing available sample of living body, ex blood, urine, stool, pus, snivel.

4. Third order information : using electro and information technology
   ECG, electromyogram, sphygmogram, X-ray image, MRI, X-ray CT etc.

Note that higher order information is also advanced health care information.

2.3 Health Care and Life Support Model

Analyzing the physician's and comedical's task in the health care life support and structuring the client information will yield a scheme as shown in figure 1. In the figure disturbance shown means inputs for client to take bad turn. The figure 2 is simplified by detector parts and treatment parts becoming each one black box. We call it "Health Care and Life Support Model".

Physician plays role of a controller in the Medical Consultation Model, i.e. he diagnoses client using the output y of detector which is originated from client, makes a treatment plan and gives directly and/or indirectly the medical treatment u to the client. The feedback from treatment block to physician block is required to confirm whether or not the client receives treatment. The r is normal health situation. The treatment is recognized as same as an operation in a control system. At this time physician verifies whether or not treatment is given.

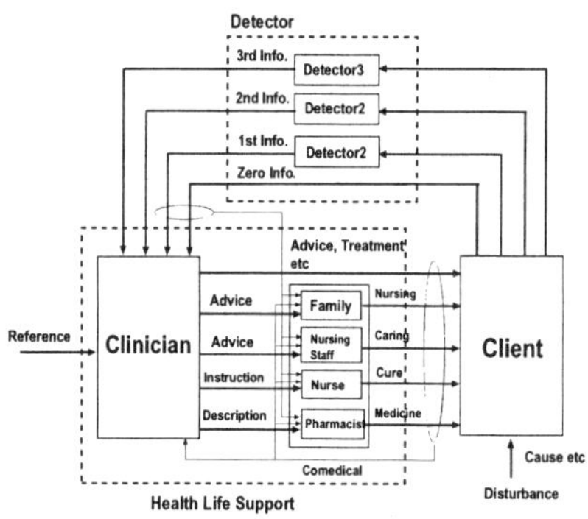

Figure 1: Information from client and task.

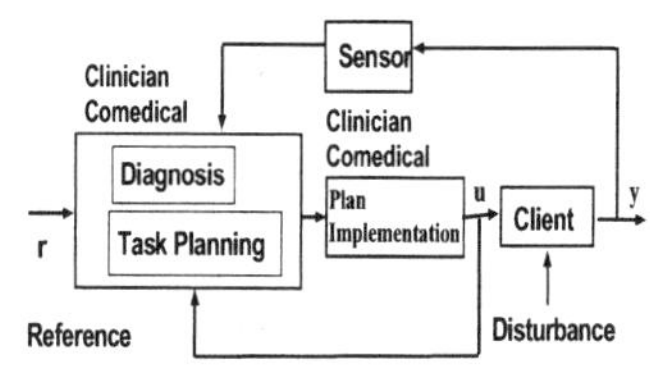

Figure 2: Healthcare Model.

3 Design of Health Care Life Support System

This section describes the modeling method of telehealth care information system based upon above the health care and life support model.

3.1 System Design

The telehealth care and life support system is regarded as setting up feedback system to share/transfer the information among client, clinician and comedical in the case of some problem of client happening. This paper defines the telehealth care information system as follows. When an irregular habitual life behavior and abnormal health condition is detected, the system confirms safety of client. And the system sends a message to clinician, nursing staff and/or neighbors depending on answer of client. In addition the system provides health advice from clinician to client.

Consequently the system has following specifications in order to perform above mentioned.

1. Obtaining the information of client

2. Transferring the information of client
3. Finding problem of client
4. Confirming client safety
5. Informing urgency to comedical, clinician
6. Providing health care advice

The fourth and the fifth mean the collaboration among client, comedical and clinician. Finally the telehealth care life support system can be designed using layer structure shown by figure 3.

3.2 Layer Structure

This section describes the relations among layers and functions of each layers.

3.2.1 Real World

The object of this system are clients, clinicians and comedical including client's family and/or neighbors.

3.2.2 Sensor Layer

The sensor layer is to gather information of client and to find urgency of client [8]. If sensor layer finds an urgency of client, the sensor layer sends a message to application layer. The message has ID of client and urgency level that client needs clinician or not, needs nursing staff or not and so on. In addition the sensor layer provides health care record to clinician via application layer. This system focuses life information (Zero order), pulse and body temperature as the third order. Architecture of sensor layer is shown in figure 4.

3.2.3 Application Layer

Application layer searches contacts of family doctor, comedical and/or client corresponding to urgency level for sending a message. With the search results application layer sends a message to interface layer. Application layer continues to send a message in order to the reply from receiver. If nobody replies, the system call an ambulance.

The application layer requests information of client to sensor layer after receiving a message of "Request : providing information of client". The application layer transfers the data to appropriate interface layer.

3.2.4 User Interface Layer

1. Clinician Interface
   Clinician interface informs urgency of client and transfers reply from clinician to the application layer. Clinician inputs the process into the system via the clinician interface. Clinician is able to retrieve health record of client.

2. Comedical Interface
   Urgency of client is informed to registered comedical via the comedical-medical interface. Comedical who received a message has to inform the condition of client and/or result of treatment to the system via the comedical interface. Also comedical retrieves health advice from the system that clinician has provided, and comedical guides client to keep health condition.

3. Client Interface(Interactive Response System)
   Client interface sends a message to confirm safety. Client can reply "No problem", "need help", "need clinician" or no answer. The client interface informs content of reply to the system.

4. System Administrator Interface
   The system administrator interface provides functions of system administrating such as registration, removing, modifying user(client, clinician, nursing staff, neighbors).

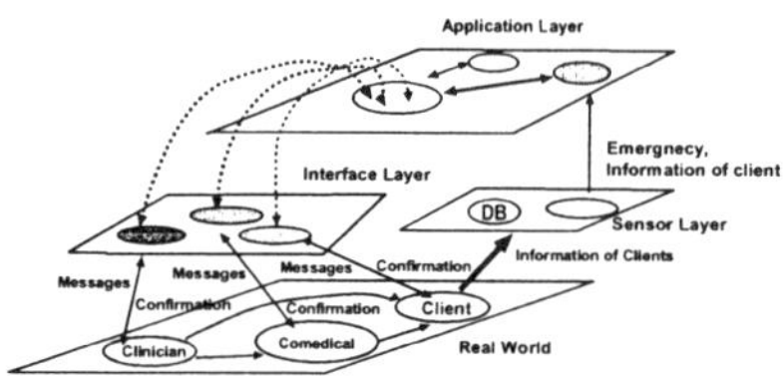

Figure 3: Layer structure for health care.

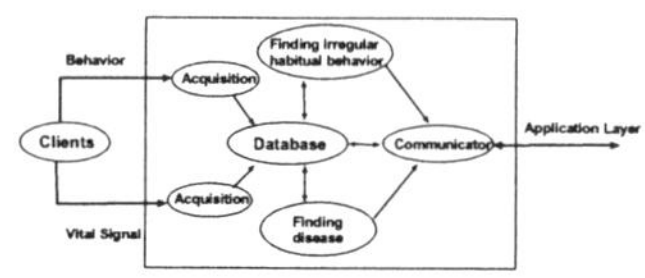

Figure 4: Architecture of sensor layer.

4 Design of Software System

In this section design and implementation of user interface as an actual example are described based on system design described in section 4 with Object Oriented Method. Software development by Object Oriented Method has some benefits as reuse, flexibility. Furthermore UML (Unified Modeling Language) can be used to design and implement the software for Object Oriented method.

4.1 Scenario

UML method suggests us to develop scenario to find use case. Because an instantiation of a use case is called a scenario, and it represents an actual usage of the system; that is a specific execution path through the system. An example for the sensor layer finding the problem of client is shown as follows.

When the sensor layer finds pathological state transition. The sensor layer sends a message to the application layer. Then the application layer decode it, simultaneously sends a message to client for confirming whether or not the client has problem. If no reply from the client, the application layer sends a message for sending a comedical to the client. Also the application layer sends a message to appropriate staff according to reply from the client.

4.2 Use Case

After developing scenario, use case could be found. Figure 5, figure 6 and figure show use cases for each interface. A use case represents a complete functionality as perceived by an actor. The actions can involve communicating with a number of actors (users and other systems) as well as performing calculations and work inside the system. The functionality of use case is described as Use Case Description.

4.3 Use Case Description

Normally Use Case Description defines a functionality of use case. This is a simple and consistent specification about how the actor and the use case (the system) interact. Two use

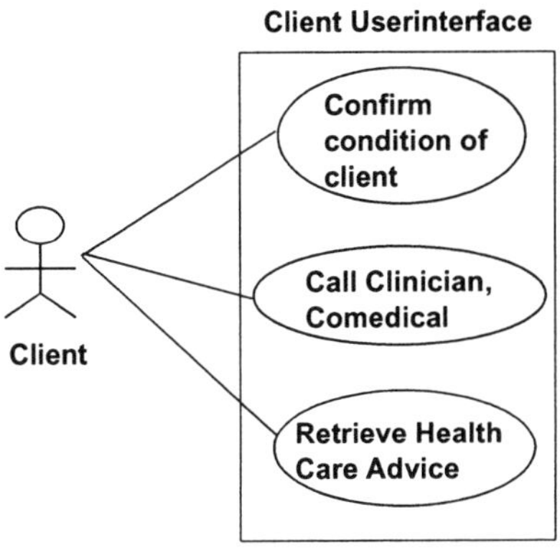

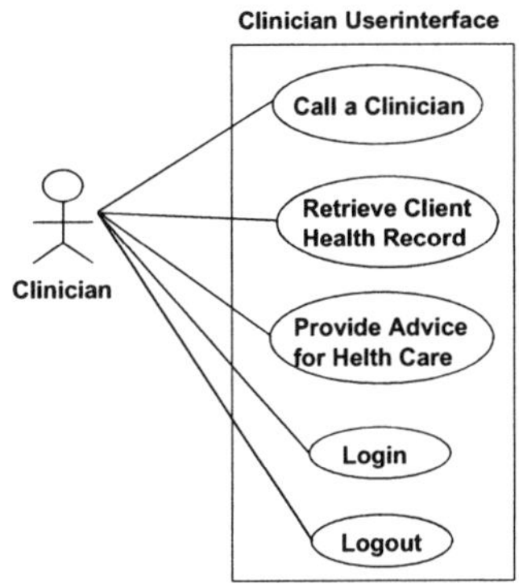

Figure 5: Use Case for Client Interface. Figure 6: Use Case for Clinician Interface.

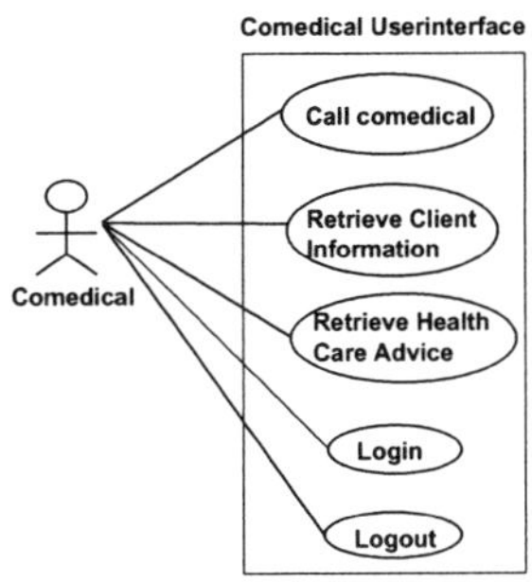

Figure 7: Use Case for Comedical Interface

ase descriptions are following as examples. Following use case description is for the system ɔ confirm safety of client.

Ɔonfirming safety of client

Use Case:

Problem happening::confirmation(ID:0011)

ummary:

When the system finds a problem of client, the system sends a message to client for onfirming saftey of client.

ctor:Client

reconditions:

A problem happens to client. Sensor layer sends a message to Application layer.

escriptions:

Basic Flow

1. Application layer sends a message of confirming safety to client via user interface.
   - Handy terminal of client shows the message.
2. The client sends a reply to the system.

Exception flow in sequence 2

If the client is not able to send a reply to the system with some reason,

1. In the case of the system receives a reply from the client in specified duration, the system call another clinician or a comedical.

Exceptions:
Communication error
Postconditions:
Communication line is set up between client and clinician and/or comedical.

Next use case description example is for the sensor layer to send a message in the case of finding emergency of the client. **Use Case:Call clinician**
Problem happens::call clinician(ID:0001)
Summary:
When some problem to client happens, the sensor layer sends a message to application layer. After the application layer receives the message, the application layer sends a emergency message to specified clinician. The system waits for reply from the clinician.
Actor:Clinician
Preconditions:
Some problem to client happens. Sensor layersends a message to application layer. The system asks the client to be safety.
Descriptions:
Basic flow

1. The application layer sends a emergency message to a clinician.

2. The clinician sends a reply to the system.

Alternative flow
In the case of no reply at above (2),

1. The system calls a clinician in priority order.

2. If any clinician no replies, the Sensor layersystem calls a medical center, nursing home and/or ambulance etc.

Exceptions:
Communication Error
Postconditions:
Communication channel is set up between the system and a clinician.

4.4 Diagrams

UML recommends the development of some kinds of diagrams to express the relation among objects and sequence of messages among objects.

A sequence diagram shows a dynamic collaboration between a number of objects. The importance aspect of this diagram is to show a sequence of message sent between the objects. Here a sequence diagrams for showing a set messages arranged in time sequence are shown as figure 8.

A collaboration diagram shows a dynamic collaboration and shows the objects and their relationships. The collaboration diagram is drawn as an object diagram, where a number of objects are shown along with their relationships using the notation in the class/object diagram. Message arrows are drawn between the objects to show the flow of message between the objects.

For convenience, a collaboration diagrams is shown in figure 9. Figure 9 shows that when sensor layer finds client problem, how the message flows between objects.

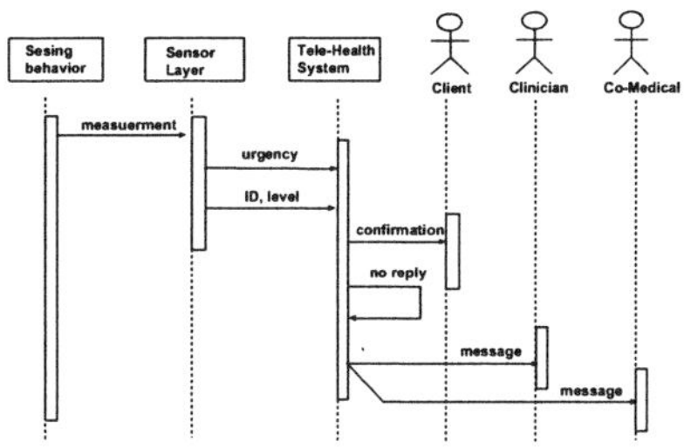

Figure 8: Information from client and task.

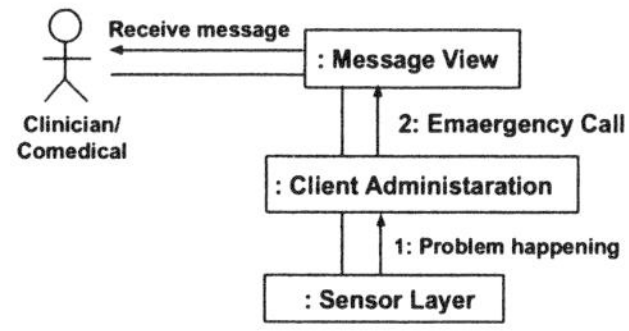

Figure 9: Healthcare Model.

5 Conclusion

This paper discussed the health care modelling and describes that tele-health support system should set up feedback loop between clinician, comedical and client on demand. As an actual example, desgning and implmentation of the system which supports collaboration and sharing information among clinician, comedical and client after finding the urgency from obtained life begavior and vital signal of client has reported in this paper. This paper does not talk the method of finding the urgency based on obtained life behavior data. We have already reported this matter[8][9]. Gathering vital signal of client is carried out by simulation.

Proposed methotology in this paper is applicable to hospital. Because physician and nursing staff are not able to continuously care the clients over twenty-four hours.

References

[1] Inada H Ishikawa K, "An experimental study on home health care support information system construction," *Proceeding of the World Congress on Medical Informatics (MEDINFO95)*, pp. 581–585, 1995.

[2] Shigeru Ohta, "Helath monitoring system for the aged, information," *Processing Society of Japan Magazine*, vol. 41, no. 6, pp. 639–643, 2000.

[3] Tanikawa Tomohiro et al, "In-house movement monitoring system for the aged living alone," *Japan Journal of Medical Informatics*, vol. 20, no. 2, pp. 270–271, 1999.

[4] S-M Yoo, H Lee, and S-Y Kim, "Medical counselling through computer communication networks," *Proceeding of the World Congress on Medical Informatics (MEDINFO 98)*, vol. 1, pp. 337–340, 1998.

[5] M Olson R. Neame, "How can sharing clinician information be made to work," *Proceeding of the World Congress on Medical Informatics (MEDINFO 98)*, vol. 1, pp. 315–318, 1998.

[6] T. Furukawa, "Clinician's diagnosis algorithm," *Mathematical Science(J)*, 1983.

[7] T. Tango, "A new statistical method for the determination of individual normal range," *JAMHTS*, vol. 9, pp. 241–246, 1982.

[8] T. Matsumoto, Y. Shimada, K. Shibasato, H. Ohtsuka, and S. Kawaji, "Creating behavior model of a senior solitary life and detecting an urgency," *Proceedings of the International ICSC Congress on Intelligent System and Applications*, vol. 2, pp. 234–238, 2000.

[9] T. Matsumoto, Y. Shimada, K. Shibasato, H. Ohtsuka, and S. Kawaji, "Developing of human behavior model at home and its application," *World Congress on Medical Informatics 2001 (to be published)*, 2001.

Toward a Human-Friendly Assistive Environment
D. Zhang and M. Mokhtari (Eds.)
IOS Press, 2004

SmartWave –Intelligent Meal Preparation System to Help Older People Live Independently

James Russo[1], Andiputranto Sukojo[1], Abdelsalam (Sumi) Helal[1], Rick Davenport[2], and William C. Mann[2]

[1] Pervasive Computing Laboratory, Computer and Information Science and Engineering Department, University of Florida, Gainesville, Florida 32611, USA
{jrusso,asukojo,helal}@cise.ufl.edu
http://www.icta.ufl.edu

[2] Rehabilitation Engineering Research Center on Aging, University of Florida
2107A Health Professions Building, Gainesville, Fl 32610-0164
{rdavenpo,Mann}@phhp.ufl.edu
http://www.rerc.ufl.edu

Abstract. As we age, simple everyday tasks become difficult to perform. Simply enjoying a hot nutritious meal may be difficult because of the natural impairments and declines in health conditions. The numerous steps required in preparing a meal and operating a microwave oven can become overwhelming due to visual, hearing, cognitive and/or neuro-motor declines. In this paper we discuss the SmartWave system, a pervasive microwave based cooking system which makes it easier for elderly people to enjoy a hot meal without having to read cooking instructions or interact with the microwave buttons. Additionally, SmartWave provides memory and coordination assistance to aid elderly with minor cognitive impairment. We describe the design and implementation of SmartWave, and discuss its integration with a smart home environment. We also describe a sample usage scenario and present the results of a study that we conducted to explore the elders' views on the usability of SmartWave.

1 Introduction

As we age, we experience normal decline in vision, hearing, cognition and movement. The cost of home health services for older persons with disabilities is increasing with the rapidly elder population. Today, one in ten elders in US suffers from Alzheimer's disease (AD) and it is estimated that 1 in 5 elders will have AD by 2050. These numbers will only increase in the future as the first of the 75.8M baby boomers begin to reach their 60s and 70s in 2008 and 2018 [1]. In 2002, AD resulted in health related expenditures of more than $61B [2] and our health and caregiver system will be increasingly stressed as those numbers increase. Hence, there is a significant need to develop innovative and cost-effective ways to help elders maintain their independence while at the same time reducing caregiver burden.

ADLs or activities of daily living are basic tasks for everyday life. They include eating, dressing and bathing [3]. In order for a person to remain independent, he/she must be able to perform these activities without assistance. For some elderly, even the simplest of tasks such as cooking a microwaveable meal can become overwhelming due to the complex cooking instructions written in small print on the cooking package and the need for memory and coordination in interacting with the microwave oven. In this paper we present SmartWave, an intelligent microwave oven integrated with a smart home environment. The system uses a commercially available microwave along with an RFID reader to allow the microwave to be automatically programmed with the correct cooking instructions. The user simply removes the food package from the freezer, places it on the counter next to the microwave, and the system then walks the user through the cooking process with visual and auditory cues from information contained within the RFID tag on the food package. The system then starts the cooking process once the food has been placed inside the microwave over and the door closed. The system could just as easily been based on the standard UPC barcodes which are currently available on food packets. However, we decided to use RFID to extend the range of usability of the system to include frail elders and elders with minor cognitive impairments, as the process of scanning a barcode is far more complex then just placing an item on the counter.

In the rest of this section, we discuss related work on intelligent kitchen systems. In section 2 we discuss the design of the SmartWave system. Technical aspects of the actual implementation are discussed in section 3. In section 4 we summarize the results of a usability study that we conduced with the help of a local focus group of older people. Finally, in section 5 we discuss our conclusion and future work.

1.1 Related Work

Future kitchen concepts have recently been explored by several industries including consumer electronics, home appliances, durable goods, and the construction industries. Some of the initiatives taken in this direction include Counter Intelligence [4], Restaurant USA [5], IBM Kitchen [6] and Siemens Smart Home [7].

Counter Intelligence introduced kitchen technologies that enable smart utensils and appliances to sense, infer, and react to the environment. Kitchen in essence, is proactively assisting the person with respect to cooking. IBM's Kitchen introduced the concept of central coordination of various appliances like microwave/stove, when one needs various appliances to prepare a recipe. SIEMENS introduced kitchen appliances that work together and gather important information from the internet (for instance, the cooking recipe).

Some of the commercially available smart kitchen appliances include: smart refrigerators [8], smart microwave ovens [9, 10, 11], and finally smart stoves [12]. To this end, TMIO [9] developed a special microwave that can immediately refrigerate your chicken once it is cooked. Another microwave from LG can be connected to PC to download recipes from Internet.

We have looked at the characteristics of Dementia/Alzheimer diseases [13,14,15,16], and looked at studies in health research laboratory [17] and among other papers [18,19,20,21] to learn the essential constraints that need to go into engineering systems for elders with these impairments. The progress report on Alzheimer disease [18] describes ongoing research in the cause, diagnosis, and treatment of AD and also ways to help caregivers support people with AD. At Intel Research Laboratory [19] a study enumerated the key themes regarding the needs and barriers to successful aging and addressed a set of design principles which apply across the stages of cognitive declines. Mihailidis [20] hypothesized that independence might be restored by using a computerized device that prompts and monitors a person as he or she completes an activity. Stanford [21] pointed out that pervasive sensors should assist residents in maintaining their independence, offering assistance only when necessary.

2 SmartWave Design

Consider the example of Maltida, the fictitious 85 year old elder woman who our Smart House is designed for. She has been living alone since her husband's death a few years ago and was recently diagnosed with Alzheimer's disease. This is in addition to common old age ailments such as impaired vision, motor skill degradation, and other cognitive impairments. Her diminished vision makes it difficult for her to read the small preparation instructions printed on food packages, her motor skill problems makes it difficult to operate the microwave oven's controls, and her cognitive ability prevents her from using more complicated kitchen appliances such as the stove. As with most elders, Maltida cherishes the independence she has in her own home, and has thus far been avoiding assisted living care. In order to maintain her independence, she must be able to perform basic ADLs including meal preparation. To support Matilda in her pursuit for independent living, we have designed an intelligent cooking system capable of helping Matilda prepare her own meals independently.

SmartWave is part of a smart kitchen which is contained within our experimental Smart House. We will describe our smart home briefly to show the interaction between the Smart House and the SmartWave. Envisioned by Mark Weiser [22] in the early 1990s, ubiquitous computing is where computation facilities embedded in the environment are available everywhere to assist users in the accomplishing their daily tasks. The computation and interaction is seamlessly and invisibly integrated into physical artifacts within the environments and is always ready to serve us without distracting us from our daily practices.

The ubiquitous vision puts an emphasis on interaction and cooperation among computational devices. This is because the limited capability of a single device to sense and control environments needs to be complemented and enhanced through cooperation and coordination. Using this vision, we designed a smart home environment which promotes successful aging and independent living. Beyond the typical home automation applications, a Smart House for the elderly must simplify and assist in the completion of every day tasks, therefore creating an assistive environment. The system continually monitors context and interprets events to assist the occupant in daily activities, one of which is meal preparation.

2.1 The Smart House Environment and Services

One of the basic services required to maximize the intelligence of a smart environment is an indoor tracking system. This system allows the smart home to make proactive decisions to better serve its occupants by enabling context awareness [23]. Presently we are using an ultrasonic positioning system which uses multiple receivers at fixed locations and transmitters located on the subject allowing location determination via time of arrival calculations.

By placing two transmitting tags on the shoulders of the residents, we are able to determine both their location and the orientation. This location and orientation is important as video cues used in conjunction with the SmartWave system will be displayed on many different monitors throughout the house depending on the residents' room location and the direction they are facing.

The floor plan of our experimental smart house is shown in Figure 1. The ultrasonic location sensors are shown in this diagram. An overhead shot of the actual smart house is shown in Figure 2.

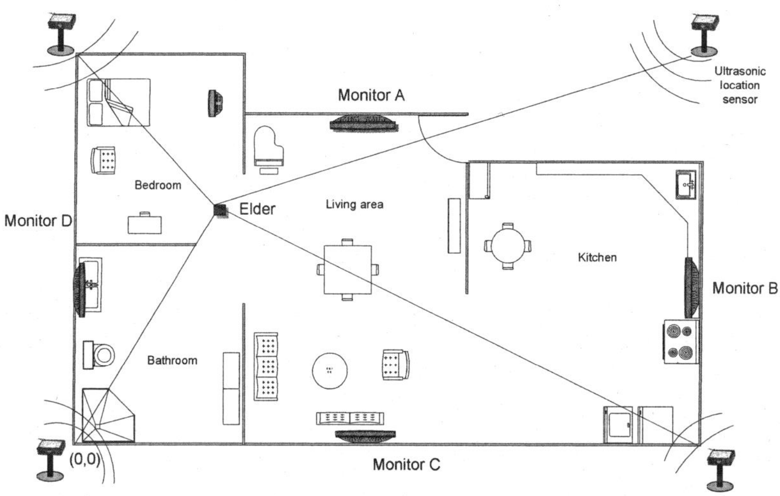

Figure 1 - Floor plan of the experimental smart house

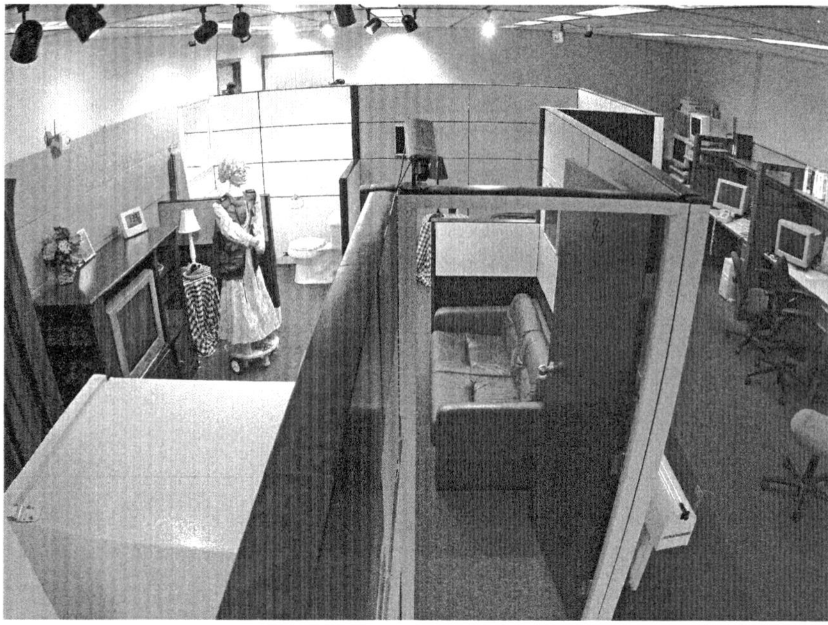

Figure 2 - Picture of the experimental smart house

SmartWave is integrated into the smart house through the Open Service Gateway Initiative (OSGi) framework [24, 25]. OSGi is an open architecture designed for the delivery of services to residential networks. Running on a residential gateway, OSGi facilitates the interaction of services from various sources in an organized and coordinated fashion. This perfectly satisfies our need for a robust framework that can support dynamic context-aware service composition using core services such as our location service. In order to provide an execution environment for services from diverse devices in a residential area, platform independence is a requirement, which is achieved by using Java.

In the OSGi framework [26], a bundle is a deliverable application packaged as a JAR (Java Archive) file. It contains zero or more services specified as a Java interface. Services are registered with Service Registry so that they can be discovered and used by other Bundles. The OSGi framework provides this execution environment for individual services and their interaction among them. We have packaged our location system into an OSGi bundle to provide the service to other services within the OSGi framework. To support rapid application development and facilitate service composition, our middleware provides a set of generic services such as:

- Indoor location and orientation service as described above.
- Voice recognition service. Provides a voice to text translation service

- Multimedia streamer service to deliver video and audio contents (e.g., cues and instructions) to monitor screens and speakers located in different rooms of the smart house.
- Database service enabling storage of various information in relational databases.

2.2 SmartWave Services

The SmartWave and the Smart Kitchen subsystem are integrated to the smart house as a set of bundles offering the following services

- *Monitoring* – by monitoring daily activities over a period of time the smart kitchen keeps track of hydration and eating events, and sends reminders and suggestions to drink or to eat a specific meal. Reminders require a great deal of coordination and the use of several prompting devices. Our reminder system is location and orientation based and makes use of both video and audio cues.
- *Prompting* – Alzheimer's disease makes it very difficult to remember the simplest sequence of steps or procedures. Even cooking a frozen food package can be a struggle. The elder might forget how to open the food package, set the microwave timer and power level, open microwave door, stir the food, or forget to remove cooked food from the microwave. Prompting is a key service offered by the smart kitchen that enhances the effectiveness of the SmartWave system.
- *Notification* – SmartWave makes no assumption about the whereabouts or the activities of the elder person while the food is being cooked. The elder could be anywhere in the house (perhaps watching television). The SmartWave uses the notification service to locate the elder and to send notification that the food is ready, or an additional step is required in the food preparation process.
- *Reassuring* – caregivers may receive special notifications to be reassured that the subject is eating her/his meals regularly.

3. Implementation

3.1 Hardware

The hardware for our SmartWave system consists of many off the shelf parts, including a standard GE microwave which was then modified to allow computer control. The microwave was examined and it was determined that the best way to control the microwave was to embed a microcontroller which would simulate the key presses of the microwave's front panel. This method of interface was chosen so that the microwave would retain all the included safety features. This microcontroller would also need the ability to determine the status of the door, so that the microwave could be programmed and cooking started once the door had been closed.

The PIC-16F628 [27] was chosen as the microprocessor used for the microwave control. The PIC-16F628 was connected to three MAX395 serially controlled switch chips. Each MAX395 [28] has 8 SPST switches on board allowing up to 8 buttons to be simulated. The three devices daisy chained together yielded 24 separate SPST switches which are used to simulate the button pushes of the front panel. Of the 24 SPST switches available, 17 have been used to control the 17 front panel buttons on the microwave model we have selected. The PIC-16F628 was also connected to an additional door switch in an otherwise unpopulated location to provide feedback on the current door status. This enables the host application to query the current door status and only send the start commands once the door has been closed by the subject.

The keypad interface in the microwave is a common row/column configuration, where each button on the membrane keypad provided an electrical connection between a row and column. The PIC-16F628 microcontroller and serially controlled switches are used to simulate the membrane keypad by electronically connecting a row and column. The input to the microcontroller was accomplished via a standard RS232 serial port, providing flexibility in the device which actually controls the microwave.

Controlling our microwave oven is the TINI processor from Dallas Semiconductor [29]. The TINI processor was chosen due to its network connectivity and how it could be easily used to interact with the existing technology in our smart home. Using this processor, we were able to seamlessly integrate the microwave and benefit from the existing technology which is present in our OSGi driven smart house. The TINI connects to the RFID reader and the microwave via two RS232 seria ports. When an RFID tag is detected, it is read, decoded and signals are sent to the smart house via the home network for video/audio cueing and also to the microwave via the serial interface for the cooking information.

A Texas Instruments RFID reader is used to determine which food packet is being scanned and to obtain the cooking instructions from that RFID tag [30], or perhaps stored in a remote database. The database could be used due to the small storage space within the RFID tag itself. In a database implementation, the RFID data would just be an identifier indicating the food packet, yielding a key into the database for the actual cooking instructions and other important information.

The work flow of the SmartWave system is shown in Figure 3. As the elder takes a frozen food packet from the microwave and places it on the countertop, the RFID tag on the back of the packet is read by the RFID reader. The packet descriptor is sent through the TINI to the home computer and then cooking instructions are sent to the PIC microcontroller within the microwave. The PIC microcontroller then electronically pushes the correct buttons on the microwave front panel. ***Figure 4*** shows snapshots of the physical components, including the RFID tags, the SmartWave with the RFID reader, the manufactured PC board installed in the microwave oven and finally the Smart Kitchen area in the Smart House.

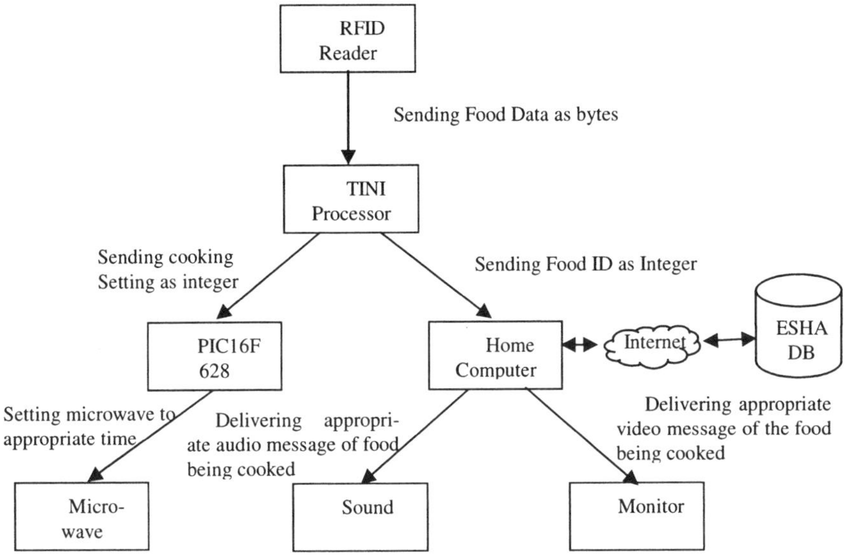

Figure 3 - Workflow and components of the SmartWave system

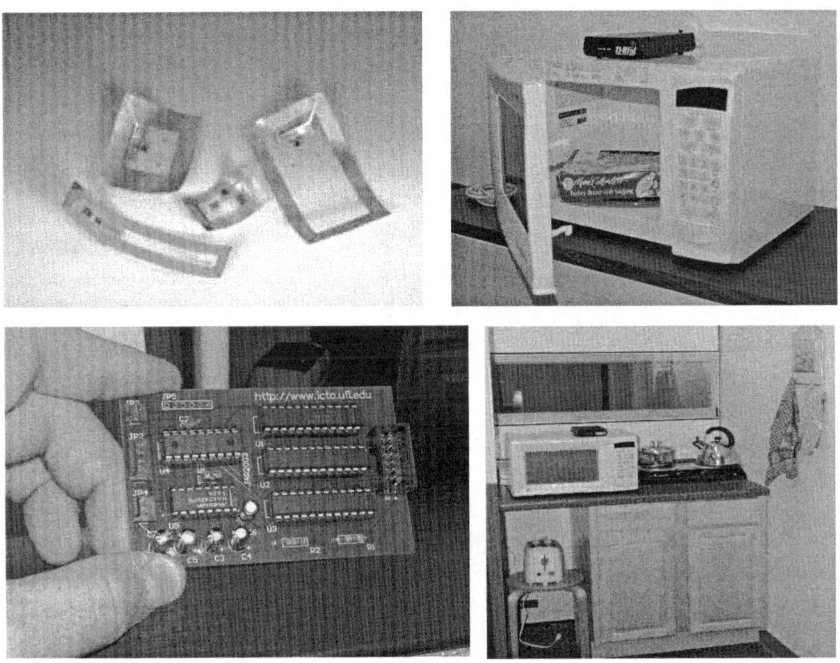

Figure 4.

3.2 Software

The OSGi framework consists of Services which can make use of other services to enhance functionality. The SmartWave service makes use of many other generic services within the OSGi framework. The service interaction flow is shown in Figure 5 below.

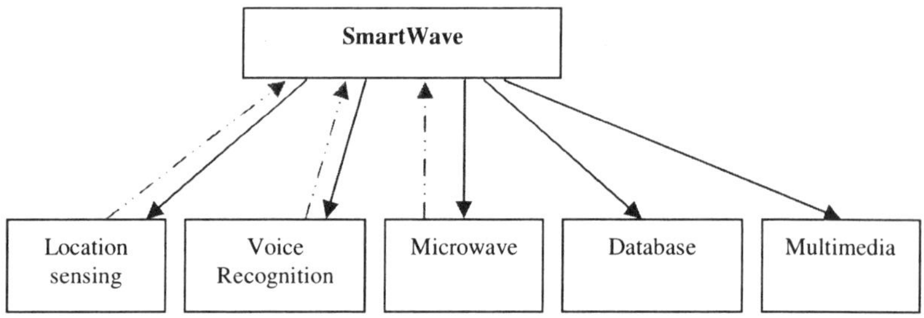

Figure 5 - OSGi service interaction flow diagram for SmartWave

The three dotted pointers to SmartWave describe an event trigger by location sensing, voice recognition and microwave service to SmartWave service. Blue pointer represent service request by SmartWave bundle to other services. There is no event generation from database and multimedia service to the SmartWave.

3.2.1 Database service

The database service, using Oracle 9i, stores various information about food nutrition, complete cooking instruction, person's diseases and health conditions, previously cooked food, personal cooking adjustments, and various sound and video clips related to the meal preparation. The food nutrition data can be downloaded from ESHA nutrition [31] and information about how to cook the food can be stored in the RFID tag. While the RFID tag can contain food description and cooking instruction, food nutritional information is downloaded via the Internet from ESHA. The database service provides access to the nutrition information and is used to potentially guard against violating diet and disease restrictions for the individual user.

3.2.2 Location service

The location service keeps track of the coordinate position and orientation of the user. With information about the house, the location service converts this low level information to higher level information such as "kitchen", "facing microwave", and "leaving kitchen". This information is used as context when displaying visual and audio cues to the user.

3.2.3 Voice recognition service

Based on the elder location, SmartWave activates certain microphones located throughout the smart home and uses certain rule grammars based on possible contexts. This will enable the user to ask for the instructions to repeat or indicate that the food was too hot. This feedback will then be stored in the database and could be used to adjust the cooking the next time this specific meal is prepared.

3.2.4 Multimedia service

The smart home has three flat LCD screens mounted on the walls in the living room, the bedroom and the kitchen. Each LCD display also contains associate speakers. They are connected to the home computer via an analog switch which controls the video and audio output to certain locations. The multimedia service provides play both video and sound directed towards a certain location within the home. To prompt the user or to send a reminder, the SmartWave requests the user location and orientation from the location service and then requests the multimedia service play the video/audio on the requested monitor/speaker.

3.2.5 Microwave Service

Microwave service represents the commercial off the shelf microwave placed in the kitchen. When the microwave bundle is activated, it attempts to establish the physical connection to the microwave. If the microwave responds, the microwave bundle will register the microwave service. Otherwise the microwave bundle will put the registration of the service on hold and continually query for the existence of the microwave. The microwave service, once registered, provides all front panel functionality as easy-to-use methods. Such methods include timeCook(time, power), isDoorOpened(), getMicrowaveState(), etc. If the microwave becomes unreachable, the microwave bundle will automatically unregister the service and wait for it to re-appear.

3.2.6 SmartWave

The following events describe the proactive operation of the SmartWave system.

- Get food id event - When the user puts the food package on the counter, the microwave will obtain the food id and send this information to the microwave service. Microwave service posts this event to the OSGi event framework to be captured by the SmartWave service. The SmartWave service then asks the database service to prepare the pertinent video explaining how to prepare this food. The video typically contains a demonstration on how to open packaging, and other simple steps required to prepare the meal. The SmartWave service requests the multimedia service to play the video on the kitchen monitor.
- Out of date events – If the food is out of date, microwave will send "Out of date event" to the microwave service. Microwave service posts this event to the

framework to be captured by the SmartWave service. The database is asked to prepare the out-of-date video and the multimedia service plays this video on the monitor in the kitchen.

- Un-microwaveable event - If the food descriptor is not of the microwaveable type such as soft drink, ice cream, the microwave will send "un-microwaveable event" to the microwave service. Again, the correct video clip will be displayed indicating that microwaving of this item is not possible.
- Stir event - Some meals require multiple steps before the considered complete. For this, an event may be required during between phases of the cooking. This event is raised when action is required by the user and the appropriate video is displayed.
- Food ready event – After the food is cooked, the microwave sends "food ready event" to the microwave service. This causes the display of the completion video to whatever monitor the user is closest to. This is done by making using of the location service in addition to the multimedia service.

4. Usability Study

The objective of our study was to explore elder views on the current usability of the microwave oven and to test the usability of our SmartWave system. The SmartWave interactive demonstration involved a general overview of the SmartWave, followed by a group demonstration of the SmartWave cooking a frozen entrée, and concluded with all study participants individually preparing their own frozen dinner entrée (Nancy's Personal Quiche Florentine) with the SmartWave. A background questionnaire was completed prior to the SmartWave demonstration and a follow-up questionnaire assessing the usability of the SmartWave system was completed once the study participant successfully cooked their own entrée.

Disability	**1**	**2**	**3**	**4**	**5**	**6**	**7**	**8**	**Results**
Low Vision	X	X	-	-	-	X	-	-	3/8 =38% have low vision
Poor Hearing	X	-	X	-	X	-	-	-	3/8=38% have poor hearing
Difficulty with hand tasks	X	X	X	-	X	-	-	-	4/8=50% have difficulty with hand tasks
Memory difficulties/learning disability	X	X	-	-	X	X	-	-	4/8=50% have learning or memory difficulties

Table 1 Summary of health impairments of the study participants

Eight elders (from the RERC-Tech-Aging consumer advisory board) participated in the interactive demonstration of the SmartWave system. Summary of the impairments of the group participants is listed in Table 1 above. The results of the background questionnaire are summarized as follows: Participants ranged in age from 66 to 82 years, with a mean of 75+5.9. fifty percent of these participants were male, and all were white. Sixty-three percent had completed college. Thirty-eight percent lived alone. Seventy-five percent of female study participants prepared three meals on a typical day, with seventy-five percent of male study participants preparing only snacks, or going out to eat, or having their spouse prepare all their meals on a typical day. All study participants had a microwave oven in their home and all reported being 'very satisfied' with their microwave. Eighty-eight percent rated their microwave as being 'very important,' with seventy-five percent using their microwave '6-10 times' during a typical week. Fifty-seven percent reported preparing a frozen food item such as a 'TV-dinner, chicken pot pie, pizza pocket 2-5 times a week.' Eighty-eight percent were 'self-taught' in using their microwave. All study participants reported microwave instructions on frozen food packages were 'not at all difficult to follow,' however forty-three percent reported that if they felt the microwave instructions were too difficult to follow they would resort to 'guessing how much time and power to use when preparing a frozen food item out of a box.' Finally thirty-eight percent reported microwave instructions on frozen food packages as 'somewhat difficult to read.'

The results of the usability of the SmartWave are summarized as follows: All study participants reported the SmartWave as 'not at all difficult to use,' with seventy-one percent rating the SmartWave as 'very easy to use when compared to their present microwave at home.' Seventy-five percent rated the difficulty level of the instructions for the SmartWave as 'just right,' with one study participant stating that the instruction level 'needed to have more steps,' with a second study participant stating 'there were too many simple steps.' Another study participant suggested that the SmartWave be outfitted with a pause button due to the fact that he had dropped his entrée and the video/audio instructions 'got ahead of him.'

One study participant ranked the SmartWave poorly commenting that the SmartWave door was hard to open when compared to her personal microwave however the SmartWave can operate with any door mechanism therefore this was not a factor of the SmartWave but rather the brand of microwave the prototype components were installed onto (she preferred a door in which she could open the microwave by pulling a handle as opposed to having to manually push in a button to open the door).

Sixty-three percent of the study participants reported that they would be 'very willing' to retrofit their home microwave with SmartWave components. The twenty-five percent that were 'not willing' stated that their home microwave works fine for their present needs however would be open to the idea of using a SmartWave in the future if the need arose. Fifty percent of the study participants stated that if they had a SmartWave oven in their home they would use it more often than they presently use their current microwave at home.

When study participants were asked if they had a SmartWave oven in their home would they buy food that was compatible with the SmartWave oven or buy what they normally purchased and seventy-five percent reported that they would buy foods that were specifically labeled 'Compatible with the SmartWave oven.' One study participant stated she would only change her purchasing habits if the food product was 'new and appealing and a second study participant had a concern regarding the possible 'comparative cost' of the SmartWave labeled food products.

This elder sample was found to frequently use and place high value on their microwave ovens at home. Although the elder sample reported both being very satisfied with their present microwave oven at home and less than fifty percent reported having problems reading or following the microwave food package instructions, once the elder group witnessed the SmartWave system they recognized the potential benefit in having this smart technology in their home. The potential benefit the elder group placed in the SmartWave was seen in the high number of elders willing to change their habits and home environment to accommodate the SmartWave oven; this was seen in the high number willing to retrofit their present microwave as well as the high number willing to change which food products they would normally buy to SmartWave labeled food.

5. Conclusion

This paper has presented the design and development of a smart microwave cooking system. The main motivation of our work is to assist the elder population live independently by creating a system that will let them prepare a meal despite age-related impairments and ailing health conditions. Our approach is to make cooking a proactive process undertaken by the smart microwave (SmartWave) by using functionality provided by the smart house. To this end, we have used RFID tags on the food packets to help attain the cooking instructions from the tag itself or from a database. Also, to incorporate great usability, we have provided assistance using video and audio to help with a step by step process of cooking the food. Finally, we have tested our prototype by conducting a study on the usability of the SmartWave system. The results were positive with respect to acceptability, usability and convenience for the end user.

References

[1] The Boomer Stats, Baby Boomer HeadQuarters. http://www.bbhq.com/bomrstat.htm
[2] R. Koppel Alzheimer Disease: The Cost to U.S Business in 2002. http://www.alz.org/Media/newsreleases/2002/062602ADCosts.pdf
[3] Joshua M. Wiener, Raymond J. Hanley et al. Measuring the Activities of Daily Living: Comparisons Across national Surveys. Journal of Gerontology: SOCIAL SCIENCES (November 1990) S229-237. http://aspe.hhs.gov/daltcp/reports/meacmpes.html
[4] Counter Intelligence by MIT. http://www.media.mit.edu/ci/
[5] Beth Panitz, Smart Kitchens: Science Fiction or High-Tech Reality? Restaurants USA. http://www.restaurant.org/rusa/magArticle/cfm?ArticleID=144
[6] IBM Kitchen Demo. http://www.ngi.ibm.com/demos/kitchen.html
[7] SIEMENS Internet House Website. http://www.siemens.com/index.jsp?sdc_pt4csuo1050417d1053184pCHNn1050417flm&sdc_sid=15177225492&
[8] LG's Internet Refrigerator. http://www.dreamlg.com/en/ref/index.jsp
[9] TMIO's Microwave oven. http://news.bbc.co.uk/2/hi/technology/2921413.stm

[10] LG's internet Microwave oven. http://www.dreamlg.com/en/cook/index.jsp
[11] Samsung's Microwave oven. http://www.samsung.com/Products/MicrowaveOven/news/MicrowaveOven_20020422_0000000846.htm
[12] TMIO's Smart Stove. http://www.tmio.com/TonightsMenuIntelligentOven.htm
[13] Dementia Information. http://www.dementia.com
[14] Alzheimer Organization. http://www.alz.org
[15] Reflection of Memory Lost Video from Alzheimer's Disease Research Center (ADRC) at Washington University School of Medicine. [video] http://alzheimer.wustl.edu/adrc2/Education/ReflectionsOnMemoriesLost/
[16] Alzheimer's disease: Unraveling the Mystery. Alzheimer Disease Education and Referral Center. http://www.alzheimers.org/unraveling/index.htm
[17] Intel Proactive Health. http://www.intel.com/research/prohealth/cs-aging_in_place.htm
[18] 2001-2002 Progress Report on Alzheimer disease. http://www.alzheimers.org/pr01-02/
[19] Margaret Morris, Jay Lundell, Eric Dishman, and Brad Needham. New Perpectives on Ubiquitous Computing from ethnographic Study of Elders with Cognitive decline. In Anind K.Dey, Albrecht Schmidt, Joseph F.McCarthy(Eds): UbiComp 2003: Ubiquitous Computing. Lecture Notes in Computer Science, Vol. 2864. Springer-Verlag, Berlin Heidelberg New York(2003) 227-242.
[20] Mihailidis, A. Fernie, G. Cleghorn, W.L. (2000). The development of a computerized cueing device to help people with dementia to be more independent, Technology & Disability, 13, 23-40. http://www.sfu.ca/~amihaili/Papers/Technology&Disability(2000).pdf
[21] Vince Stanford. Using Pervasive Computing to Deliver Elder Care. In Pervasive Computing January-march 2002. http://www-robotics.usc.edu/~gaurav/CS599-IES/elder-care.pdf
[22] M. Weiser," The Computer for the 21st Century," Scientific American, vol.256, no.3, (1991) 94-104
[23] A. Helal, B.Winkler, C.Lee, Y.Kaddoura, L.Ran, C.Giraldo, S.Kuchibhotla, and W. C. Mann. Enabling Location-Aware Pervasive Computing Applications for the Elderly. In Proceedings of the first IEEE International Conf. Pervasive Computing & Communications, Dallas-Fort Worth, Texas (2003) 531-538.
[24] D. Marples, and P.Kriens, "The Open Service Gateway Initiative : An Introductory Review," IEEE Communications Magazine, 39(12), (2001) 110-114.
[25] Sun Microsystems. Java Embedded Server. http://www.sun.com/software/embeddedserver/
[26] John Barr.OSGI Specification and Roadmap. http://www.osgi.org/resources/docs/JohnBarr_Workshop-JRB=Slides.pdf, HomeNet 2001 (2001)
[27] Microchip Microcontroller www.microchip.com
[28] Maxim IC Switches www.maxim.com
[29] TINI http://www.ibutton.com/TINI/
[30] Texas Instrument RFID. http://www.tiris.com
[31] ESHA Research. http://www.esha.com

Toward a Human-Friendly Assistive Environment
D. Zhang and M. Mokhtari (Eds.)
IOS Press, 2004

Home Monitoring and Control Applications via SMS

Dr. Zhongming MA
School of EEE, Singapore Polytechnic
500 Dover Road, Singapore 139651
Tel: 65-68790698, Email: mazhongm@sp.edu.sg

Abstract: This paper described our work on a SMS (short message service) based control and monitoring system. It is a Microcontroller based portable system, able to carry out two-way communication. The device can transmit and receive message (SMS). After receiving message, it is able to display the message locally on LCD or carry out the commands extracted from SMS to control relays, fans, lights, etc. Sending message: send local status of switch/sensor, analog input values from sensors, such as pressure, temperature, ECG etc, to other parties. Possible applications: Home Security system, Warehouse control, Remote HVAC, Remote metering, Tele-assistance, medical data collection and processing, etc.

Introduction

SMS is getting very popular and widely used now. It will be very convenient to use SMS doing some remote control and monitoring. In our project, we combine a GSM modem and a microcontroller system together, to build a device which is capable of sending and receiving SMS, able to send the local digital and analogue parameters to remote party for monitoring, and receiving SMS for displaying and carrying out the control commands embedded in the message.

1. About SMS

Short Messages are two-way alphanumeric messages and binary messages that can be sent and received by GSM modems / modules or server equipment with Short Message Service (SMS) capabilities. The SMS service is provided by the Global System for Mobile Communications (GSM). Short Messages sent from GSM units are called mobile originated, while messages received by GSM units are called mobile terminated. Short messages are stored and forwarded by the Short Message Service Centres (SMSC).

An SMSC is identified by a Global Switched Telephone Network (GSTN) number, which has to be known to the sender of a mobile originated message. The availability of the SMS service over different mobile networks depends on roaming agreements of the networks, as well as on a mechanism to deliver the messages. It is the network operator responsibility to inform the user about the success or failure of the message delivery.

The Short Message Service SMS, as defined within the GSM 900 / 1800 / 1900 digital mobile phone standard has several unique features:

A single short message can be up to 160 characters (7bit coded) or 140 characters (8 bit coded) of text in length. Those 140 / 160 characters can comprise of words or numbers or an alphanumeric combination. Non-text based short messages (for example, in binary format) are also supported. More about that binary mode you will find at the link PDU mode.

The Short Message Service is a store and forward service, in other words, short messages are not sent directly from sender to recipient, but always via a SMS Center (SMSC) instead. Each mobile telephone network that supports SMS has one or more messaging centers to handle and manage the short messages.

2. System Hardware

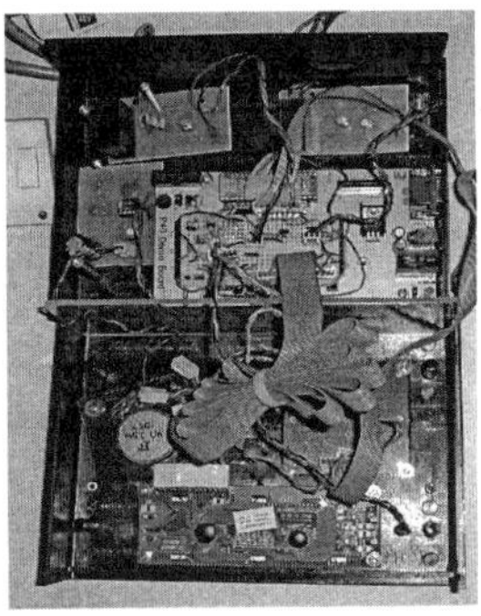

Figure 1 The device hardware

The microcontroller used in this project is BasicStamp MCU BS2p40-Pin Module (shown in Figure 2), known as BS2P40.[1]

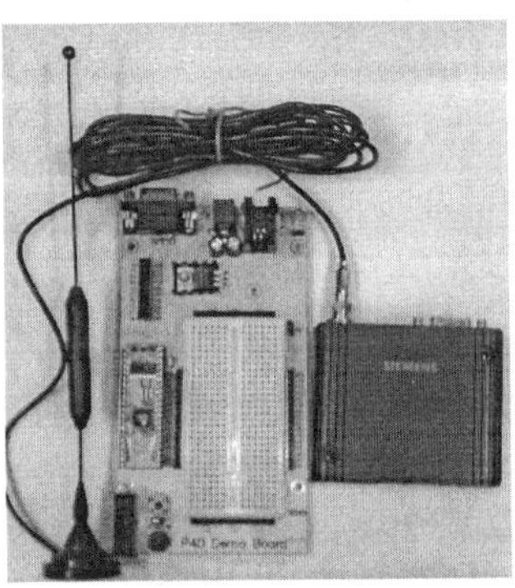

Figure 2 MCU with GSM modem

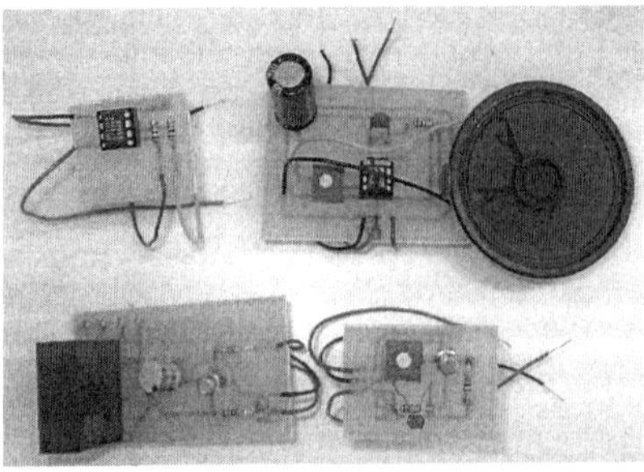

Figure 3 Some sensors and actuators

We choose this MCU as it is easy to program. All BasicStamp MCUs programs are written using the PBASIC code.

2.1 GSM Modem [2]

The GSM modem has the same function as a mobile phone and is commonly used in Communication Company. A SIM card is inserted into the modem to perform various functions. The GSM modem uses AT-command to perform various functions.
The GSM modem use in the project is the SIEMENS TC35 GSM Modem. At a basic level, it will interpret SMS messages, verifying the incoming password and controlling the output relays and sensors through the micro-controller. On the other hand, the micro-controller stored the user information of that particular message and sends an outgoing message back to the sender. In this way we achieve a two-way communication between the sender and the system itself.

2.2 Other Hardware

LCD: It is a parallel LCD with a 2-line by 16 characters for local message display.

- *Light Dependent Resistor*

We are using the light dependent resistor (LDR) to detect the brightness of the room or used for security detection.

- *Temperature Sensor*

The temperature sensor used is a digital sensor, DS1624.

- *Motion Sensor (PIR)*

A PIR (passive infra-red) sensor from Nicera and a custom-made surface mount movement detector IC for intruder detection.

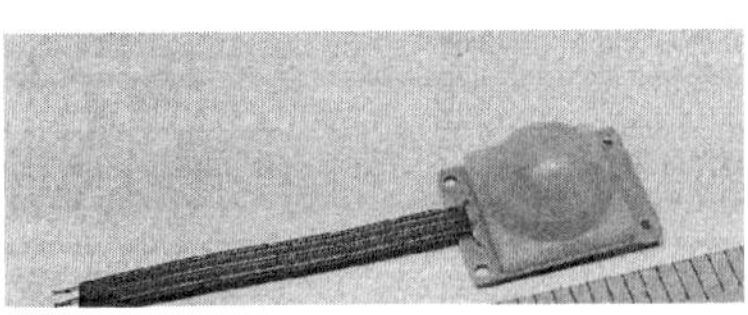

Figure 4 Motion Sensor

3. Software Design

3.1 SMS Format [3]

The Short Message Service features confirmation of message delivery. This means that unlike paging, users do not simply send a short message and trust and hope that it gets delivered. Instead the sender of the short message can receive a return message back notifying them whether the short message has been delivered or not. The default factory parameter of this acknowledge from the transmitter of a SMS to the receiver of a message by most GSM modem is OFF, so that you will get no confirmation from the receiver. If you turn it on, then you get an conformation that the SMSC has got the message and after the delivery of the short message to the receiver you will get an additional, second message (SMS backward) that the message is delivered to the a GSM phone or modem. In this automatic generated message is the data and time of the delivery coded. The acknowledge, coding scheme the time of storage of a short message in the SMSC and a lot of more will be set with the command **AT+CSMP**.

A other way is to send a prefix with the text message. This prefixes are not equal by the different GSM operators in the world. By the German GSM operator Vodafone you have to add *N# and by the GSM operator T-Mobil you have to add *T#. The notation with AT+CSMP is equal in all SMSC. The handling with the prefix *T# or *N# was or is necessary if you would like to get an acknowledgement by the send of a SMS with a mobile GSM handset. Not all mobile phones can switch on the bit for an acknowledgement.

If you would like to understand the 3 parameters of this command, you have to understand the SMS in PDU mode. Another important command is AT+CNMI. It tells the GSM modem how to handle an incoming short message.

The SMS message, as specified by the ETSI organization (documents GSM 03.40 and GSM 03.38), can be up to 160 characters long, where each character is 7 bits according to the *7-bit default alphabet*. Eight-bit messages (max 140 characters) are usually not viewable by the phones as text messages; instead they are used for data in e.g. smart messaging (images and ringing tones) and OTA provisioning of WAP settings. 16-bit messages (max 70 characters) are used for Unicode (UCS2) text messages, viewable by most phones. A 16-bit text message of class 0 will on some phones appear as a Flash SMS (blinking SMS or alert SMS).

There are two ways of sending and receiving SMS messages: by text mode and by PDU (protocol description unit) mode. The text mode (unavailable on some phones) is just an encoding of the bit stream represented by the PDU mode. Alphabets may differ and there are several encoding alternatives when displaying an SMS message. The most common options are "PCCP437", "PCDN", "8859-1", "IRA" and "GSM". These are all set by the at-command AT+CSCS, when you read the message in a computer application. If you read the message on your phone, the phone will choose a proper encoding. An application capable of reading incoming SMS messages can thus use text mode or PDU mode. If text mode is used, the application is bound to (or limited by) the set of preset encoding options. In some cases, that's just not good enough. If PDU mode is used, any encoding can be implemented.

Using either test mode or Protocol Description Unit (PDU), one can send or receive SMS messages through GSM modem. In our system, text mode is chosen as it is much simpler to work with. When the GSM modem receives an incoming message, it will first check the

message's contents. If it contains the correct password, the microcontroller will extract other parts of the message.
If the message is not beginning with the correct password, then an invalid message will be send back to the sender.

3.2 SMS Handling

The following two instructions set the GSM modem to "text mode".

List 1 Modem setting

```
SEROUT 10, 18447, ["AT+CMGF=1", CR]
 //  'set text mode pin2 to A10
SERIN 11, 18447, [WAIT("OK")]
 //  'wait for text mode ok reply (pin3 to A11)
```

Following commands are to read the SMS message:

List 2 Reading SMS message

```
SEROUT 11, 18447, ["AT+CMGR=",DEC i , CR]
   // 'read message memory locations
SERIN 10,18447,1000, start1 ,[WAIT ("+CMGR:"),
WAIT("UNREAD"), WAIT(","), SKIP 4, STR
MessageAddress\8\0]
```

Whenever there is an incoming message, the modem will inform the BasicStamp MCU by interrupt to view the message. Upon viewing the message, the BasicStamp MCU could decide whether the message is a command with password or just a normal message. If the message is a command with password, it will thus activate the different applications.

We assign the message codes for the different applications as follows:

- *Relay A – zona, zoffa*
- *Relay B – zonb, zoffb*
- *Both Relays – zon all, zoff all*
- *Check status – zstatus*

After every task is fulfilled, the controller will send a confirmation message back to the sender. If the message is a request for checking field status, the controller will get all the data of ambient temperature, both relays' and light's status and send them to the requesting party.

List 3 Sending local status

```
SEROUT  10, 18447, ["AT+CMGS=", 34,"+65", STR
MessageAddress\8, 34,CR]
// 'send msg command
SEROUT 10, 18447, ["Successful", 26]
   "'Temp=", DEC DAT," Degree Celsius ","
R1=",DEC ko," R2=",DEC ko2 ," LDR=",DEC LDR,
PAUSE 100
SERIN 11, 18447, [WAIT ("+CMGS:"),
```

List 4 Analog data capturing

```
//   'fetches temperature result.  Value returned in
T_HI and T_LO
    GOSUB START
    I2COUT 8,$90,[$AA]
    GOSUB START        'read
    O_BYTE= $91
    GOSUB OUT_BYTE
    GOSUB NACK
    GOSUB IN_BYTE      'fetch the two byte reading
    GOSUB ACK          'acknowledge each byte
    T.BYTE1 = I_BYTE   'high byte
    GOSUB IN_BYTE
    GOSUB ACK
    T.BYTE0 = I_BYTE
    GOSUB SSTOP
    RETURN
```

However if the message is not of the above, the BasicStamp MCU will send an "invalid password" message back to the sender. It is noted that the GSM modem does not store the sender information, therefore, the microcontroller has to store the sender's information such as the cell-phone numbers. By doing so, we have successfully achieve a 2-way communication between the system and the sender.

After every task is fulfilled, the controller will send a confirmation message back to the sender. If the message is a request for checking field status, the controller will get all the data of ambient temperature, both relays' and light's status or any other inputs such as bio-signals like ECG, and send them to the requesting party.

3.3 Local hardware control

The MCU has connected to a few buttons, LCD, sensors, keypad and Modem. User can set the receiver's mobile phone no. using the keypad, and use the buttons for local I/O control. The LCD normally displays the status of the various devices such as relays, LDR and the temperature in the room.

4. Conclusion

SMS based system for remote control and monitoring is a new technical approach. The whole system has been tested working very well. It is portable, economic, reliable and flexible. The system can be extended easily to have many inputs and outputs, either digital or analogue.

References

[1] Pbasic MCU datasheet, www.parallax.com
[2] Siemens TC35 GSM modem datasheet.
[3] PDU format of SMS, http://www.gsm-modem.de/sms-pdu-mode.html

Chapter 3

Context Awareness and Activity Monitoring

Toward a Human-Friendly Assistive Environment
D. Zhang and M. Mokhtari (Eds.)
IOS Press, 2004

Moving Telematics from the Laboratory to a Truly Enabling Technology within the Community

Anthony P. GLASCOCK, Ph.D. and David M. KUTZIK, Ph.D.
Department of Culture and Communication.
Drexel University
Philadelphia, PA 19104
USA

Abstract. The intent of all care for the frail elderly and persons with chronic diseases, whether provided formally by professionals or informally by family members, is the delivery of the appropriate intervention, by the appropriate person, at the appropriate time. To achieve this goal, a clear and accurate knowledge of a person's performance of functional tasks in her/his home environment is absolutely necessary. It is vital to know on a daily basis if a frail older person is getting out of bed, preparing breakfast, using the bathroom, taking her/his medication and performing other fundamental tasks necessary for independent living. To this end, a behavioral monitoring technology has been developed and tested in the residences of volunteers in both New York City and Philadelphia. An analysis of data collected during this test indicates that the monitoring system is highly reliable and that the information that results is highly valid.

Introduction

As part of research conducted in Ireland during the late 1980's, the senior author interviewed over 200 individuals during which the question, "have you ever helped or provided care for an older person?" was asked. If the respondent answered yes, the follow-up was, "please explain in what way". Sean, a man in his forties responded yes, he looked after an older man named Paddy and when asked how, Sean replied, "well, every morning I look across the valley to Paddy's house to see if there is smoke coming from his chimney." When asked for details, Sean continued, "you know, if there is smoke coming from Paddy's chimney by seven thirty I know that he is up, making his tea and about his business; if there isn't, I walk across to his house to see if he is himself". This answer gained increased significance in the early 1990's when both authors were faced with caring for an increasingly frail parent. It became clear that there was a need for a technological equivalent of smoke from Paddy's chimney, a technological solution that could work over distances much greater than the valley that separated Paddy's house from Sean's, but one that retained the features that made the smoke so attractive--non-obtrusive, simple and inexpensive.

Thus, the smoke metaphor became the guiding principle from which the current monitoring system emerged. From the start, the key was the usability and acceptability of the system by both the individual being monitored and by the caregiver; it had to be easy to install and use, and it could not be threatening. If a system required people to change their behavior, or it required major modification of their residence or if they were fearful that the system was "big brother", it would not be accepted and widely used. From this belief came the eight principle comprising the overall design philosophy: 1) the design should be based on the needs o individuals, not on the existence of a technology; 2) it should use existing technology, nothin new should be invented, but instead off-the-shelf components used; 3) it should be invisible t the person being monitored; 4) its use should require no change in the normal behavior of th monitored individual, it should be passive rather than active; 5) the installation should require n retrofitting to the residence; 6) it should monitor objects in the environment, not the individual 7) it should be software driven so that monitored activities could be easily added and removed a the needs of the individual changed; and 8) it should be cost-effective, similar to the cost of cabl TV.

1. What to Monitor

However, even with these design principles in place, the question of which activities t monitor remained and it took almost a decade to answer this seemingly simple question. Ove fifty formal caregivers--geriatricians, case managers, geriatric nurses, hospital discharg planners, managers of assisted living and congregate housing facilities and geriatric socia workers were interviewed and over 200 individuals were surveyed, at national and internationa meetings, as to what activities should be monitored. Their responses, in rank order, were: 1 medication adherence; 2) stove use; 3) eating; 4) overnight toileting; 5) wake up time; 6) genera up-and-around; 7) bedtime and overnight sleep disturbance; and 8) bathtub use. The inclusion o some of these activities is obvious, but others require some explanation. Bathtub use is really check on bathtub overflow, and up-and-around, although not a "specific task oriented behavior' was seen by many caregivers as a proxy for a person undertaking normal if somewhat non specific activities. There were different "number one" activities to monitor depending on th profession of the respondents. Geriatricians ranked overnight toileting as the most importan activity, hospital discharge planners ranked up-and-around as number one, case managers ranke medication adherence as most important, while managers of assisted living and congregat housing facilities ranked bathtub overflow at the top.

Given these findings, it was apparent to us that any monitoring system had to be able t monitor these eight task oriented behaviors. In addition, the analysis of the responses indicate that any effective monitoring system had to be structured in such a way that monitored activitie could be easily added and/or subtracted depending on the needs of individual clients, the contex in which the system was installed, and changes in the needs of the client over time. Monitorin bathtub overflow might be essential in an assisted living facility, but not necessarily in a on story single-family dwelling. In other words, a cost effective system had to be able to "switc on" and "switch off" activities easily and quickly.

2. System Development

A fully functional scale model that monitored five activities and recorded the events on remote computer terminal was in place by early 1993. This work culminated in the filing for patent in the fall of 1994 that was granted in November of 1997.[1] In early 1995 the first full operational system was taken from the laboratory and placed in a "residence", an activity of dail living suite at a major medical center outside of Philadelphia: a one bedroom apartment with full kitchen, bedroom, living/dining area and bathroom. Elderly patients spent the night in th uite in order to be assessed as to their ability to function independently. The monitoring system, long with a video camera, was installed in the suite to record activity during the overnight stays. n addition, all patients were interviewed prior to and after they spent the night in the room. The nstallation of the video camera and the interviews allowed for a systematic cross-validation of he monitored behavior.

Two findings emerged: first, do not place sensors near heating and air conditioning vents; nd second, less is often more. Initially, every appliance—microwave, dishwasher, stove, elevision—and every cabinet and drawer in the kitchen was monitored. Also, multiple motion letectors were placed throughout the living/dining room, bedroom, bathroom and kitchen. The esult of this was that much of the data proved to be redundant and that the large amount of data ctually confused the "caregiver"/researcher and concealed important patterns. Consequently, ensors were turned off in a systematic way until it was able to accurately "observe" the task riented behavior with the use of the smallest number of sensors.

The next phase of development was limited sequential home testing which lasted almost wo years and involved the installation of monitoring systems, one at a time, into the homes of lderly or chronically ill individuals[2]. The installations ranged from one to three months and luring this period, participants were interviewed on a regular basis to determine the validity of he recorded activities and the acceptability of the system. Perhaps the most important finding of his stage of research was how quickly participants accepted the system and "forgot" that it was resent. Participants stated that after two to three days the system became invisible and they did ot think about it until we visited. Finally, a website to which the data collected could be sent, utomatically translated into information and displayed in an appropriate manner for a specific aregiving environment was developed, resulting in VirtuCare™[3].

3. Technological Description

The culmination of this development was the Everyday Living Monitoring System ELMS) that presently consists of two main components: 1) the residential system consisting of notion detectors and a base station; and 2) a website that provides for processing of the sensor lata converting them to behavioral information displayed with graphics and text for caregivers.

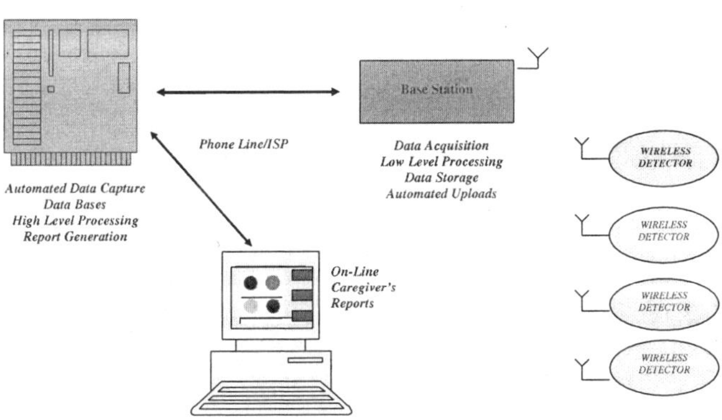

Figure 1: System Diagram

3.1 Residential system

The wireless motion detectors are Xanboo units. that combines a passive infrared motion detector with a 420 MHz wireless transmitter capable of reliably sending programmable unit identification code for up to 120 feet to the base station. The base station unit collects and transmits sensor data to the remote monitoring site through the Internet. The base station presently used are comprised of a wireless Xanboo compatible receiver, a microprocessor and flash memory, for data storage, low level processing and Internet upload control, plus a burst modem. The unit is approximately 10 x 6 x 3 inches and is connected to the phone line through a RJ-11 jack and plugged into a standard AC receptacle. The base station firmware is designed to record and time stamp all incoming sensor signals, store them in memory, format them to an XML file and upload periodically to the web server via a burst modem at programmable time intervals. To minimize the effects of power and/or phone line failure, the base stations are designed to archive days or even weeks of data and to automatically reboot and upload when power and phone lines are restored.

3.2 Web-based remote monitoring site

The web-based remote monitoring site consists of a PIN secured server designed to receive behavioral data from the base units and translate them into information. The server currently used is made up of: the web-based front end for the caregiver and administrators; the SQL based relational database management system; the automated scripts; and the Java based collector software. The server operating system is a Red Hat Linux installation running on Intel hardware.

Once in the server, the raw data are translated into information through the application of specific algorithms that take the individual data points corresponding to sensor events and create composite variables representing specific human activities. Both status and trend analysis rules are used by the server. Status rules analyze sensor events collected during the same day to infer if a particular human event has occurred. For example, signals from the bathroom motion detector are examined for their time stamp and compared with data from the other motion detectors to determine if a person may have fallen. Trend analysis rules, on the other hand, search for change in the state of the present day's activity in relation to expected frequencies and timings of activities based on a continuous baseline analysis.

The information that results from the application of these two rules is further distilled to provide easily interpretable and timely advice to the caregiver. Thus, the web site's PHP pages transform the information on each activity into icons and clear narrative statements that relay the most important trends as simply as possible. Current day information is automatically compared to previously collected activity data in order to determine changes in activity. Green indicators are displayed when the data show no significant deviation in the frequency and/or timing of data for a given activity; yellow status indicators are displayed when the frequency and timing of a given activity is higher or lower than expected; and red status indicators are displayed when a still higher threshold of deviation is recorded.

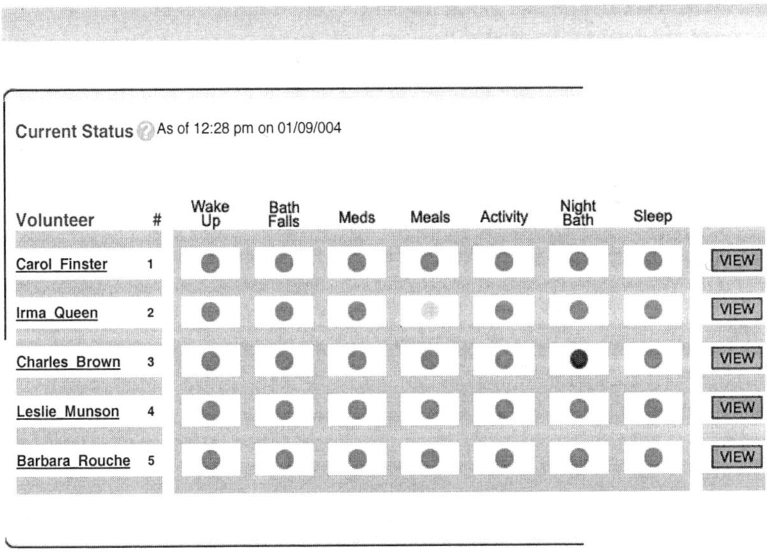

Figure 2. Web shot of Activity Summary Data

4. Field Tests

To test the usability and acceptability of the ELMS, two field tests have been undertaken in: 1) a high-rise, independent living senior building of one and two bedroom apartments in New York City; and 2) independent households in and around Philadelphia. A special secure website was established for each of the settings that allowed professional staff members and caregivers access to the information on the volunteers on a 24/7 basis. The web pages provided a daily summary for each of the volunteers for six activities: waking time; bathroom falls; the taking of medication; meal preparation, overall level of activity; and nighttime bathroom use, and ambient temperature. The volunteers were interviewed prior to the installation of the monitoring system to obtain information on demographic background, health status, self assessed functionality, and formal and informal care. In addition, each volunteer was asked to sketch a "typical" day's routine. Repeat interviews were undertaken approximately every six weeks to update health and functional status and to obtain the views of the volunteers on the system.

The characteristics of the volunteers from the two field sites are basically the same. The average age of the volunteers at the high-rise, independent living senior building in New York City is 79 and for those living in and around Philadelphia 77. Both groups are predominantly female (77%); African American (67%); and economically depressed (all but two individuals living in subsidized housing). The most important difference between individuals in the two groups is in level of impairment: the volunteers in Philadelphia are much more impaired than those in New York and as a result, 75% of the volunteers in Philadelphia are home-bound, whereas only 20% of the volunteers in New York are home-bound. The ELMS has been installed in the New York City residences since October 2003, while it has been in the residences of the Philadelphia area volunteers since March 2004.

5. Reliability and Validity

Results from the field tests indicate that ELMS is extremely reliable, produces vali information and is accepted by both the volunteers and their caregivers. This is crucial becaus without a high level of reliability and validity, the system will not meet the needs of the clien nor the expectations of the caregiver. A large number of "false positives", i.e., indications that a individual did not wake-up, will result in needless worry, disturbing phone calls or even th notification of emergency personnel. Just as damaging are "false negatives", i.e., the lack of th recording of an increase in overnight bathroom use, which could indicate a change in healt status that needs to be addressed. Consequently, one of the main purposes of the field tests wa to determine the overall reliability of the system and validity of the information produced.

5.1 Reliability

Although the main objective of the field tests was to assess the reliability of the dat generated by ELMS, at the same time, the reliability of the information collected through th interviews of the volunteers is also of concern. For example, if the information collected durin the interview on the number of days and amount of time a home health aide is in the residence i unreliable; the interpretation of daily activity may be invalid, causing caregivers to misinterpre activity level. Overall this information is highly reliable, by our estimate well over 95% However, there are challenges associated with the continued reliability of this information Perhaps the biggest challenge is how to update information on medication, given the frequenc of changes in the number and type of medication the frail elderly and chronically ill individual are prescribed. But, methods to update changes in other activities need to be developed as well, i the reliability of the information is to remain high.

In order to conclude that ELMS itself operated reliably for a single event the followin had to occur: 1) the detector successfully triggered; 2) the signal received by the base station; 3 the data recorded and time stamped; 4) the data uploaded to the website; and 4) the informatio depicted in the proper format. That is, that the color shown on the chart (see Figure 2) was th result of the system operating reliably. An example of an error is a red showing on the chart fo "Bath Fall" when no fall occurred. In this instance something went wrong with the system: eithe the bathroom sensor recorded the participant's entry into the bathroom, but not her exit; or th signal did not reach the receiver; or the signal was not uploaded to the website. To date, ther have been over 10,000 such "events" and the overall reliability of the monitoring system i slightly over 98%.

A second even more rigorous test of reliability was employed in which every recorde "event" for each day was examined to determine if there were inconsistencies, that is, if an even was recorded, e.g., medication taken, when the detailed activity chart indicated that there was n activity in the residence. If the crosscheck showed such a contradiction, an error in the reliabilit of ELMS occurred. This examination resulted in more than 38,000 data points being cros checked and a reliability level of slightly less than 98%.

An attempt was made to determine the cause for the errors found in both of the tests of ·liability. The most frequent reasons in the first test, accounting for 80% of the errors, was: 1) ulty sensor placement e.g., placing a motion detector within the refrigerator to register each me the refrigerator door was opened and closed did not work well resulting in intermittent gnals being received; and 2) human tampering, e.g., a volunteer removing a motion detector om the wall because she did not think that it was working. The most common cause of errors in e second test of reliability was the appearance of activity, specifically meal preparation, when general activity was recorded. This was the result of the way general activity is timed and ploaded to the website, and an adjustment to the algorithm appears to have corrected this berration.

2 Validity

In contrast to the determination of reliability, it is more difficult to present a precise level validity of the information produced. This is because of the nature of validity itself and the troduction of human interpretation into the calculations. In the context of our test, validity is garded as the truthfulness of the information produced by the monitoring system, that is, that e system truly measures the selected activities. The system may be highly reliable, but the formation is only valid if it can be correctly interpreted; that a red actually means that omething is wrong.

To aid in our analysis, we have divided validity into two components: machine validity nd caregiver validity. Machine validity is a combination of the system's reliability and the alidity of the interpretive algorithms that determine the patterns of behavior of the participants nd continuously look for change in the patterns. Thus, the colors displayed on the event chart e entirely the result of the monitoring system's hardware and software functioning properly. It reasonable to argue that underlying this functioning is a set of assumptions about the selected ctivities, e.g., the opening and closing of the refrigerator is a valid "proxy" measure for meal eparation, but once these assumptions have been programmed into the system, it is relatively asy to determine the level of machine validity.

This level is 95%. Since, as stated above, the system's reliability is a determinant of achine validity, it is, by logic, impossible for machine validity to be greater than the systems liability (98%), the remaining errors must be the result of problems with the algorithms used to roduce the color indicators. All but a tiny number of these errors are "threshold errors", e.g., the olor indicator showing red for meal preparation because of a decline in "events" from 22 the eceding day to 14. The algorithm that calculates the running average is placing too much eight on the 22 events and not enough on the overall pattern, thus resulting in the threshold for d to be crossed when it should not have been. This is a machine validity error; one, however, at can be easily corrected by an adjustment in the appropriate algorithm.

Caregiver validity is not as easily calculated and yet, it is the reason for the entire onitoring system to be developed. People, who are making decisions based upon the "advice" at the system produces, must have confidence that what they see is valid, or they will not take ction. If a caregiver is not completely confident that a red truly means that an action must be ken, the system has little utility. An extensive study of caregiver validity that examines the tual use that caregivers make of the monitoring system is presently underway and although nly preliminary findings are available, these results do suggest the way that the monitoring ystem will be used in actual caregiving environments.

6. The Pyramid

The challenge associated with the introduction of any new caregiving practice, let alon one dependent on the use of an innovative technology, is how to engage practitioners to use i And, even if practitioners are willing to try to use it, an equally daunting challenge is t incorporate the new technology into existing caregiving models without having the caregiver' fear of being replaced by a machine or unease associated with technology or dread of appearin dim-witted defeat the attempt before it even begins. To meet this challenge it is essential th practitioners grasp the underlying structure of ELMS.

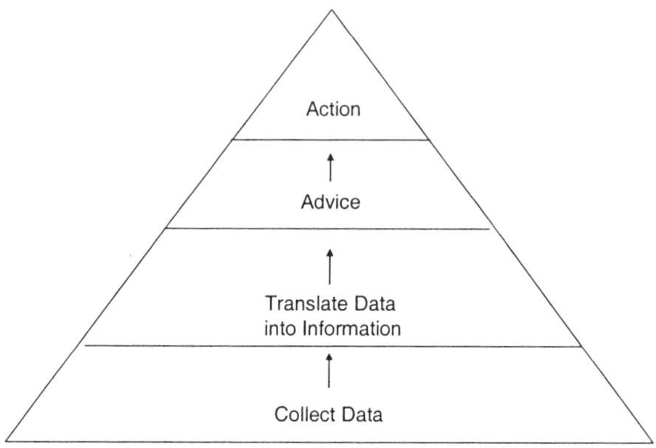

Figure 3. General Caregiving Model

The pyramid depicts a general caregiving model that begins, at level one, with th collection of data on a client. In the context of behavioral monitoring, these data would be abou functional tasks, e.g., overnight toileting, medication adherence. In existing caregiving models these data are usually collected by various forms of retrospective interviewing, perhap supplemented by pill counting or questioning a caregiver about the client's behavior. Th reliability of these data is always a concern because of timeliness and the accuracy of responses If the data are unreliable, the information that results, level two of the pyramid, will not be valid Validity entails the human interpretation of the data and, in a caregiving context, is usually th result of some protocol combined with experience. In other words, the data, whether reliable o not, are subject to interpretation that translates the data into information. An example of invali information is an alarm generated by a personal emergency response system indicating that ther is a fall when no fall has occurred. This is a false positive and is both expensive and dangerous given that frequent such false positives could result in the assumption that there is no emergenc and thus lack of response.

However, all information, in a caregiving context, is ultimately distilled into some forn of advice—level three on the pyramid. This advice may be quite specific, as illustrated in the fal example above, a client has fallen or more general, medication needs to be reviewed with th client because there are too many pills left at the end of the month. Whether general or specifi the advice leads directly to action, level four, by the caregiver—phone 911, speak to client abou medication adherence. The action is taken because the caregiver is confident in the advice, th advice is regarded as accurate because the information on which it is based is valid and the information is valid because the data are reliable. Thus, we have come full circle. If the data are not reliable, the base of the pyramid, the action taken by the caregiver may not be appropriate or the timing may be inappropriate or even the caregiver taking the action may not be the most appropriate person for the required action. Enter ELMS.

7. The Advantages of the Everyday Living Monitoring System

ELMS was designed to collect more reliable data and to more effectively and efficiently translate the data into valid information than existing caregiving models. If the ELMS can achieve these twin goals, the advice given will be more accurate and timely and the action taken by the caregiver more appropriate, thus providing better care, saving money and providing peace of mind to the client and her loved ones.

The field tests, reported upon above, have convincingly demonstrated that the system collects extremely reliable functional data (98% level of reliability) that compares favorably with data collected by any other caregiving model. In addition, the data are much more timely, being collected and analyzed continuously compared to the infrequent data gathering devices employed in other caregiving models. Moreover, the resulting information has an extremely high validity (95%) and an undeniable advantage over the information collected by any other caregiving model. The information generated by ELMS is continuously interpreted, both on a daily basis and through trend analysis, to pinpoint changes in behavior that could indicate a problem before it can become a crisis. The key, of course, is how this information is distilled into advice and then action taken by the caregiver. However, there is every indication that the action taken by the caregiver is more appropriate and more timely than actions taken without ELMS.

References

Kutzik, D. and Glascock, A.P. United States Patent #5,692,215- "System for Generating Periodic Reports, Generating Trend Analysis, and Intervention in Accordance with Trend Analysis from a Detection Subsystem for Monitoring Daily Living Activity." United States Patent Office, Washington, DC, November 25, 1997.

Kutzik, D. and Glascock, A.P. Canadian Patent #2,208,594 -"User Monitoring System" Canadian Patent and Intellectual Property Office, Ottawa-Hull, Canada, 2000.

Kutzik, D. and Glascock, A.P. United States Patent #6,108,685- "System for Generating Periodic Reports, Generating Trend Analysis, and Intervention in Accordance with Trend Analysis from a Detection Subsystem for Monitoring Daily Living Activity--2." United States Patent Office, Washington, DC, August 22, 2000.

Glascock, A.P. and Kutzik, D. "Behavioral Telemedicine: A New Approach to the Continuous Non-Obtrusive Monitoring of Activities of Daily Living." Telemedicine Journal 6(1), Spring, 2000, pp. 33-44.

Kutzik, D. and A.P. Glascock, "Monitoring Household Behaviors to Enhance Safety and Well-Being." In Gerotechnology: Research and Practice in Technology and Aging, edited by Sunkyo Kwon and David Burdick. New York, NY: Springer Publishing Company, In Press.

Towards a Common Context Model for Virtual Community Applications

J. Indulska[1], K. Henricksen[2], T. McFadden[2], and P. Mascaro[2]
[1] *School of Information Technology and Electrical Engineering, The University of Queensland*
Email: jaga@itee.uq.edu.au
[2] *Distributed Systems Technology Centre*
Email: {kmh,mcfadden,mascaro}@dstc.edu.au *

Abstract. Instrumentation of home appliances and devices with sensors and actuators enables the creation of smart, context-aware environments which can intelligently support users in a variety of tasks, including tasks that support independent living of the elderly. This paper describes how the complexity associated with designing and implementing context-aware applications can be reduced through both context reuse and programming methods that allow context evaluation to be decoupled from applications. The paper describes a family of applications for smart homes that fall into the category of virtual community applications for the elderly, and demonstrates that these applications can be supported by a common, evolvable set of context and preference models.

1 Introduction

Homes are equipped with a variety of appliances and devices, and can be further instrumented with sensors and actuators. This, coupled with a variety of wired and wireless communication technologies, creates a heterogeneous computing and communication infrastructure suitable for enabling the creation of context-aware home environments which can intelligently support users in a variety of tasks. This support may range from hiding heterogeneity of devices and communication technologies (e.g., by providing common and self-explanatory interfaces to entertainment units and appliances) to complex support for independent living of the elderly. The latter may not only include seamless control of sensors, actuators, appliances and other devices, but also a variety of context-aware applications supporting daily activities (and remote help with these activities from family members or the local community), health monitoring, and building of virtual communities [1, 2].

Due to the variety of user activities which should be intelligently supported by a smart home, and the heterogeneity of devices, communication technologies and interaction protocols between devices, most smart home applications require a rich set of context information in order to re-configure and self-adapt when the context or user preferences change. Such

*The work reported in this paper has been funded in part by the Co-operative Centre for Enterprise Distributed Systems Technology (DSTC) through the Australian Federal Government's CRC Programme (Department of Education, Science and Training).

context information may include information about device characteristics, device location, user location, and user activity.

Many challenges in designing smart home environments are akin to those faced when designing pervasive systems in general. Mobility of users, a variety of user activities, heterogeneous communication technologies and heterogeneous devices introduce similar requirements for context-awareness as those seen in other application domains of pervasive systems. Such systems require models for describing and evaluating context, adaptability methods which can be applied in response to context changes (or context-aware applications which can adjust their behaviour when notified about context changes), and appropriate middleware/infrastructure responsible for context gathering, management, evaluation and dissemination [3, 4].

It is commonly acknowledged that the design and implementation of context aware applications are difficult tasks, and that new approaches are required which can support developers of context-aware applications. Context-aware applications often need to evaluate similar context facts and, more often, contextual situations built from context facts. Therefore, techniques that allow reuse of situations have the potential to considerably simplify the development of new applications. It should also be noted that most of the current context-aware applications have context evaluation hardwired into the application logic, which implies that any changes in the context model or user preference model require re-programming of the applications. If context and preference evaluation logic can be separated from the applications it is possible to create evolvable applications which will work with modified types of context information or user preferences.

In this paper, we discuss applications for smart homes that fall into the category of virtual community applications, and demonstrate that these applications can be supported by a common, evolvable set of context and preference models. In defining the common models, we draw on our previously developed modelling techniques [5, 6], which are sufficiently rich to allow us to capture diverse types of context information, including imprecise, incomplete and ambiguous information, and to describe context-dependent user requirements and preferences. We demonstrate benefits that arise from context and preference reuse, which include reduced complexity associated with constructing new virtual community applications, reduced effort required for customisation and fine-tuning of applications, and more consistent behaviour across a user's set of applications.

The structure of the paper is as follows. Section 2 shows example virtual community applications and provides an informal description of the context information needed for such applications. This description provides insight into the potential for context reuse when building such applications. Section 3 introduces a formal common context model for the applications, while Section 4 presents a common preference model. Section 5 briefly describes how our infrastructure for context-aware computing allows evolution of the context and preference models without re-programming applications that rely on these models, and Section 6 concludes the paper.

2 Example virtual community applications

The virtual community applications that we consider have diverse goals, but are primarily concerned with providing support for independent living in communities of elderly people. They include applications that support:

- assistance for the elderly with everyday tasks by remote family or community members;
- dynamic formation of groups of people who are interested in activities such as shopping or playing chess, based on their preferences and availability; and
- awareness of the activities of others in nearby smart homes using abstract visual representations, helping to minimise isolation and provide assurances of others' well-being.

2.1 Selected applications

The following three example applications have been selected for discussion in this paper:

1. Instant communication with a family member, friend or health worker, achieved using context-aware choice of communication channel (telephone, SMS, e-mail, etc.) according to the current activity, devices (and their communication modes) and preferences of communicating persons.
2. Servicing of sensor-based alarms/events by family members, community members or health workers. Any event/alarm which requires external help (e.g., a burnt out light bulb or the elderly person lying on the floor) is evaluated based on the current context and policies/preferences to determine who should be informed. Context-aware communication (described above) is used to deliver information about the event.
3. Organisation of social activities (e.g., shopping, theatre, or a bridge game). When an elderly person wants to organise a social activity, context information is used to determine which people are preferred for the activity, and context-aware communication is used to contact them.

An informal characterisation of the context information required by these three applications is presented in the following subsection.

2.2 Required context information

The simplest of the three applications, application 1, requires context information about family members, health workers, and community members, including information about their activities, locations, and communication devices. Context information about devices should include modes of operation (types of communication channel) and location. The information about the elderly person's communication devices and the callee's activities and devices are the basic context facts used in this application. These basic facts must be supported by additional information about both the elderly person's and the callee's preferences for communication devices and communication modes.

Application 2 is more complex as it requires all of the context information used by application 1 (to support context-aware communication), as well as information about a variety of sensors available in the house, their types and states, and their positions within the house. Context facts (e.g., sensor states) can be used to define more complex contextual situations (expressions built from context facts). One example is an emergency health situation (e.g., person lying on the floor in the kitchen and not moving), which needs to be deduced from the states of several sensors. Such situations need to trigger some help actions, and therefore the set of preferences defined for application 1 also needs to be extended for application 2 to include preferences about recipients of alarms or notifications about particular situations.

Application 3 requires all of the context information defined for application 1, as well as additional information about people's hobbies and interests and preferred social groups.

2.3 *Other applications*

The next section presents a formal context model for the described three applications, discussing reuse of context facts and context situations in the applications. Due to space limitations we cannot formally show that this context model can be used for a much larger number of virtual community applications. However, even from the informal model described in the previous subsection, it can be clearly seen that further applications of this type can be based on the same context model (with some small extensions). Additional applications that we have considered include:

- An application providing cooking advice from a family member or health worker. This application may be triggered by the elderly person or the smart home (the latter in the case when a medical evaluation of the cognitive abilities of the elderly shows that the person needs help with particular activities in the kitchen). It is assumed that there is a video camera allowing the helping person to observe activities in the kitchen. When the application is triggered, a person able to help is found based on the current context, and context-aware communication is used to communicate the request.

- An application supporting a distributed activity (e.g., remote bridge game). The application uses context-awareness to adapt to location/device changes of the participants.

- Ambient communication which provides awareness of the activities of others. When some community members are involved in particular popular activities (e.g., walking a dog), others are informed using a mode of delivery (e.g., a visual representation on an "ambient community screen" or a scrolling message at the bottom of a TV) that is appropriate to the current context and the recipient's preferences.

3 Common context model

A common model of context fact types for applications 1-3 is presented in Figure 1. The notation used is discussed in [5], and is an extension of the Object Role Modeling (ORM) notation [7]. The context information has various origins and quality. It can be sensed from physical or logical (software) sensors, derived from other context information or defined by users. It is important that context models address the issue of context imperfection, incompleteness and ambiguity, as this allows developers to create robust and reliable context-aware applications that are able to deal with conflicting context information or temporary lack of sensor data. The presented model captures context facts (e.g., person using device, home contains room) of various types (static, profiled, derived, sensed), and also quality, histories and relationships of context information.

Based on the defined context facts, more complex situations can be described. Both facts and situations can be reused in other applications. Figure 2 shows some example situations from application 1 which are reused in applications 2 and 3. Figure 3 presents examples of

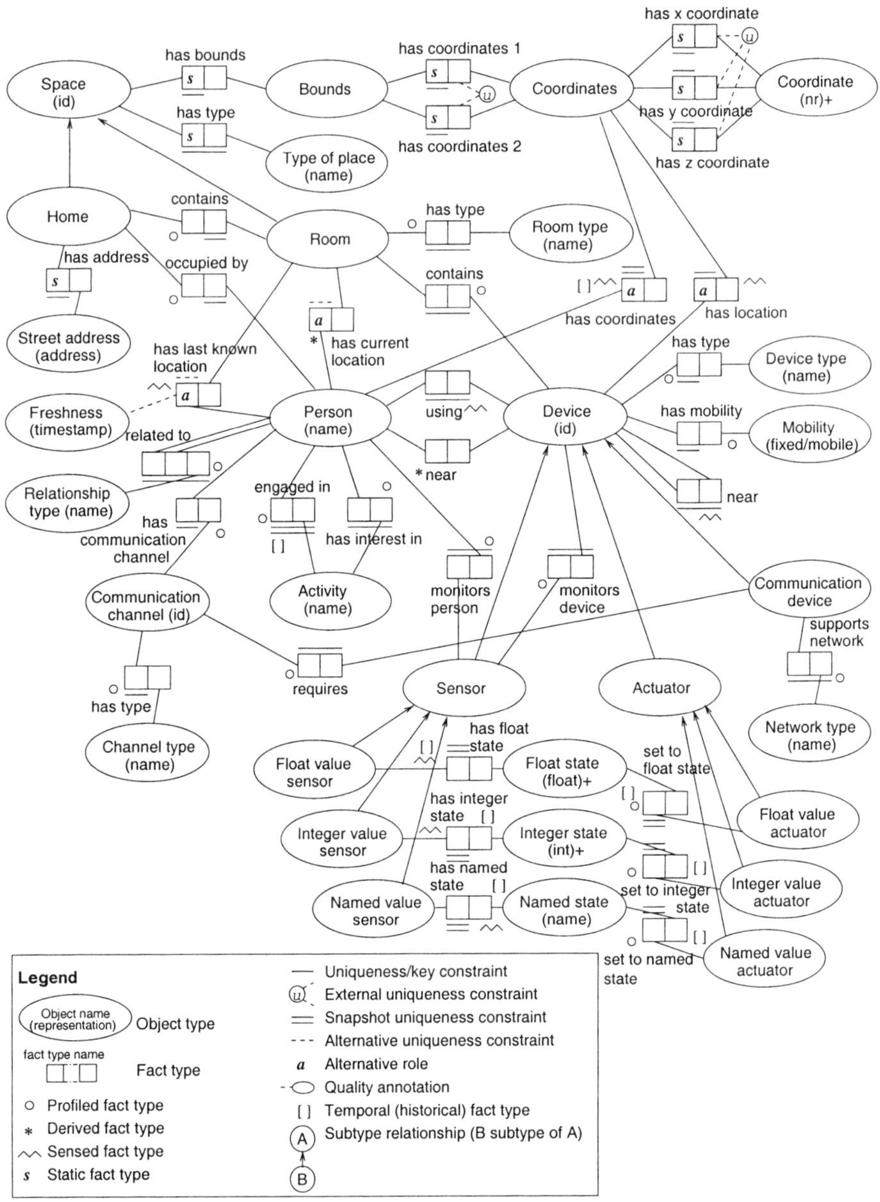

Figure 1: Common context model.

additional situations which are required for application 2. The examples are of two kinds: a situation which should trigger a home maintenance notification (when a light bulb is not working) and a situation which should trigger a health emergency alarm (person lying down

```
• IsChildOf(child, parent):
    PersonRelatedTo[child, parent, 'relation.son'] or
    PersonRelatedTo[child, parent, 'relation.daughter'] or
    PersonRelatedTo[parent, child, 'relation.mother'] or
    PersonRelatedTo[parent, child, 'relation.father']

• CanUseChannel(person, channel):
    forall device
        . CommunicationChannelRequires[channel, device]
        . PersonNear[person, device] and
          not exists sensor
              . SensorMonitorsDevice[sensor, device]
              . SensorHasType[sensor, 'device.status.busy']
                and SensorHasNamedState[sensor, 'device.status.busy.true']
```

Figure 2: Example situations for application 1.

```
• RoomLightBurnedOut(room):
    exists lightSwitch
        . RoomContainsDevice[room, lightSwitch]
        . DeviceHasType[lightSwitch, 'light.switch']
          and ActuatorSetToNamedState[lightSwitch,'light.on']
          and not DeviceHasSensedNamedState(lightSwitch, 'light.on')

• PersonHasFallen(person):
    PersonIsHorizontal(person) and not PersonMoving(person, 5) and
    exists coordinates
        . PersonHasCoordinates[person, coordinates]
        . exists space
              . SpaceHasBounds[space, bounds]
              . BoundsContainsCoordinates(bounds, coordinates) and
                not SpaceHasType[space, 'space.rest.position']
```

Figure 3: Example situations for application 2.

and not moving and not in a typical rest space). The situations `DeviceHasSensedNamedState` (used in the `RoomLightBurnedOut` situation), `PersonIsHorizontal` and `PersonMoving` (used in the `PersonHasFallen` situation) are omitted due to space limitations.

4 Common preference model

The goal of our preference model is to address a need for new techniques for capturing user requirements and preferences in a context-dependent fashion. The model is based on the situation abstraction and enables candidate choices (such as communication channels that can be used for interactions between users in the case of a communication application) to be rated according to their suitability for the current context. Figure 4 presents example preferences for the context-aware communication application, which forbid the use of communication channels when the required devices are not available, and assign higher precedence to telephone than email when the elderly person is contacting one of their children about a matter of high priority. Application 2 can reuse these preferences, but also requires preferences that describe how each type of event should be handled. Some examples are shown in Figure 5 for the `RoomLightBurnedOut` and `PersonHasFallen` situations. Application 3 requires ad-

```
• when not CanUseChannel(callee, channel) or
       not CanUseChannel(caller, channel)
  rate forbid

• when IsHigh(priority) and IsChildOf(callee, caller) and
       IsTelephone(channel)
  rate 1

• when IsHigh(priority) and IsChildOf(callee, caller) and
       IsEmail(channel) and AtWork(callee)
  rate 0.5
```

Figure 4: Example preferences for application 1.

```
• when RoomLightBurnedOut(room) and IsChildOf(contactPerson, occupant)
  rate 1

• when RoomLightBurnedOut(room) and IsNurseOf(contactPerson, occupant)
       and WorkingHours()
  rate 0.8

• when RoomLightBurnedOut(room) and IsNurseOf(contactPerson, occupant)
       and not WorkingHours()
  rate forbid

• when PersonHasFallen(room) and IsNextOfKinFor(contactPerson, occupant)
  rate oblige

• when PersonHasFallen(room) and IsDoctorFor(contactPerson, occupant)
  rate oblige
```

Figure 5: Example preferences for application 2.

ditional preferences about social groups and activities, but these are not shown here because of space limitations.

5 Support for context evolution

Context-aware applications have to be supported by an infrastructure able to gather, process, and evaluate context and preference information. This infrastructure must provide powerful context and preference query capabilities as well as notification mechanisms. We have developed an infrastructure for context-aware applications that meets these requirements, and allows modelling and evaluation of context facts (and their quality, ambiguity, history, and dependencies), situations and user preferences [5]. Context and preference information can be discovered and reused in newly created applications. This support for reuse simplifies the development of context-aware applications and allows for highly flexible behaviour.

Most of the current approaches to construction of context-aware applications assume that context evaluation constitutes a part of the application logic. Applications built in this way must be re-programmed for any changes in the context model (and/or preference model), which means that they cannot gracefully evolve as the context and/or preference model evolves.

The novel programming model supported by our software infrastructure [5] allows insertion of context- and preference-dependent decision points into the normal flow of application logic. These decision points are implemented as calls to an API which supports context-dependent choice amongst sets of alternatives (e.g., available communication channels). User preference information forms the link between the context and the chosen action(s). Preferences assign ratings to the alternatives according to the context and other application parameters, and, based on these ratings, the application selects and invokes one or more associated actions. This solution is very flexible and enables modification and fine-tuning of context and preferences when required (even at run-time).

6 Conclusions

This paper presented a common context and preference model designed for a family of context-aware, virtual community applications which can support elderly persons. Our modelling approaches allow us to capture a rich and diverse set of context information, including ambiguous and otherwise imperfect information. They also enable reuse of context facts, contextual situations built from facts, and user preferences. Moreover, our approach to programming context-aware applications separates the application from the underlying context and preference information, allowing the latter to be easily evolved over time to support changes in user requirements and environment resources (e.g., addition of new sensors) with minimal impact on the application.

The presented virtual community applications require a rich set of contextual information about a number of persons (the elderly, family members, friends, health workers and community members). Some of these types of context information naturally raise privacy concerns, and, to address these, we are currently developing extensions to our context modelling approach to incorporate ownership information and context-dependent privacy preferences (expressed using the preference model described in this paper).

References

[1] E.D. Mynatt, J. Rowan, S. Craighill, A. Jacobs, Digital family portraits: Providing peace of mind for extended family members, Proc. of the ACM Conference on Human Factors in Computing Systems (CHI 2001), Seattle, ACM Press, 333–340.

[2] M. E. Pollack, L. Brown, D. Colbry, C. E. McCarthy, C. Orosz, B. Peintner, S. Ramakrishnan, I. Tsamardinos, Autominder: An Intelligent Cognitive Orthotic System for People with Memory Impairment, Robotics and Autonomous Systems, **44**(3-4), (2003), 273–282.

[3] Anind K. Dey, Daniel Salber, Gregory D. Abowd, A Conceptual Framework and a Toolkit for Supporting the Rapid Prototyping of Context-Aware Applications, Human-Computer Interaction, **16**(2-4), (2001), 97–166.

[4] Guanling Chen, Ming Li, David Kotz, Design and Implementation of a Large-Scale Context Fusion Network, Proc. of the 1st International Conference on Mobile and Ubiquitous Systems: Networking and Services (Mobiquitous), Boston, (2004).

[5] K. Henricksen, J. Indulska, A Software Engineering Framework for Context-Aware Pervasive Computing, Proc. of the 2nd IEEE International Conference on Pervasive Computing and Communications (PerCom), Orlando, (2004), IEEE Computer Society, 77–86.

[6] K. Henricksen, J. Indulska, A. Rakotonirainy, Modeling Context Information in Pervasive Computing Systems, Proc. of the 1st International Conference on Pervasive Computing (Pervasive), F. Mattern, M. Naghsineh (eds). Lecture Notes in Computer Science, Springer Verlag, LNCS **2414**, (2002), 167–180.

[7] T. A. Halpin, Conceptual Schema and Relational Database Design, Prentice Hall, Sydney, 2nd edition, (1995).

Toward a Human-Friendly Assistive Environment
D. Zhang and M. Mokhtari (Eds.)
IOS Press, 2004

Monitoring Elderly People Using a Multisensor System

Marie CHAN*, Eric CAMPO*,**, Daniel ESTÈVE*
**LAAS-CNRS, 7 avenue du Colonel Roche, 31077 Toulouse cedex, France*
***ICARE-IUT Blagnac, 1 place Georges Brassens, 31703 Blagnac cedex, France*

Abstract. Within the framework of a monitoring project named PROSAFE, LAAS-CNRS has developed a multisensor system designed to monitor elderly living at home with as much safety as possible by diagnosing any abnormal event relative to previously recorded normal situations. The system consists of a number of motion sensors, a Personal Computer (PC) and a communication network linking sensors and the computer. A data acquisition and processing software is used to complete the system. The aim of this paper is to present the method used for detecting abnormal situations and the results obtained by using an unsupervised algorithm to process elderly trajectories. The trajectory classes obtained represent typical displacements of the elderly. Any situation deviations relative to such typical trajectories are viewed by the system as abnormal.

Introduction

Detecting things or people or keeping track of people usually require a video camera or the use of Global Positioning System (GPS), and even a mobile phone based on the degree of precision needed and the applications sought. In this field, LAAS-CNRS has been involved in the PROSAFE project and has developed a multisensor system designed to monitor the elderly. This system does not feature the common drawbacks of a video camera that necessitates large data storage systems while failing to respect intimacy, or a GPS and a wireless telephone that has to be worn by people. The multisensor system has been devised to help the elderly and disabled people living alone, to stay at home with as much safety as possible. It passively observes individuals moving and not necessarily wearing electronic devices in the house. It learns the person's activity patterns from those observations. Thus, the system typically performs such key operations as people detection, keeping track of people, activity classification and event detection. So far emphasis has been placed on detecting people in a room. To do so, current duration on a local site is compared with a statistical evaluation of previous stays on that same local site using the multisensor system [1]. In real time, in case of situation deviation relative to previously recorded normal situations, and also in case of emergency, or to avoid anything going wrong, the system warns formal or informal caregivers.

In this paper, a dynamic dimension has been added by including people moving in the house and we have focused on keeping track of people. It has been shown that the classification of the observed patient's motion allows activity patterns to be learnt. These patterns represent the usual movements of patients, and therefore, any movement deviation relative to previously memorized common behavioural patterns will prompt the system to warn caregivers. The method used is based on an unsupervised learning algorithm processing raw data collected by the multisensor system. Each class of trajectories has got characteristics in frequency, mean duration and mean distance.

1. Material and Methods

1.1 Multisensor System

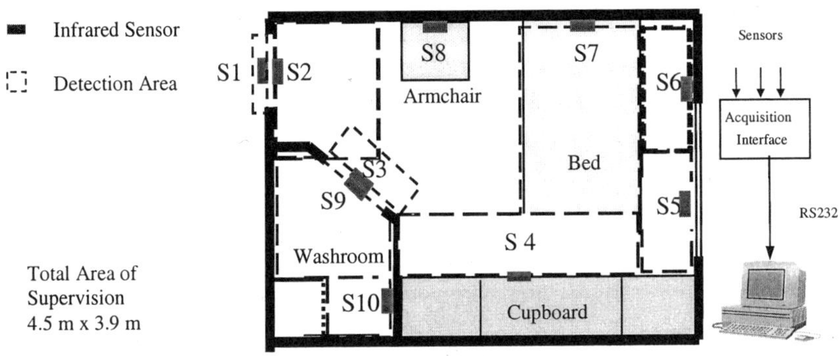

Figure 1. Multisensor system

An experimental multisensor system has been installed in a patient's housing (bedroom and washroom), its consists of a set of infrared motion sensors located on the ceiling of the elderly room in an institution, a communication linking the PC to the sensors in the wire version using an industrial type (RS485) bus, a digital to analog converter and a (RS232) serial link [2]. ADAM acquisition boards are equally used to complete the system allowing for data collection [3]. The PC hosts the data acquisition and processing software [4].

1.2 Subjects Involved in the Study

A number of persons decided to enrol in the study. The aim was to simulate trajectory classes in accordance with specific motion scenarios.

1.3 Data Acquisition Process

The system is used to observe the motion of a subject in the room divided into several zones as shown in Figure 1. When a subject moves in the room, several zones are crossed. One or several sensors are, therefore, becoming involved. In the latter case, the number of zones in the elderly room can be in excess of 10. Sensors are maintained live for 0.5 seconds and the acquisition period lasts 0.5 seconds. When a person stands still, no sensor is triggered. Raw data are in the form of a file including a set of data lines. Each line is composed of a set of 1 bits (0 or 1) according to the sensor status, time and date of the event. A raw data file exampl is created that reads as follows:

0010000100 07/09/2003 23 :43 :05.0
0010000000 07/09/2003 23 :43 :05.5
0000000010 07/09/2003 23 :43 :07.5
0000000000 07/09/2003 23 :43 :09.5
0000000001 07/09/2003 23 :43 :27.6
0000000000 07/09/2003 23 :43 :29.1
0000000001 07/09/2003 23 :44 :13.1
0000000010 07/09/2003 23 :44 :16.6
0010000000 07/09/2003 23 :44 :19.6
0011000000 07/09/2003 23 :44 :20.6
0010000000 07/09/2003 23 :44 :22.6
0000000000 07/09/2003 23 :44 :41.2
0000001000 07/09/2003 23 :44 :46.2
0000000000 07/09/2003 23 :44 :47.7
0000001000 07/09/2003 23 :45 :09.7

This file shows that the patient moves towards the bathroom, stays there for a while and the goes back to bed.

1.4 Trajectory Extraction

Each patient's trajectory in the room as shown in Figure 1 is a succession of sensors bein triggered or points (x, y, t). The room size is 4.5 m by 3.5 m. We transformed the room into plan with x and y coordinates, whose origin (0,0) is the bottom left corner of the room a shown in Figure 1. Each point in the trajectory consists of 3 coordinates, 2 coordinates in spac x and y and a time coordinate t. Looking back at the previous file, each data line can b referenced with a point in the plan x y previously defined. Where a single sensor is activated the point is the zone centre. When several sensors are triggered, the point is the barycentre o the different corresponding zones. Taking a time origin at 9 pm for example, the time t expressed in second, of each event is marked using this initial time. To extract a trajectory, parameters are chosen, the starting point, which is in one of the room's zones (Figure 1), an the length or the trajectory's number of point. In this study for each trajectory, two consecutiv points always have got different time and space coordinates.

1.5 Motion Scenarios

A volunteer has simulated a set of trajectories including eight separate classes. Simulation ha been based on the study according to [5], dealing with the travel behaviour of nursing hom residents perceived as wanderer and nonwanderers and demonstrating that the trajectories ca include pacing, direct, lapping and random travel patterns. Each trajectory class i characterized by the trajectory start and end or by the trajectory form. The characteristics of th eight classes simulated by the volunteer are shown in Table 1. Each class consists of about 3 different trajectories. The total number of trajectories is 240, with duration of approximatel one minute, and with a number of variable points according to the volunteer's moving speed for each trajectory.

Table 1. The eight simulated trajectory classes

Class	Characteristics	Sensors most often triggered
a	Bed-window	S7, S6, S5
b	Lapping	S7, S8, S3, S4, S5, S6
c	Pacing	S7, S8, S3, S4, S5, S6
d	Zigzagging	All sensors
e	Bed-armchair	S7, S8, S3
f	Bed-bathroom	S7, S8, S3, S9, S10, S4
g	Bed-cupboard	S7, S8, S3, S4 or S6, S5, S4
h	Bed-exit	S7, S8, S2, S1 or S3

1.6 Unsupervised Classification Method

In previous study, we detected abnormal events based on the person standing still in a local position [1]. A history of the patient standing still was recorded during a reference period. For each local position, a summary of the time spent was given. A duration threshold was defined for each local position, and an excess time was defined to trigger an alarm. To account for changes in mobility habits, duration thresholds were periodically readjusted for alarm triggering purposes. However, we want our diagnosis to be based on the notion of trajectory and not on local position detection only. In this study, a new dimension is provided through the use of people indoor moving trajectories. Thus, the way the patient moves in the room and the trajectory created are considered, the aim being to keep track of a person in the room. The diagnosis method is based on:

- The learning of normal situations through classes of elderly repetitive indoor trajectories,
- The diagnosis of abnormal situation based on comparison between real time current situations and previously recorded normal learning database.

In this study, we have focused on the normal situation learning database. An unsupervised method based on the "k-mean" method has allowed obtaining distinct classes of trajectories [6], each class of trajectories has been characterized by a typical trajectory. The method used is composed of several steps:

- Initialization, choice of a high number of prototypes or typical trajectories,
- Computation of a distance value between the presented trajectory tp and each prototype trajectory, determination of the nearest typical trajectory and update of the typical trajectory using the following formula:
  $n = n + pas * (tp - n)$
- All k iterations, till the minimum desired number of typical trajectories is obtained, and deletion of a typical trajectory,
- When the minimum desired number of typical trajectories has been reached, the worst 20 % individuals in each class are deleted.

At each iteration, the sum of distances between each trajectory and its typical trajectory is computed and the process is discontinued when the sum obtained is fairly low relative to the previously computed value. With this algorithm, classes of trajectories are discarded if they have got few representatives of their class (standing too far). Thus, the consistency of each class can be enhanced, by removing marginal elements. Also, the least interesting typica trajectories are deleted to obtain the desired number of typical trajectories. Classes that hav been left out are selected in accordance with two criteria. Classes that look too much alike ar first deleted, from a certain number of iterations, and classes with limited number o representatives are equally discarded. In the first case, all pairs of possible typical trajectorie that look too much alike are checked. Then one of the two is discarded. In the second case, w check whether a typical trajectory must be discarded if at least one of the classes comprise fewer individuals than a minimum number. If this is the case, the class with fewer individual is deleted; in the opposite case we are back to the first case and a redundant typical trajectory i deleted. To initialize the process, a large number of typical trajectories are used. They mus look sufficiently like the trajectories observed so that right from the start all classes ar allocated a certain number of individuals. The following notation is used, x_i, y_i, t_i and x'_i, y'_i, t' respectively stand for the coordinates of both trajectories, and the measurement of the distanc separating them is as follows:

$$D(tr_1,tr_2)=\min_{\substack{0<j<N/3\\0<k<N/3}} \sum_{i=1}^{i<2N/3} (x_{i+j}-x'_{i+k})^2+(y_{i+j}-y'_{i+k})^2+(y_{i+j}-y'_{i+k})^2+(\log t_{i+j}-\log t'_{i+k})^2$$

Not only does this measurement introduce the notion of distance but also that of time by usin the decimal logarithm of time or duration of each point, the latter being measured in second, it value is high relative to the distance in meter. The use of a decimal logarithm leads to a smalle distance-duration ratio.

2. Results

Using the trajectory length that varies from 4, 5, 6, 7, 8, 9, 10, to 12 points, the unsupervise classification method has been used to test the database of simulated trajectories. The bes results are obtained with trajectories including more than four points and less than nine points With the unsupervised classification method we have got the simulated classes. We discarde those short trajectories made up of two or three points. These can be looked at as agitation i bed or in other zones already reported [4]. We present the results obtained for five poin trajectories in Figure 2, where A is the starting point of the trajectory and B the end of it. I this study a preliminary extraction of trajectories including a precise zone (zones 10, 5 or 2) i carried out using the unsupervised method. For trajectories with five points, a classificatio leading to five classes is sought, plus three so-called extra classes including specific point (zones 10, 5 or 2). The number of trajectories or frequency, mean distance and duration for th classes obtained are shown in Table 2. For all trajectories with 5 points, classes exhibit number of trajectories between 58 and 15, a mean distance between 3.54 m and 0.94 m, and mean duration between 3.8 s and 72.06 s. The three classes including a specific poin (bathroom, window in zone 5 or exit) have been retrieved. The longest mean duratio corresponds to the class of trajectories including a point of the bathroom. The different classe correspond to the characteristics of the simulated trajectories. They correspond to classe simulated by volunteers as shown in Table 1. Trajectories through the window of zone 6 are i class 1. Class 2 includes trajectories starting in zone 3, toward zone 4 and ending in zone 8 Class 3, 4, and 5 include trajectories located mainly on the left in the room. The last three

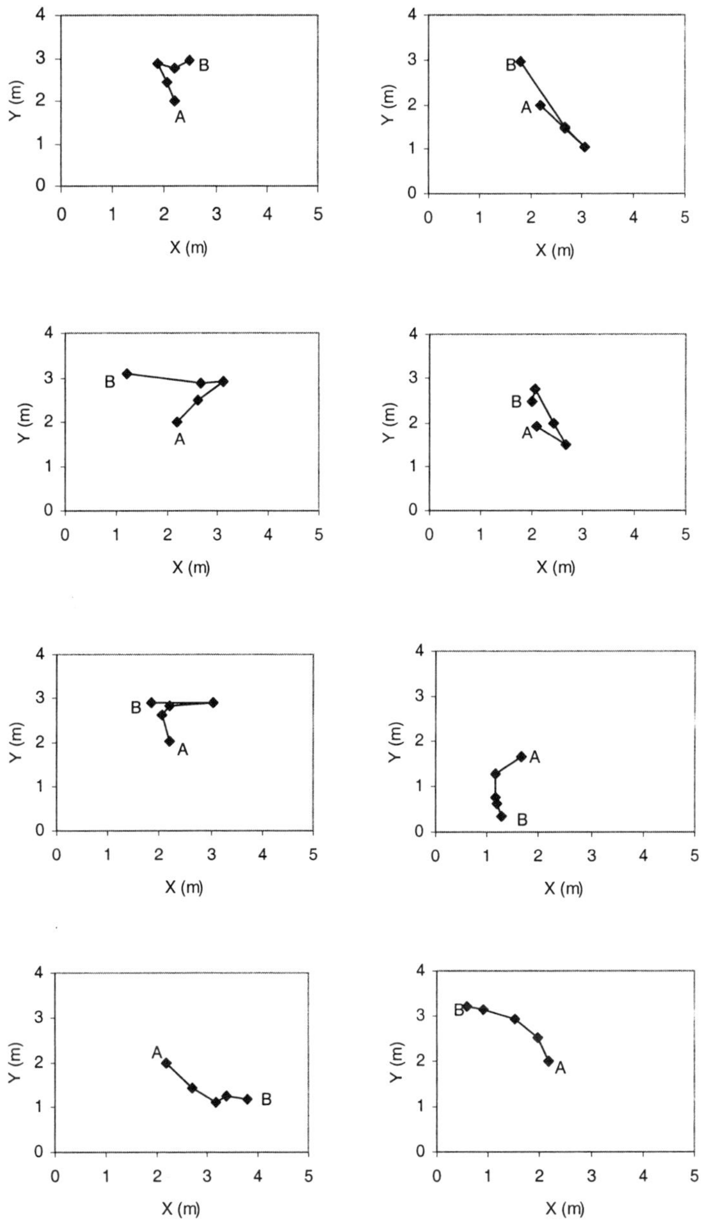

Figure 2. Results of unsupervised classification
A: start of trajectory
B: end of trajectory

classes originate from preliminary extracted trajectories including specific points in the bathroom, zone 5 or zone 2.

Table 2. Unsupervised classification results

Class	1	2	3	4	5	6	7	8
Number of trajectories	58	44	15	24	20	15	23	20
Mean distance in m	1.63	3.54	3.17	2.41	2.91	0.94	1.2	1.58
Mean duration in s	4.1	4.42	4.29	3.34	7.7	72.06	3.8	6.6

Discussion

The unsupervised classification method has been used to retrieve the simulated trajectory classes. Certain classes have been fully retrieved while others only partially. The results reflect the characteristics of the simulated database. Classes most easily retrieved feature homogeneous items in the class as shown in the examples of the last three classes, the one starting from zone 3 to exit the room, this being the most direct, just like for the trajectory class that involves the bathroom and those including a point of the cupboard zone 4. It was found that with the longest trajectories, classes are more easily retrieved but short trajectories (i.e., the bed to window) are not found and cannot be separated from the longest trajectories. It is not possible to classify different length trajectories with this unsupervised method. In addition it has been found that with classes 2, 3, 4, and 5 most trajectories aim at a point located in the left hand part of the room. Unsupervised classification calls for the user to specify the number of final classes desired. This problem will influence the results. Indeed, the user must have an idea of the approximate number of underlying classes in the database. Also, the data must be consistent, as zigzagging class includes trajectories from and to the bed, and the results obtained only reflect part of the trajectories of this class. The last three classes of Figure 2 are the most representatives of the corresponding simulated classes. For this method it is necessary to have consistent items and an adequate number of prototypes for each class.

Prospects

In this study we have reviewed the results of a trajectory classification based on an unsupervised method. The aim is to use repetitive classes for real time trajectory deviation detection purposes versus previously recorded situations considered as normal. The different aspects of the multidisciplinary PROSAFE project are being developed. We are putting the emphasis on the following points:

1. Trajectory extraction depending on the sensor system used.
2. Enriching the trajectory database through simulation.
3. Improving the results by initializing the classification process.
4. Using other unsupervised classification methods.
5. Using other methods: bayesian, probabilistic, for classification.

6. Setting up the real time alarm diagnostic module in the event of an abnormal situation.
7. Setting up an outdoor trajectory detection system to supplement the indoor trajectory detection system.

Acknowledgements

The authors gratefully acknowledge the support of the French MENRT through grants allotted to the project and Hospital of Muret for the experimental site and their helpful support.

References

[1] Chan, M., Campo, E. and Estève, D. (2003). PROSAFE, a multisensor remote monitoring system for the elderly or the handicapped. 1st International Conference On Smart homes and health Telematics (ICOST'2003), Paris France, 24-26 September: *Independent Living for Persons with Disabilities and Elderly People* (edited by Mounir Moktari), pp. 89-95. Amsterdam: IOS Press.

[2] Chan, M., Bocquet, H., Campo, E., Val, T. and Pous, J. (1999). Alarm communication network to help carers of the elderly for safety purposes: a survey of a project. *International Journal of Rehabilitation Research*, **22**(2), 131-136.

[3] Advantech, Total solution for PC-based industrial automation, *Solution Guide*: 61: 7.2-7.7 and 8.1-8.8.

[4] Chan, M., Campo, E., Laval, E. and Estève, D. (2002). Validation of a remote monitoring system for the elderly: Application to mobility measurements. *Technology and Health Care*, **10**, 391-399.

[5] Martino-Saltzman, D., Blasch, B.B., Morris, R.D. and Wynn McNeal, L. (1991). Travel Behavior of nursing home residents perceived as wanderers and nonwanderers. *The Gerontologist,* **31**(5), 666-672.

[6] Diday, E., Lemaire, J. and Testu, F. (1983). *Eléments d'analyse de données*, Dunod, Paris.

Toward a Human-Friendly Assistive Environment
D. Zhang and M. Mokhtari (Eds.)
IOS Press, 2004

Empowering the User to Build Smart Home Applications

Tao ZHANG, Bernd BRÜGGE
Technische Universität München
Institut für Informatik/ I1, Boltzmannstraße 3
85748 Garching b. München, Germany

Abstract. *Recent research has shown that end-user programming will form an important part of any general purpose context-aware computing system, since the system behavior of existing context-aware systems does not reflect the situation the end-user intended. This paper is concerned with end-user programming and modification of context-aware application behavior. We present a three-tier approach to build context-aware applications, which separates context collection and distribution from rule-based inference that controls application behavior. Prototypes were created to evaluate our approach. The primary focus was directed towards the rule conflict management and user interface issue, that are related to defining rules. We conclude this paper with a short usability case study based on these prototypes and an outlook into future work.*

1. Introduction

Beginning with Mark Weiser's [17] vision of *ubiquitous computing*, new technologies like *tangible interfaces*, *wearable computing*, *mobile computing* elevate the style of interaction beyond the traditional desktop environment and are becoming important in the everyday life. The foremost objective in building context-aware applications is to create a sensor rich environment that responds specifically to people, place and time. The user is not tied to one particular device but interacts with a network of intelligent devices embedded in the environment.

To develop a context-aware application, developers currently have two options: Either they build a system that hypothesizes system behavior using an inference engine [11,15], or they predefine a specific system behavior [2]. Recent research has shown that both of these approaches have not proven long term compatibility with the end-users' expectations [7].

- The system behavior cannot be predicted by an inference engine, since there are many human or social aspects of context that cannot be sensed or even inferred by sensors or devices available today [1]. There is no ascertained way for a system to infer a correct contextual state just by collecting sensor information. At best, the system can provide an approximation or an educated guess of the real context.

- The behavior of the context-aware system and its applications cannot be recognized and hardcoded by the developer, since it is very difficult for the developer to foresee what information and sensors are necessary to infer a contextual state. Moreover he cannot foretell whether the results produced by the system are meaningful to the end-users [7].

Currently, a variety of systems have been built, that are hardcoded [2]. The behavior of these systems has become a routine matter of recognizing states and triggering corresponding activities. While this approach can work in situations with well-defined social expectations (e.g. turning off a mobile phone in a theater), it fails for situations in which end-users' behavior is less predictable (e.g. at home). People feel like they are loosing control of the system and begin to fight the system, because the system view of context does not match what was actually happening.

We believe that the only way a system can agree with the users' expectations is to have the user program the system behavior. To accomplish this, we would like to empower users to build own applications in a most simple way.

This paper is concerned with end-user programming and modification of context-aware environments, where an end-user is referred to as a person who has had experiences with handheld devices like mobile phones or PDAs, but cannot program in JAVA or C++. We present an architecture composed of three separate but interrelated layers – a context layer for capturing and handling physical sensors, a rule layer providing high-level behavior specifications, and an user interface layer providing user interfaces supporting end-user control and modification.

2. Related work

Most context-aware research has focused on building infrastructures to support developers in building applications and on the applications themselves [2], not enough emphasis has been placed on empowering end-users to build their own context-aware applications.

Humble et al [8] presented the development of a user-oriented framework to support the user reconfiguration of ubiquitous domestic environments. They present a lightweight component model that allows users to interconnect a range of devices easily. The framework discovers available ubiquitous components and presents these to users as jigsaw pieces that can be dynamically recombined. However, the emphasis is on reconfiguration rather then programming and the approach does not seek the richness of programming expression. *iCAP* [16] is focused on helping developers rapidly prototype, test, and iterate their context-aware applications. It is based on previous work in ubiquitous computing applications, specifically those that involve the development of rule based conditions. Some of these include AgentSheets [14] and Stick-e notes [12].

In his most recent work, Dey presented a new prototype environment called *a CAPpella* [3] for end-users. In this environment, tools are available to end-users in order to demonstrate and change the system behavior without any programming skills. However, to build simple applications, end-users must first learn how *a CAPpella* works and then spend time extracting information from the sensor data manually. After that, an inference engine teaches a model based on annotated logs. For the system to work predictably users have to refine the system behavior many times. Both scenarios introduced in his paper (meeting scenario and medicine taking scenario) [3], discovered that the average users have to still spend a lot of time and effort to achieve an often very limited benefit.

3. A three-tier Architecture

This paper is concerned with end-user programming and modification of context-aware application behavior using a rule-based approach. We present a three-tier approach to building context-aware applications, which separates context collection, distribution from rule-based inference that controls application behavior [18]. While the software developers are primarily responsible for the context layer and rule layer, end-users use a graphical user interface to modify and control the overall system behavior.

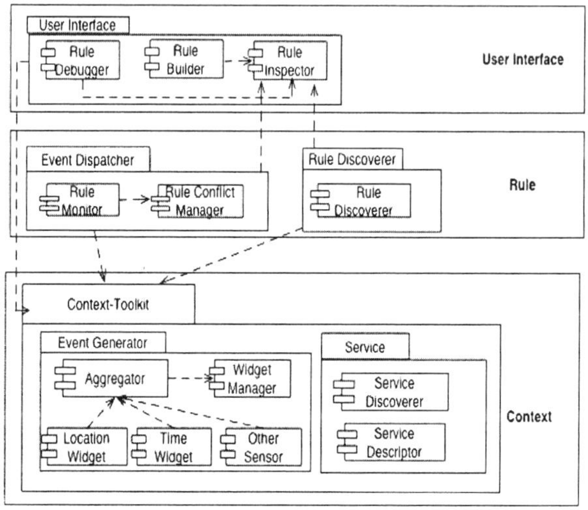

Figure 1: Three-tier architecture for context-aware systems

In the architecture shown in *figure 1*, we select the context-toolkit, a framework developed by Dey [2], which separates the acquisition and representation of context from the delivery and reaction to sensor context by a context-aware application, as our low-level communication infrastructure.

The system behavior is specified through an ECA Rule Specification Language. Each rule is composed of an **E**vent part, a **C**ondition part, and an **A**ction part. The ECA concept is based on past research in active databases, where application developers specify with the help of a powerful ECA Rule Specification Language sophisticated conditions over events, supplied by diverse event sources and associate to them actions [13]. In the past, ECA rules were applied to conventional databases, which can only carry out actions concerning database operations. A smart home may not only use this resource database in the ECA rule definition but can also trigger home services.

Depending on incoming *Sensor Events* from the *Context Layer,* the *Rule Monitor* evaluates initially all the ECA-rules which *Event parts* that match the actual situation. These selected rules may conflict with each other if the *Event parts* of more than one rule are matched concurrently or if the services to be executed are exclusive. The *Rule Monitor* delegates those conflicting rules to a component called *Rule Conflict Manager,* which solves the rule conflicts before calling the corresponding *Services* of the *Context Layer. Rule Discoverer* is a software component that discovers user behavior patterns using the *frequent pattern discovery [9].* For example, if the user did the same action several times in a same situation, the system will remember it by observing the actions of the user and automatically generate new rules. Since it is quite challenging to provide good rules by just collecting sensor information, users are still expected to refine the rules by removing noise information from sensors.

Using handheld computers like PDAs, end-users are then allowed to define high-level ECA rules. With these rules, the end-users can "program" different personal context-aware applications without special programming skills. They can not only read the rules, but also modify them, delete them, make each of them active or inactive *(Rule Builder & Rule Inspector).* Using this model, each end-user is now able to personalize the rules to suit his needs and notions for how the environment should react to his actions. Rules that are effectively executed are listed in chronological order. In case the user has difficulties to understand the system behavior, the user is able to track any executed rules in the past and figure out its rationale, he can then eventually undo, redo some actions, or overwrite some rules *(Rule Debugger).*

4. Scenarios

Our first scenario deals with a remote antenna station for a high-power transceiver at a remote location like the top of a mountain, the middle of the desert or an oil rig. Exceptional situations such as transistor fail or temperature fail are automatically detected by sensors embedded in the environment. The antenna station is connected with a maintenance and installation information system, which gives the technician context-aware help, depending on the exceptional situation and the skill level of the technician. When an exceptional situation occurs and the technician is not on site, he is informed immediately and can monitor the situation in the antenna station with his UMTS mobile phone. A rule for this scenario can be defined as follows:

Scenario:	*Remote Maintenance*
Event part:	*When LED transistor fail OR temperature fail,*
Condition part:	*(and) the technician is NOT in the antenna station,*
	(and) the skill level of the technician is very low,
Action part:	*(then) turn on the video recorder to capture the whole exceptional situation,*
	(and) send the captured Video clip to the technician's UMTS mobile Phone,
	(and) send the SMS " Please exchange transistor, and align quiescent current"

Our approach can also be used in a smart home to assist the elderly and individuals with disabilities. Users can specify personal activities they would like the house to automate (temperature control, control of hard-to-reach devices, etc.). For a grandmother sitting in a RFID-tagged [10] wheelchair, who usually has her breakfast between 7am and 8 am, the following rule could be defined by her caretaker or discovered by the system:

Scenario:	Having Breakfast
Event part:	*When the wheelchair with RFID-tag is detected in the kitchen,*
Condition part:	*(and) it is the first time between 7 am and 8 am,*
Action part:	*(then) turn on the kitchen light,*
	(and) turn on the kitchen coffee maker,
	(and) displays the morning news on the kitchen video screen.

5. *Status*

To evaluate our approach, different prototypes have been realized such as the component of the rule tier responsible for rule conflict management, as well as the user interface responsible for defining rules.

5.1 Using JESS for the Rule Layer

We have implemented the *Rule Monitor* and *Rule Conflict Manager* using JESS [5] – a rule-based expert system written in Java.

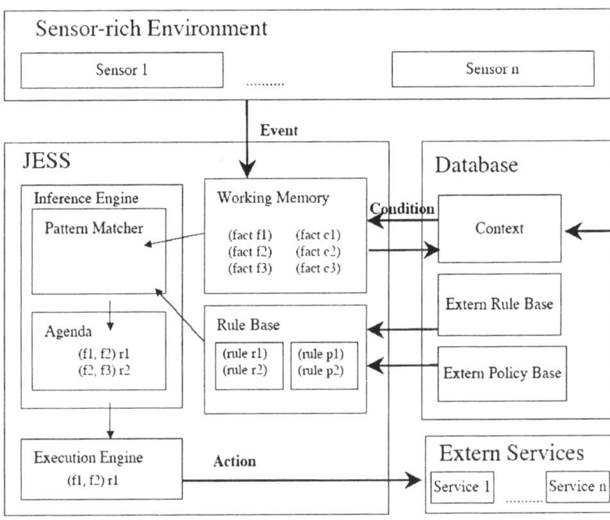

Figure 2: Using JESS for the Rule Layer

End-user defined rules and policies are stored in a relational database (mySQL) and will be uploaded into the JESS internal rule base at runtime. Depending on the incoming events captured by sensors and context (e.g. state of system component), the facts in the JESS *Working Memory* will be updated. *Pattern Matcher* then searches automatically through vast amounts of combinations of facts to find those combinations that satisfy rules to figure out which rules should be fired, while *Agenda* is responsible for using the conflict strategy to decide which of the rules, out of all those that apply, have the highest priority and should be fired first. This approach is suitable for our task, since the built-in inference engine implements the *RETE* algorithm [4], a very efficient mechanism to solve the difficult many-to-many matching problem. The *Execution Engine* component fires the rules. It calls the external services, which eventually change the context (see figure 2).

The advantages of JESS are the following: (1) JESS consists of a rule specification language that can be used to define ECA rules. (2) JESS works well with the context-toolkit, since both are implemented in Java. (3) Low-level rule conflict resolution strategies are by default integrated in JESS. While the end-users define the priority of the rules, JESS is responsible for triggering rules in the right order at runtime.

5.2 *User Interface Prototypes for defining personal rules*

The JESS syntax is not easy to understand. Therefore, prototypes of the *Rule Builder* and the *Rule Inspector* were implemented to evaluate different user interface concepts for defining rules.

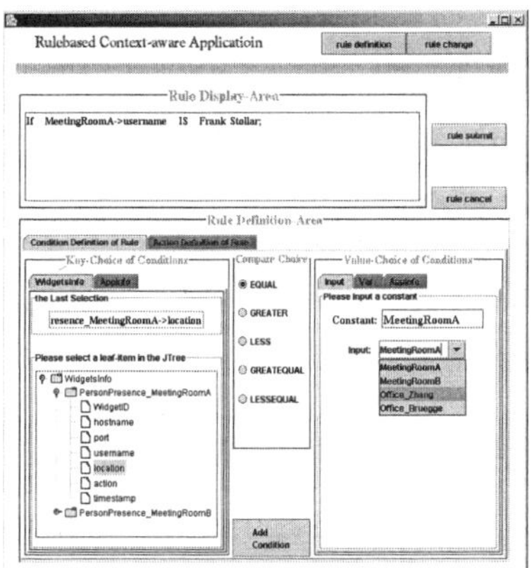

Figure 3: Rule Builder (version 1)

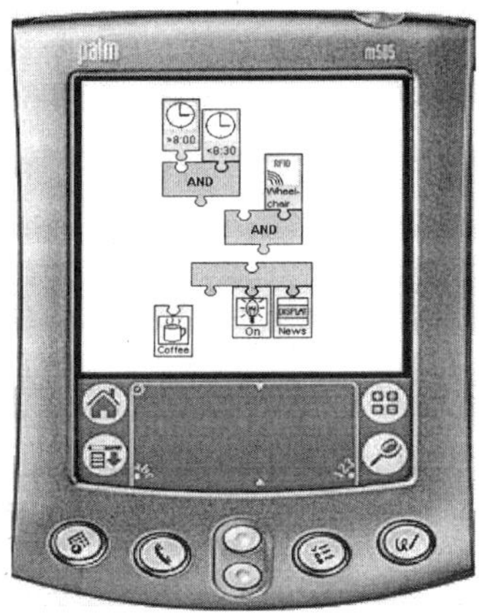

Figure 4: Rule Builder (version 2)

The first prototype *(figure 3)* provided a graphical representation of the JESS concept of rules. The second prototype was based on exemplar-based approach using puzzle-like pieces *(figure 4)*. In this approach, end-users simply copy and refine existing rules - either predefined by the developers, or partly recommended by the *Rule Discoverer (see 3)*. Since the behavior pattern is highly individual, end-users are expected to modify the system behavior by adding or removing conditions and actions with the drag and drop feature.

6. Evaluation and next steps

We evaluated our prototypes in a laboratory-based intelligent environment with two *smart boards, Java iButtons, PDAs* as well as Bluetooth-enable mobile phones.

We have built context-aware applications as follows: *Just after the user enters his office in the morning, his personal emails will be showed automatically on the smart board, at the same time, the music program iTunes starts playing his favorite classic music. As soon as the user get unexpected visit, emails will disappear immediately and the music turns automatically down.*

The first graphical user interface prototype has been tested during winter semester 2003/04. Ten computer science students were asked to build their own applications using the *Rule Builder* (Version 1). Most of the students commented, that user control over the environment increases by using personal rules, because they can change the system behavior in run mode. Nevertheless, only three students were ready to spend time for building rules from scratch as the first user interface prototype is still too complicated to use. The second user interface prototype is now implemented and has been currently tested by fifteen computer science students. To define the same rules, students using the second prototype need about 75% less time, require substantially less help and make fewer mistakes than those using the first prototype. Therefore we believe an exemplar-based user interface can significantly improve the usability. In order to find out if non-computer scientists are capable of precisely specifying personal ECA rules, we plan to do more evaluation work with non-computer scientists in the future.

7. References

1. Bellotti, V. & Edwards, K, Intelligibility and Accountability: Human Considerations in Context Aware Systems. Human-Computer Interaction, 16. 2001
2. Dey, A.K. et al. A conceptual framework and a toolkit for supporting the rapid prototyping of context-aware applications. HCI Journal 16(2-4), 2001, 97-166.
3. Dey, A.K. et al. a CAPpella: Programming by Demonstration of Context-Aware Applications, CHI 2004
4. Forgy C.L. "Rete: A Fast Algorithm for the Many Pattern/ Many Object Pattern Match Problem", Artificial Intelligence 19, pp. 17-37, 1982
5. Friedman-hill, E., Jess in Action - Rule-based Systems in Java, Manning Publications Co., 2003.
6. Gajos, K. et al. End user empowerment in human centered pervasive computing. Proc. Pervasive 2002, 134-140.
7. Greenberg, S. Context as a dynamic construct. Human-Computer Interaction, 16, 2001
8. Humble, J, et al, "Playing with the Bits" User-configuration of Ubiquitous Domestic Environments, Ubicomp 2003.
9. Hand D.J, et al, Principles of Data Mining, The MIT Press, 2001
10. LARAN RFID, A Basic Introduction To RFID Technology and its Use in the Supply Chain, White Paper, 2004
11. Mozer, M.C. The neural network house: An environment that adapts to its inhabitants. Proc. AAAI Spring Symposium on Intelligent Environments 1988, 110-114.
12. Pascoe, J. ''The Stick-e Note Architecture: Extending the Interface Beyond the User.'' In Proceedings of Intelligent User Interfaces, pp. 261-264. 1997.
13. Paton N.W. and Díaz O. "Active Databases Survey", ACM Computing Surveys, Vol. 31 No.1, pp. 63-103, March 1999
14. Repenning, A. ''Creating User Interfaces with Agentsheets.'' In Proceedings of Symposium on Applied Computing, pp. 190-196. 1991.
15. Schmidt, A. and Van Laerhoven, K. How to build smart appliances. IEEE Personal Communications 8(4), 2001, 66-71.
16. Sohn, T. and Dey, A.K. iCAP: An Informal Tool for Interactive Prototyping of Context-Aware Applications. Extended Abstracts of CHI 2003, 974-5.
17. Weiser, M., Some computer science issues in ubiquitous computing, Communications of the ACM, 1993.
18. Zhang, T., An Architecture for Building Customizable Context-Aware Applications by End-Users, Pervasive 2004 Doctoral colloquium.

Segment extraction using wavelet multiresolution analysis for human activities and fall incidents monitoring system

Myo Naing Nyan, Francis E.H. Tay and K. H. W. Seah
Department of Mechanical Engineering
National University of Singapore

Abstract. Segments related to fall incidents and daily activities from continuous accelerometer record were extracted using wavelet multiresolution analysis. The acceleration signal from a vertical accelerometer is sufficient for segment extraction. Segments were extracted from different reconstructed details or approximated levels by using different mother wavelets. It can be shown that wavelet multilevel decomposition and reconstruction is a useful technique to extract the signal patterns of fall incidents and daily activities.
Keywords: Segment extraction, wavelet multiresolution analysis, fall incidents, daily activities.

1. Introduction

Singapore has one of the fastest aging populations in the world, with an anticipated increase in the proportion of older persons above 65 years of age from 7.3% in 1999 to 18.9% in the year 2030 [1]. Moreover, the aging of the population and the related increase in the burden of chronic diseases have already had a major impact on most western health care systems [2]. The burden of falls is likely to increase with the growing proportion of older persons who will be spending significant portions of their daily routines either alone or with an equally elderly and frail spouse. Locally, Ministry of Health data shows that injury arising from trauma was the commonest cause of death in Singapore in the year 2000. While it is clear that falls are important cause of serious injury in the elderly, it is important to remember that falls also result in a fear of falling, loss of confidence, and restriction of mobility and independence, which may be either self-imposed or imposed by care-givers. The ability to monitor a person's posture and movement may help to both identify persons at risk of falls and guide interventions to reduce risk of falls for individuals who have been identified to be at risk. Detection or identification of human activities in daily life is important not only for safety but also for monitoring people living under free-living conditions. This surveillance can also be the detection of major incidents such as a fall, or a long period of inactivity in their daily environment.

Moreover, the assessment of posture and motion is an essential issue in ambulatory monitoring because physiological responses, such as changes in heart rate or blood pressure, may result from changes in body position and physical activity [3]. Estimation of the momentary metabolic rate (energy expenditure), rehabilitation treatment, kinematic analysis of body movement are other criteria for the assessment of daily physical activity. There are mainly two types of motion detection in previous research work, home-based visual or position sensors analysis [4-7] and body-fixed sensors detection [3], [8-11]. The visual instruments may not be suitable in a private space for a privacy reason. Moreover, such kind of indoor monitoring devices are essentially fixed at a single location. If the subject is to venture beyond the designed sensor range, as in the case of wandering patients suffering from dementia, the effectiveness of the sensors will be compromised. Therefore, body-fixed devices are more feasible in free-living environment. In the past, ambulatory assessment was based on various motion sensors such as pedometers, actometers and accelerometers at various locations as waist, wrist, thigh and lower leg. Using two or more different sites of evaluation is burdensome for the elderly in long-term monitoring because of cable connection. In our detection system, in view of the emerging emphasis on better and more comfortable activity monitoring system for the elderly, inertial sensors (accelerometers and angular rate sensor) are attached on a garment to get a wearable system. Patterns related to fall incidents and activities from inertial sensors are extracted and classified in our detection method. Unlike EEG, ECG signal classification or speech recognition, constant time window cannot be applied within selected time duration of the signal for feature extraction in our classification process. Moreover, segment lengths are varying even for same type of activities. The performance of the system in classification greatly depends on the accuracy of length of the extracted segment. Therefore, in our activity identification process, extraction of segments related to activities from a continuous accelerometer record is one of the key issues. This paper will contribute to segment extraction from the accelerometer outputs based on the wavelet multi-resolution analysis for human activities monitoring system.

2. Methods

2.1 Experimental Design

In the experimental set-up, ADXL105 (Analog Devices) single axis accelerometers were arranged in medio-lateral and vertical at sternum position and in medio-lateral and antero-posterior at shoulder position. For antero-posterior information at sternum and vertical information at shoulder, MMA1220D (Motorola) low G micromachined accelerometers were used. Even though two sets of accelerometers were distributed at sternum and shoulder, only the set at sternum was used in this study. Yaw rate sensor (ADXRS150, ±150°/sec) was attached at the waist level to get the sagittal plane information of the body Fig. 1. The amplifier gain of sensors was set to give the sensitivity of 250mV/g and approximately 3mV/deg/sec. Gyroscope was placed at the inner surface of the garment. Bluetooth™ facilitated wireless communications from the shirt to PC for signal processing. The transmitter 90 x 50 x 20 mm, 200 g and DC power supply were placed inside the pocket. The receiving part was connected to the serial port and power was supplied from the USB port. In this way, signals were digitized at 256-Hz sampling rate and recorded by a PC.

2.2 Wavelet multiresolution analysis

The wavelet transform is a tool that cuts up data or functions or operators into different frequency components, and then studies each component with a resolution matched to its

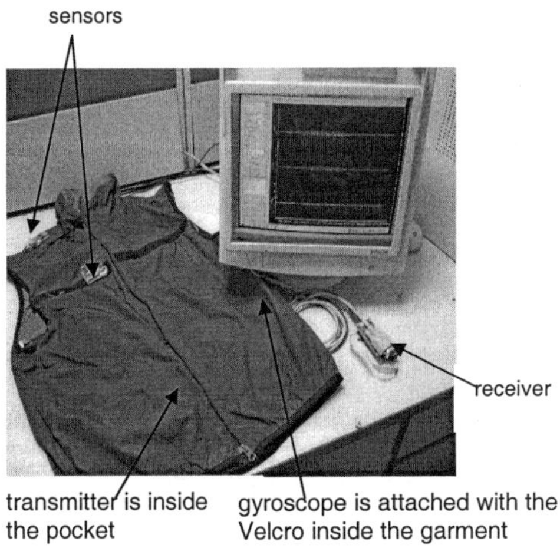

Fig.1. Experimental setup

scale [12]. While it provides the time at which frequency components occurred in construct to Fourier transform, wavelet processing supplies good frequency resolution at both low and high frequency. This is useful information for analyzing nonstationary signal, where the frequency content changes over time. In decomposition, the original signal $f(x) \in L^2(R)$ is measurable and has a finite energy and A_{2^j} is a linear operator and a projection operator on a particular vector space $V_{2^j} \subset L^2(R)$. Moreover, $A_{2^j} f(x)$ is the approximation of a function at a resolution 2^j and it can be characterized by 2^j samples per length unit in which j is the level of decomposition $j \in Z$. More precisely, the close subspaces V_j satisfy

$$\ldots \subset V_2 \subset V_1 \subset V_0 \subset V_{-1} \subset V_{-2} \subset \ldots \quad (1)$$

$$\overline{\bigcup_{j \in Z} V_j} = L^2(R), \quad (2)$$

$$\bigcap_{j \in Z} V_j = \{0\}. \quad (3)$$

Equation (2) makes certain that $\lim_{j \to -\infty} A_{2^j} f(x) = f(x)$ for all $f \in L^2(R)$. All the spaces are scaled versions of the central space V_0 is the additional requirement according to equation (4).

$$f \in V_j \Leftrightarrow f(2^j \cdot) \in V_0 \quad (4)$$

The detail signal at the resolution 2^j, $D_{2^j} f(x)$, is the difference of information between the approximation of a function $f(x)$ at the resolutions 2^{j+1} and 2^j. It is derived by the orthogonal projection of the original signal on the space O_{2^j} which is the orthogonal complement of V_{2^j} in $V_{2^{j+1}}$. In numerical characterization of these approximation and differentiation operator, a unique function $\phi_x \in L^2(R)$, called a scaling function, such that if it

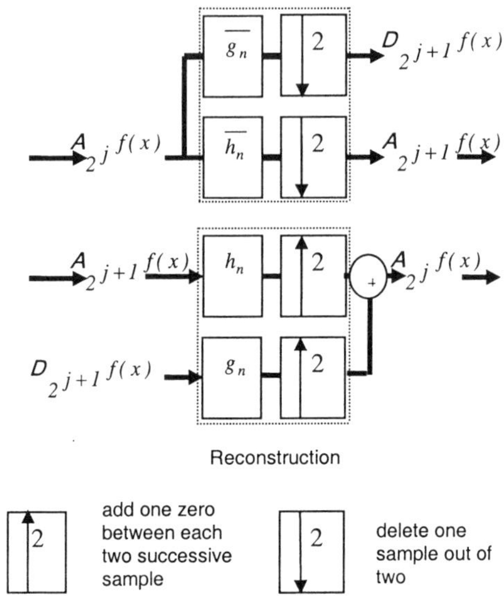

Fig.2. Multilevel decomposition and reconstruction

is set as $\phi_{j,n}(x) = 2^{-j/2}\phi(2^{-j}x - n)$ in which $j,n \in Z$ is an orthonormal basis of V_{2^j} and another unique function $\psi_{j,n}(x) = 2^{-j/2}\psi(2^{-j}x - n)$ where $j,n \in Z$, called a wavelet function, is an orthonormal basis of O_{2^j}. Let $h(n)$ be the discrete scale filter coefficients whose impulse response is $h(n) = \langle \phi, \phi_{-1,n} \rangle$ and $g(n)$ be the discrete wavelet filter coefficients whose impulse response is $g(n) = \langle \psi, \phi_{-1,n} \rangle$ with $g(n) = (-1)^n h_{-n+1}$. In practice, the measuring device gives only a finite number of samples: $(c_n^0)_{1 \le n \le N} = \langle f, \phi_{0,n} \rangle$ and which is the starting point of decomposition and each decomposed level has $2^{-j}N$ samples for $j \ge 1$ and the total number of samples in decomposed levels is the same number as the original approximated signal $(c_n^0)_{1 \le n \le N}$ because of the orthogonal representation. Wavelet coefficients can be derived by equations $c_k^j = \sum_n \overline{h_{n-2k} c_n^{j-1}}$ and $d_k^j = \sum_n \overline{g_{n-2k} c_n^{j-1}}$, where $\bar{h} = (\overline{h_{-n}})_{n \in Z}$. Therefore, c^0 can be decomposed as $d^1, d^2, d^3, \ldots, d^J$ and a coarse approximation of c^J. Moreover, reconstruction can be accomplished by the equation

$$c_n^{j-1} = \sum_k \left[h_{n-2k} c_k^j + g_{n-2k} d_k^j \right].$$

The procedures followed in decomposition and reconstruction are shown in Fig. 2.

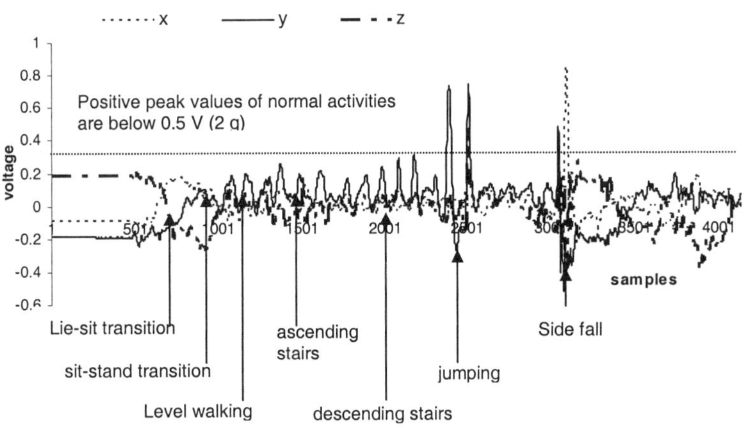

Fig.3. Series of activities from accelerometers arranged in medio-lateral (x), vertical (y) and antero-posterior (z) directions

2.3 Segment extraction using wavelet multiresolution analysis

Generally, fall incidents and activities accepted as fundamental for daily routines are forward fall, backward fall, side fall, sit-stand/stand-sit transition, sit-lie/lie-sit transition, level walking, ascending stairs and descending stairs. Actually, sitting, standing and lying postures happen at the end of their transitions. Therefore, the classification of these transitions is sufficient to recognize the postures instead of using additional sensors in activity identification. A flowchart of our algorithm can be seen in Fig. 4. Even though accelerometer signals related to three directions are applied in classification, only signal from vertical accelerometer is enough to be utilized in segment extraction. Therefore, discussion in the following is related to vertical acceleration signal.

Firstly, the signal was segmented into 10 sec duration. Since the maximum length of segments among activities is around 1.2 sec, 10 sec duration is appropriate to be executed. Actually, fall incidents to any direction have highest amplitude among activities in time domain vertical acceleration signal. Even for side fall, the positive peak value is above 2 g (0.5 V). Moreover, it never reaches above 2 g (0.5 V) for normal activities like sit-stand/stand-sit transition, sit-lie/lie-sit transition, walking, ascending stairs and descending stairs. Fall segment was extracted from the reconstructed detail signal at level five by using “Symlets order three (sym3)”. After the fall incident detection and extraction, signals before and after the fall incident were separated into two parts to detect the remaining activities. The

DWT decomposition into eight levels by "Daubichies order 3 (db3)" mother wavelet was used for the remaining of the data. The approximation signal corresponding to level eight (0-1Hz) was reconstructed. The vertical accelerometer measures approximately 1g in sitting or standing position and almost zero g in lying posture. Therefore, the orientation of the accelerometer distinguishes the lying posture from sitting/standing positions. Sit-lie and lie-sit transitions were detected by an appropriate threshold level and excluded from the ten second segment including the data before and after these transitions. Therefore, the remaining segments to be extracted yet are those related to sit-stand/stand-sit transitions and

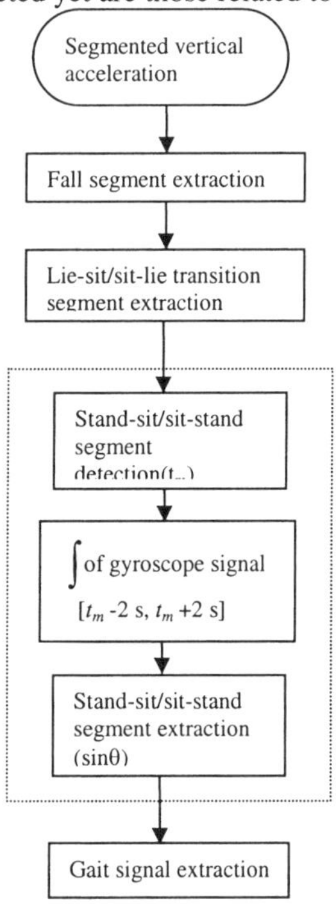

Fig.4. A flowchart of segment extraction for fall incidents and daily activities

gait patterns. In the approximated signal, all minima points (including the global minimum point) of the remaining data lower than half of the global minimum point were considered as the locations of sit-stand and stand-sit transitions. Even though we can detect the locations, sometimes it is not possible to locate break points for the start and end of these transitions especially for sit-walk and walk-sit transitions. sine(θ) of the gyroscope signal for time duration [t_m -2 s, t_m +2 s] was used to find the start and end of these transitions [13]. t_m is the minimum point of the approximated signal for one location. sine(θ) was derived according to equation (5) and peak points P1 and P2 were considered as the start and end points of sit-stand and stand-sit transitions [13]. In this case, actual angle θ was not necessary in peak points detection. Therefore, initial condition was set zero in equation (5).

$$\theta = \int_0^t g dt \qquad (5)$$

Therefore, gait patterns are the remaining part of the vertical acceleration signal in our segment extraction procedure.

3. Results

Fig.3. shows the series of activities from accelerometers arranged in medio-lateral (x), vertical (y) and antero-posterior (z) directions. Even though jumping is not included in the activities to be identified, it is shown to see the comparison of the positive peaks among

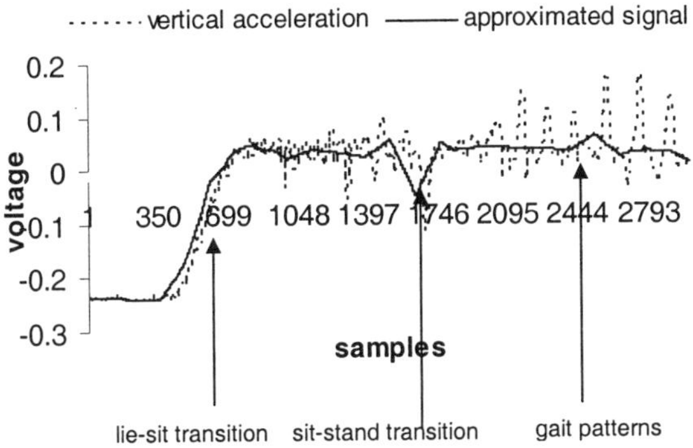

Fig.5. Vertical acceleration signal and the approximated signal at level eight (0-1Hz)

activities. Fig.5. shows the vertical acceleration signal and its approximated signal at level eight by using "db3" mother wavelet. Minimum voltage difference between lying posture and sitting or standing posture is 0.2 voltages and no minimum point in other postures is as low as any point in lying posture in approximated signal. Therefore, extraction of sit-lie/lie-sit transition was accomplished by using appropriate threshold voltage. After sit-lie/lie-sit transition segment extraction, sit-stand/stand-sit segment was extracted by using another threshold level. Wavelet decomposition and reconstruction was applied to enhance the gait patterns and to reduce noise. The approximated signal at level six by using "Discrete Meyer" mother wavelet was considered.

4. Discussion

We can see that the signal patterns related to activities are very close to each other and very troublesome to be extracted in time domain as shown in Fig. 3. Frequency domain transformation cannot display the time information of activity patterns as in time-frequency transformation. Actually, fall is also posture transformation from standing up position to lying down position and the effect of the orientation changes at the vertical accelerometer

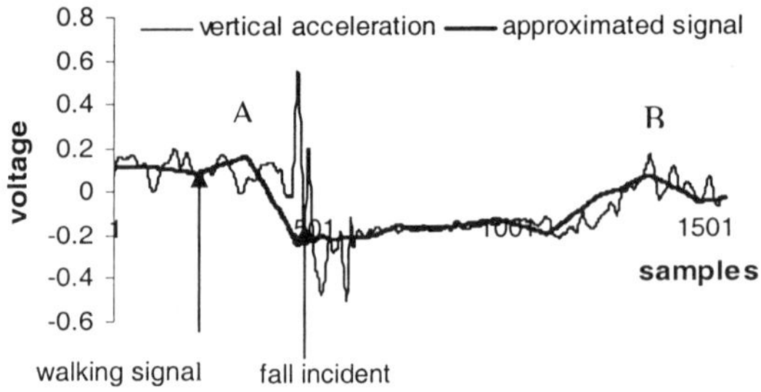

Fig.6. Vertical acceleration and approximated signal for fall incident

causes the complication in sit-lie/lie-sit transition detection. Therefore, it is necessary to exclude the entire signal related to fall incident from point A to point B as shown in Fig. 6. Detection is the same procedure as the sit-lie/lie-sit transition detection as expressed above. However, sometimes slippery backward fall on the hip does not vary the orientation of the vertical accelerometer.

In conclusion, the segments related to daily activities and fall incidents from a continuous vertical acceleration signal were extracted using wavelet multiresolution analysis and we could show that wavelet multilevel decomposition and reconstruction is a useful technique to extract the signal patterns of fall incidents and daily activities.

References:

[1] Health Facts Singapore 2001.

[2] B. Najafi, K. Aminian, A. Paraschiv-Ionescu, F. Loew, C. J. Bula, P. Robert, 2003. Ambulatory system for human motion analysis using a kinematic sensor: monitoring of daily physical activity in the elderly. Biomedical Engineering, IEEE Transactions on, Volume: 50 , Issue: 6, 711 – 723.

[3] F. Foerster, M. Smeja, J. Fahrenberg, 1999. Detection of posture and motion by accelerometry: a validation study in ambulatory monitoring. Computers in Human Behavior, Volume 15, Issue 5, 571-583.

[4] A. Yamaguchi, M. Ogawa, T. Tamura, T. Togawa, 1998. Monitoring behavior in the home using positioning sensors. Engineering in Medicine and Biology Society, 1998. Proceedings of the 20th Annual International Conference of the IEEE , Volume: 4 , Pages:1977 - 1979 vol.4.

[5] H. Mori, J. Hoshino, 2002. Independent component analysis and synthesis of human motion. Acoustics, Speech, and Signal Processing, 2002. Proceedings. (ICASSP '02). IEEE International Conference on , Volume: 4 , Pages:IV-3564 - IV-3567 vol.4.

[6] Ge Wu, 2000. Distinguishing fall activities from normal activities by velocity characteristics. Journal of Biomechanics, Volume 33, Issue 11, Pages 1497-1500.

[7] N. Noury, T. Herve, V. Rialle, G. Virone, E. Mercier, G. Morey, A. Moro, T. Porcheron, 2000. Monitoring behavior in home using a smart fall sensor and position sensors. Microtechnologies in Medicine and Biology, 1st Annual International, Conference On. 2000, Pages:607 – 610.

[8] G. A. L. Meijer, K. R. Westerterp, F. M. H Verhoeven, H. B. M. Koper, F. ten Hoor, 1991. Methods to assess physical activity with special reference to motion sensors and accelerometers. Biomedical Engineering, IEEE Transactions on , Volume: 38 , Issue: 3 , Pages:221 – 229.

[9] C. V. C. Bouten, K. T. M. Koekkoek, M. Verduin, R. Kodde, J. D. Janssen, 1997. A triaxial accelerometer and portable data processing unit for the assessment of daily physical activity. Biomedical Engineering, IEEE Transactions on, Volume: 44, Issue: 3, 136 – 147.

[10] M. Sekine, T. Tamura, M. Ogawa, T. Togawa, Y. Fukui, 1998. Classification of acceleration waveform in a continuous walking record. Engineering in Medicine and Biology Society, 1998. Proceedings of the 20th Annual International Conference of the IEEE , Volume: 3 , Pages:1523 - 1526 vol.3.
[11] P. H. Veltink, Bussmann, B. J. Hans, W. de Vries, W. L. J Martens, R. C. Van Lummel, 1996. Detection of static and dynamic activities using uniaxial accelerometers. Rehabilitation Engineering, IEEE Transactions on, Volume: 4, Issue: 4, 375 – 385.
[12] I. Daubechies, 1992. Ten lectures on wavelets. Philadelphia, Pa.: Society for Industrial and Applied Mathematics.
[13] B. Najafi, K. Aminian, F. Loew, Y. Blanc, P. A. Robert, 2002. Measurement of stand-sit and sit-stand transitions using a miniature gyroscope and its application in fall risk evaluation in the elderly. Biomedical Engineering, IEEE Transactions on, Volume: 49, Issue: 8, 843 – 851.

Toward a Human-Friendly Assistive Environment
D. Zhang and M. Mokhtari (Eds.)
IOS Press, 2004

Aware home understanding life activities

Katsunori MATSUOKA
Living Informatics Group, Institute for Human Science and Biomedical Engineering
National Institute of Advanced Industrial Science and Technology
1-8-31 Midorigaoka, Ikeda, Osaka 563-8577, Japan

Abstract. A home monitoring technology was developed under the national research project in Japan. It enables to monitor daily life activities seamlessly and find automatically unusual conditions caused by illness of living persons or home accidents. Two kinds of aware home technology were developed; one is based on a large sensor network system with 167 sensors installed in a house, and another is based on a simple sensor system using only two kinds of sensors. In the first case, the developed system understands individual living behaviors and finds unusual conditions by comparing current behavioral sequence with an ordinary one. In the second case, it detects a moment when unusual condition occurs in a house by evaluating the "ordinariness of living". Performance of the developed systems is discussed with some experimental results.

Introduction

In Japan, home accidents are increasing year by year with the increase of elderly people in our society as shown in Fig.1 [1]. Especially it becomes serious problem that death accidents of the elderly persons over 65 years old due to home accidents have been increasing by 1.7 times as many as death traffic accidents. Moreover, the birthrate in Japan is decreasing quickly while the number of elderly people is increasing. In this situation, it becomes important to develop a home monitoring system, which monitors everyday life activity of a person and finds unusual conditions caused by illness or accidents.

In the national research project carried out from 1999 to 2003 in Japan, two kinds of an aware home technology were developed. One is based on a large sensor network system with 167 sensors. Another is based on a simple system with two kinds of sensors. In both cases, they can detect unusual conditions in a house.

In this paper, these systems developed in the project are reported and its performance is discussed with some experimental results.

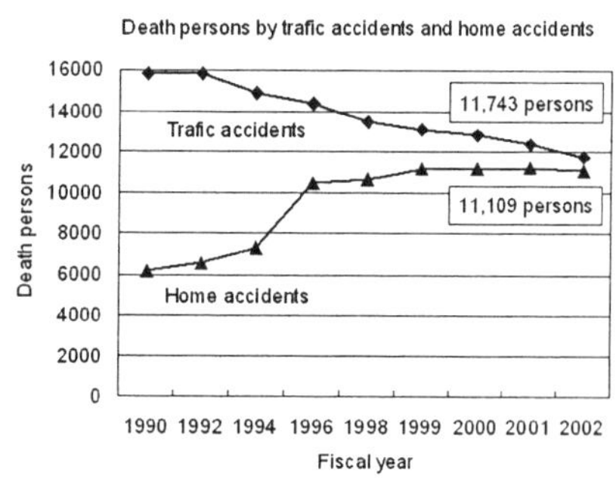

Fig.1 Death persons by traffic accidents and home accidents in Japan [1]

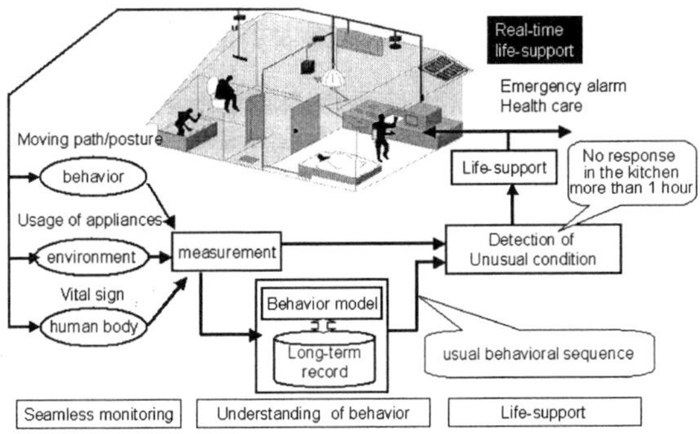

Fig.2 The concept of aware home technology in the research project

1. The concept of aware home technology

The style of living in a home is different individually. Thus, in the research project, an unusual condition was defined as a situation deviating from the ordinary living state. Then it becomes important to develop a method to extract an ordinary living state with multiple sensors installed in a house and an evaluation for discriminating a usual/unusual situation by a comparison of a current living state with the ordinary one. In order to get an ordinary living state, it is necessary to record living activity seamlessly and in a long term.

The concept of aware home system developed in the project is illustrated in Fig.2. Multiple sensors installed in a house detect the behavioral information and a usage of home appliances. A wearable sensor detects vital signs such as heart rate. All sensor data are accumulated and recorded. Then the ordinary living state is extracted from the long-term record and unusual condition can be detected by comparing a current living state with the ordinary one. When unusual condition is detected, an alarm is transmitted to a hospital to be rescued, or information about illness of a person is notified to a family or the person.

2. Understanding of a life activity as a personal behavioral sequence

2.1 Monitoring system for individual living activity

An experimental house named "Smart House Osaka" with 167 sensors (15 kinds of sensors) was built, which understands "who did what, when, and where" in real time [2,3]. The sensors described in Table 1 were installed in it. It was designed to monitor individual activity of five persons simultaneously.

Table 1 List of sensors installed in the house

sensors installed in the house	1	infrared sensor	20
	2	passage sensor	15
	3	sensor in appliance	17
	4	light sensor	33
	5	RF-ID generator	13
	6	bed sensor	4
	7	sensor in toilet	2
	8	Opening/Closing sens	28
	9	water flow sensor	12
	10	CCD position sensor	7
	11	hand rail sensor	3
	12	force plate	1
	13	position sensor	2
wearable sensor	14	acceleration sensor	5
	15	heart rate sensor	5
Total number			167

appliances with sensor	
Pot	1
refrigerator	1
air-conditioner	6
microwave oven	1
hot-water supply system	1
TV	2
gas range	1
washing machine	1
video	1
rice cooker	1
audioapparatus	1
Total number	17

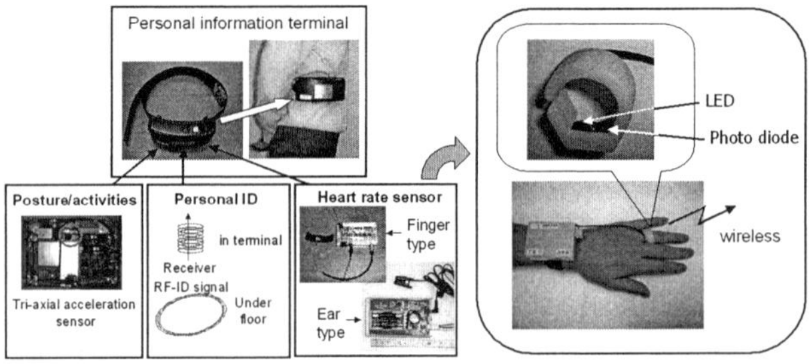

(a) Personal information terminal (b) Heart rate sensor

Fig.3 Wearable sensors to detect five kinds of postures and a heart rate in sleeping

Identification of a person is carried out by detecting a signal from the RF-ID (Radio Frequency Identification) generator installed in each floor with a wearable terminal carried on each person. By the video image processing in every room, a moving path of each person is extracted in real time. The usage of home appliance and an open/close state of window or door are detected with a switch sensor installed in it. An infrared light sensor in each room monitors human body movements.

Two types of wearable sensors were developed as shown in Fig.3. An acceleration sensor detects five kinds of body postures, which are standing, sitting, walking, lying, and falling down. Its detection accuracy was verified to be more than 90 percent by experiments. A ring type optical sensor detects a heart rate at a finger during sleeping.

2.2 Translation of sensor signals into a personal behavioral sequence

Sensor signal patterns are always different according to a human behavior even in a same behavior. Therefore it is hard to extract a useful difference from raw sensor data. Then we proposed a method to translate sensor signals into behavioral information [2,3].

The fundamental behaviors necessary for the description of everyday life were selected as twelve behaviors in Table 2. The developed translation algorithm consists of three stages. In the first stage, sensor signals are assigned to a person who locates in a detection area of sensor. In the second stage, sensor signals are clipped by a time-window of 10 seconds and translated into a candidate of behavior according to the relations between sensor signals and behaviors. In the third stage, the candidate of behavior is replaced with the more probable behavior when a behavioral context is not feasible.

By shifting a time window at every second in the second stage, a real-time translation into behaviors can be performed with a delay of about 10 seconds. Figure 4 shows an example of real-time translation into a behavioral sequence.

Table 2 List of fundamental behaviors

	behavior		behavior
1	sleeping	7	relaxing
2	washing face	8	bathing
3	meal	9	toilet
4	meal preparation	10	going out
5	washing	11	desk work
6	cleaning	12	movement

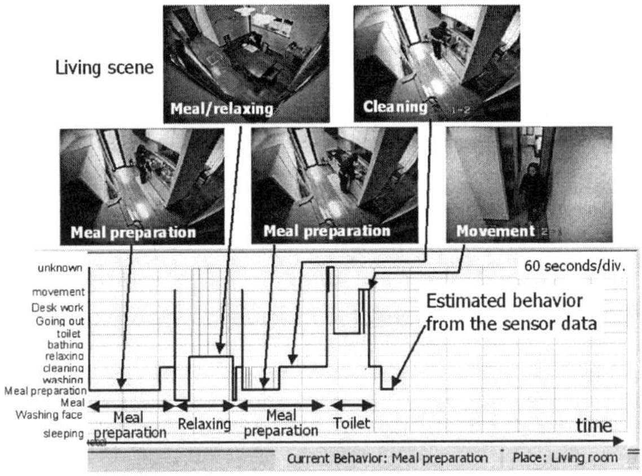

Fig. 4 An example of real-time translation into the fundamental behaviors from sensor signals

2.3 Experimental results obtained by an actual long stay

To verify the function of real-time translation into behaviors, we had an experimental stay of a four-person family during a month. The family consists of a father, a mother, and two children, whose ages were in the level of 40 years old, 40 years old, 20 years old and 10 years old, respectively. The stay was carried out after receiving the approval of the Ethical Committee on Human Research at AIST Kansai and obtaining a subject's informed consent.

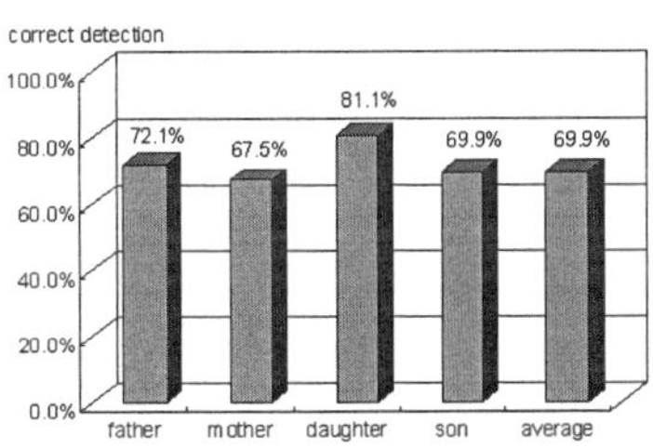

(a) Percentage of correct detection of behaviors

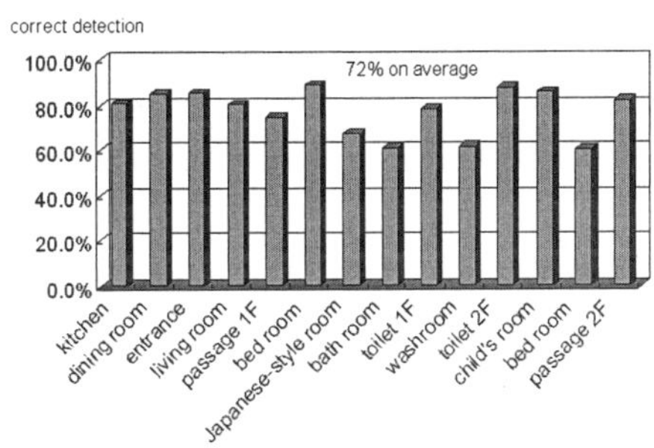

(b) Percentage of correct detection of staying room

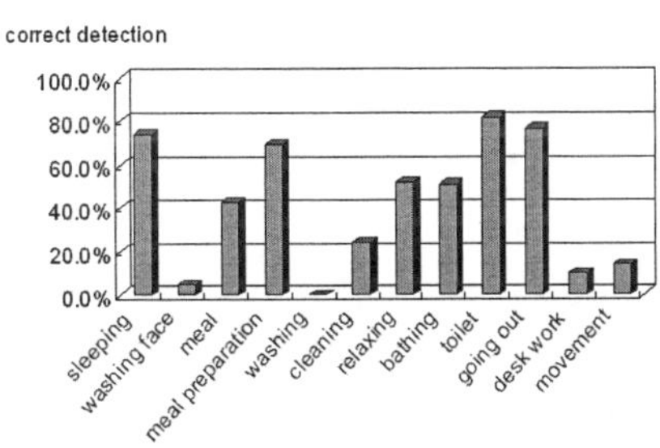

(c) Percentage of correct detection of each behavior

Fig.5 Verification results of the developed algorithm for the data obtained in the one-month stay in the experimental house.

In the verification, a behavioral sequence obtained by the algorithm was compared with that obtained with a video analysis by a human observation. A video image was recorded during 5:30-23:00 in every room except for a toilet, a bathroom, and a washroom.

It was verified that the developed system detected each person's behavior correctly at about 70% of living period as shown in Fig.5 (a) and each staying room correctly at about 72% as shown in Fig.5 (b). However the percentage of correct translation into each of 12 fundamental behaviors was obtained as 36% as shown in Fig.5(c). It was a low performance compared with the former result obtained in a short stay experiment [3], in which 70% was obtained. It is supposed that the reason of this poor result is depending on the individual difference in behaviors.

2.4 Detection of unusual situation by using behavioral sequence

In the experimental stay, it was verified to detect three types of unusual situations; in which (1) too long time is spent for a behavior, (2) the rhythm of living activity worsens, and (3) unusual behavioral sequences occur. In the case (1), it was verified that unusual situation was found within 56 minutes in the system. It is useful to provide an early recognition of danger situations such as a home accident. In the case (2), it became possible to evaluate the daytime activity in 7 stages by the acceleration sensor and the quality of sleep in 4 stages by the heart rate sensor. By combining them, a circadian rhythm of living activity can be evaluated in 18 stages and provide support in the recovery of rhythm by applying light stimuli or advices. In the case (3), it became possible to detect a disordered sequence of behaviors or too frequent behaviors. That is supposed to be a sign of mental illness such as a depressive mood disorder or a senile dementia. It would be helpful to inform it to a family at an early stage and to undergo an early medical treatment.

3. Understanding overall activities of family with simple sensors

3.1 Monitoring system for family activity with simple sensors

A simple system for monitoring a family activity was developed [4], which consists of two kinds of sensors: an infrared light sensor and an electric power sensor as shown in Fig.6. Infrared light sensor mounted on a lighting appliance is put on every room and detects a body movement. In a small room, another infrared light sensor in Fig.6 (b) is placed. An electric power sensor in Fig. 6 (c) is connected with an electric appliance and detects its power consumption. The sampling rate for an infrared light sensor is one second and that for an electric power sensor is one minute. All signals from sensors are transmitted by wireless.

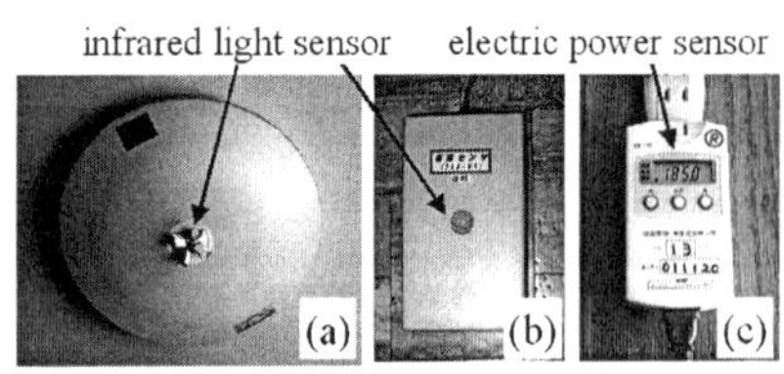

Fig.6 Sensors for detecting family living activity

3.2 Understanding of life activity

To compare the living activity, we proposed a method that transposes each time-segment of sensor signals into one of a limited number of living states and evaluates the similarity of transposed series [4,5,6].

The proposed method consists of two steps as shown in Fig. 7 [4]. The first step extracts principal components from all segments of sensor signals clipped by a time window. The second step finds a limited number of clusters by classifying the vectors of principal component loadings for each segment. These steps are performed only with two parameters; a number of principal components and a distance between clusters.

Figure 7 (d) shows an example of transposed cluster series for the data obtained with a four-person family. The cluster series expressed well a tendency of change of living activity. In this case, each segment was clipped with a time-window of two minutes at every ten seconds. The most significant ten principal components were used for the cluster analysis and the normalized distance between clusters was decided as a value of 0.6.

3.3 Evaluation of "ordinariness of living"

By using the occurrence probability $P(t,c)$ of cluster c at time t, the index $O_T(t)$ of "ordinariness of living" for a evaluation period of T can be defined as

$$O_T(t) = \sum_{c=0}^{N-1} \int_{\tau=0}^{T} P(t-\tau,c)\, Q(t-\tau,c)\, d\tau, \qquad (1)$$

where $Q(t,c)$ has a value of one when the cluster c appears and otherwise zero, and N denotes the total number of clusters.

While the index $O_T(t)$ with T=*24 hours* was useful to detect unusual day [4], the index $O_T(t)$ with a short evaluation time is not good for a real-time evaluation because its

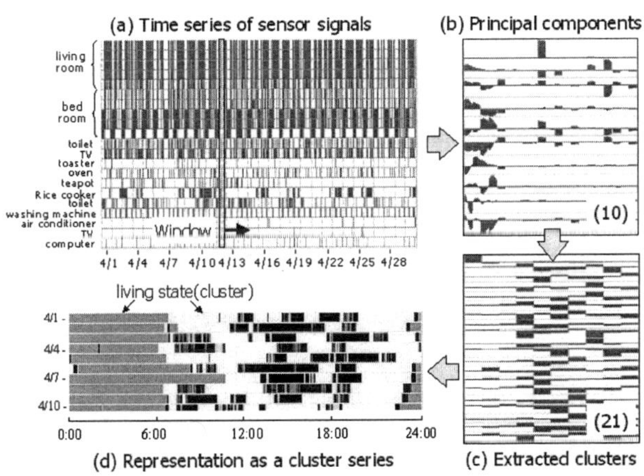

Fig.7 Processing flow of transposing sensor signals into a series of living clusters

statistical property varies with time [6].

Then a evaluation index *R(t)* with the normalized-deviation score $\hat{O}_T(t)$, which has a constant variance at any time, was proposed for a real-time evaluation of ordinariness of living [6]. They are defined as

$$\hat{O}_T(t) = \frac{O_T(t) - \overline{O}_T(t)}{\widetilde{O}_T(t)} + \overline{O}_T(t), \tag{2}$$

where $\overline{O}_T(t)$ and $\widetilde{O}_T(t)$ denote the mean and the standard deviation of $O_T(t)$, respectively, and

$$\begin{cases} R(t) = \int^{t} \hat{O}_T(\tau)\, d\tau, & \text{if } \hat{O}_T(\tau) < 0 \\ R(t) = 0, & \text{if } \hat{O}_T(t) \geq 0 \end{cases} . \tag{3}$$

The evaluation index *R(t)* has a large negative value when a current living state deviates from the ordinary living state. Then unusual situations can be detected by discriminating an evaluation index value.

The most important feature of the proposed analysis is that it does not need any information about room layout, sensor type, sensor position, or number of people living in.

3.4 Experimental results obtained for one-year data

To verify the performance of the real-time evaluation of ordinariness of living, the data obtained with a four-people family during one year was analyzed by the proposed method.

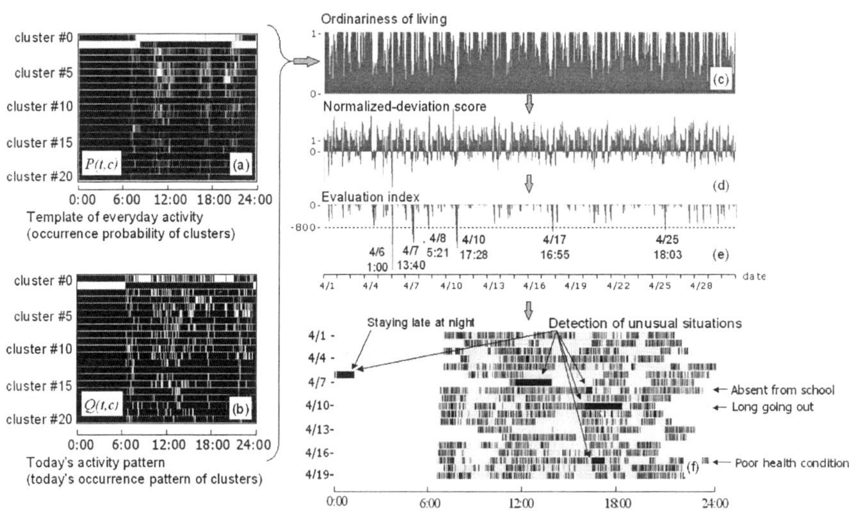

Fig.8 Evaluation process for ordinariness of living and detection of unusual situation: (a) Occurrence probability of each cluster at each time, (b) current occurrence of clusters, (c) ordinariness of living, (d) normalized-deviation score, (e) evaluation index, and (f) detection of unusual situation (dark regions) superposed on the cluster series of living.

The flow of data processing is shown in Fig.8.

By the evaluation of ordinariness of living, 73 times of unusual states was detected. By the comparison with the declaration of family, it was found that 19 times of unusual states were agree with the declaration but there is no declaration in the other case. For example, in the cases of getting agreement, it was detected situations of staying late at night, long going out, absent from school, poor health condition and etc. as shown in Fig.8 (f).

Conclusion

The research work on the development of aware home technology carried out in the national research project in Japan was introduced. The key concept is to detect unusual situations from the ordinary living state extracted by the long-term record.

Finally, I would like to describe about the concept of privacy protection in the developed system. It is indispensable to make a closed system in which all information acquired in a house should not leak to others. A part of information allowed by a user can be sent to the pre-decided person such as families or a medical doctor when unusual situation is detected. All living information should be under the management of a user.

Acknowledgments

This research work was carried out in collaboration with the Matsushita Electric Industrial Co., Ltd., Matsushita Electric Works, Ltd., Sorex Co. Ltd., Osaka Gas Co. Ltd., the University of Tokyo, and the Research Institute of Human Engineering for Quality Life under the national research project named as "Behavior-based Human Environment Creation Technology" operated by the Ministry of Economy, Trade and Industry and the New Energy and Industrial Technology Development Organization. I would like to express my appreciation to all members cooperating with this research work.

References

[1] The Ministry of Health, Labour and Welfare, Japan, Report on the investigation of population movement statistics: http://wwwdbtk.mhlw.go.jp/toukei/ kihon/ indexy_1_2.html, 2001.

[2] K. Matsuoka, Measuring behavior in a house, Proc. of SICE Annual Conference 2002, pp.856-859, 2002.

[3] K. Matsuoka, Development of real-time life support system based on living behavior understanding, *Proc. of IEA 2003*, vol.4, pp.470-473, 2003.

[4] K. Matsuoka, Detection of unusual behavioral condition based on the long-term record of life activity in a house, *Technical Report of IEICE*, MBE2002-128, pp.65-68, 2003.

[5] K. Matsuoka, Detection of unusual condition based on the long-term record of life behaviors in a house, *Proc. of BPES2003*, pp.279-282, 2003.

[6] K. Matsuoka, Understanding of living activity in a house for a real-time life support, Joint 2nd International Conference on Soft Computing and Intelligent Systems and 5th International Symposium on Advanced Intelligent Systems, 2004 (in press).

Toward a Human-Friendly Assistive Environment
D. Zhang and M. Mokhtari (Eds.)
IOS Press, 2004

OSGi Surveillance Service for Smart Home

ZHENG Song[1], ZHANG Daqing[1], G. MOHAN[2], NI Xiao[1],
1: Institute for Infocomm Research, Singapore
{szheng, daqing, nixiao }@i2r.a-star.edu.sg
2: Electrical and Computer Engineering Department, National University of Singapore, elegm@nus.edu.sg

Abstract. This paper illustrates a novel Web-based surveillance service built upon the OSGi framework and the JMF technology. The surveillance service bundle can be downloaded from the Web and installed in an OSGi-compatible residential gateway. The service is able to provide real-time video and 24-hour stored video to the Internet. Different from most commercial surveillance systems, the proposed method transmits the video stream via HTTP so that the video is enabled to penetrate the firewalls. In order to reduce the HTTP transmission delay, an intra-stream synchronization mechanism is introduced to improve the efficiency of each HTTP connection. The OSGi-based solution also enables compound services realization through multiple services collaboration. The benefits of building applications upon OSGi framework suggest that OSGi will be a very useful framework in the smart home environment.

Introduction

The pervasive connectivity of the Internet has created a great demand for conducting ubiquitous video surveillance through the Internet. A home surveillance system can be used not only as a security guard, but also to monitor the elders at home. With the number of networked homes, as well as the number of networked devices within the home proliferated at an accelerated pace, Web-based surveillance system becomes easily available at home.

We have also seen some commercial tools in the market which can function as a Web-based surveillance system, such as the MSN Messenger which is a default component of Windows XP. A Messenger running on a home PC can transmit real-time video over the Internet to another Messenger running on an office PC. Another example is the Java Media Studio (JMStudio) which is able to transmit or multicast video data to an Internet address. However, these solutions have some limitations.

- In order to minimize the transmission delay, these solutions employ real-time transport protocol (RTP) to transmit video data. Since RTP is a protocol running on top of UDP which may not be fully supported by firewalls, a user may have problems in receiving the video without manually configuring the port forwarding on the firewall [1].
- Due to the privacy consideration, it is not desirable to multicast the home video to the public. It is better to be accessed only by family members.
- Though multicasting by JMStudio is able to transmit video from one to a group simultaneously within the LAN, multicasting is still in its infancy in the Internet presently [2].

- These solutions have higher requirement on the media server and thus higher cost as a result. Two PCs are required to run the same software. Otherwise, interoperability issue arises between PCs running MSN Messenger and JMStudio.

The emergence of Residential Gateway (RG) technology brings a new solution to the Web-based surveillance system. The RG further brings down the cost, making home surveillance system affordable and accessible in every home. The gateway, acting as a central connection point in the residential network, is able to coordinate many devices, such as video camera and printer, and enable compound services through multiple services collaboration.

Aiming at integrating the RG technology with a smart home environment, an Open Service Gateway Initiative (OSGi)-based full service RG is developed in our institute with the sponsorship of Infocomm Development Authority of Singapore (IDA). Built upon Linux platform, the most distinguished feature of the RG is its ability to run OSGi services. This paper presents a Web-based OSGi surveillance service running on the RG. Different from above-mentioned commercial Web-based surveillance solutions, the proposed mechanism enables the video data to penetrate the firewalls and to lower the cost. The service can be downloaded from the Web and installed in an OSGi residential gateway. Java Media Framework (JMF) is implemented to capture real-time video frames. The OSGi HTTP service is used to transmit video stream. An intra-stream synchronization for HTTP streaming is introduced to reduce the HTTP transmission delay.

The rest of this paper is structured as follows. Section 1 presents an overview of OSGi and JMF. Section 2 describes the architecture of the surveillance service. Section 3 describes the details of the intra-stream synchronization for HTTP streaming. Section 4 illustrates the benefits of the proposed mechanism. Section 5 summarizes this paper.

1. Overview of OSGi and JMF

1.1 Open Service Gateway Initiative (OSGi)

Found in March 1999, the OSGi creates open specifications for the delivery of a wide array of services to end users. The OSGi specifies a framework upon which services execute. The specification allows the deployment and management of services in a coordinated fashion [3]. Several basic services, such as HTTP service, log service, permission administrator and so on, have been included in the specification. The key benefits of OSGi are the followings:

- Platform independent. Based on Java technologies, the OSGi gateway can run on most operating systems.
- Multiple network technology support. Home network technologies, such as Jini and UPnP, facilitate device and service discovery in OSGi gateway [4].
- Security. OSGi defines SSL service for secure network communication and enforces policy-based fine-grained control mechanisms to permit local resource access [5].
- Multiple services support and service collaboration. Multiple applications from different service providers are able to run on a single service platform and provide functionality to other services.

An OSGi service platform is an instantiation of a Java Virtual Machine (JVM), an OSGi framework and a set of bundles, as shown in Figure 1 [6]. The framework provides a concise and consistent programming model for application developers. Consistent interfaces ensure that the software components can be mixed and matched, and still result in a stable system. These components are called as bundles. The framework allows bundles to select an available implementation at runtime through the framework service registry [2]. A bundle is a Java Archive (JAR) file that contains Java class files to implement zero or more services, a manifest file and resources such as HTML pages, help files, icons, and so forth [7]. By using JAR to store applications and their resources in a standard ZIP-based Java file format, a bundle's size is smaller. Thus the bundle is faster to be downloaded from the service provider and easier to be deployed in an OSGi gateway through the Internet. A bundle can register or unregister services with the OSGi framework service registry. Bundles can discover services offered by each other by querying the service registry using a simple service discovery interface.

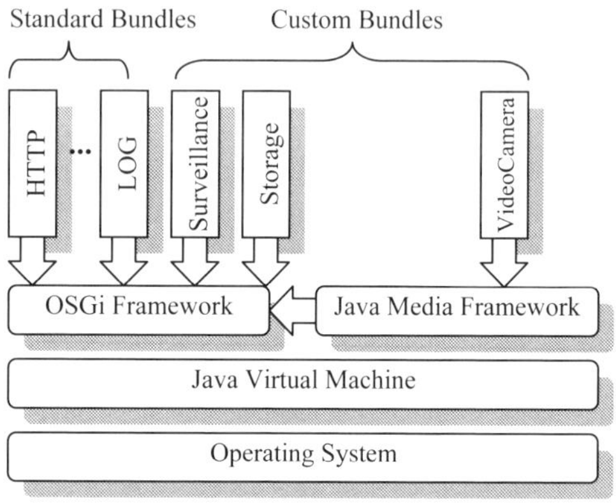

Figure 1. OSGi Architecture for Home Surveillance

1.2 Java Media Framework (JMF)

JMF API specifies a simple, unified architecture, messaging protocol and programming interface for media recording, transmission and playback. Currently at version 2.1.1, JMF is Sun's initiative to bring time-based media processing to Java. Time-based media is data that changes meaningfully with respect to time, such as audio and video clips, and animations. Also a complete reference implementation, JMF 2.1.1 enables users to do anything imaginable with multimedia, such as playing various multimedia files in a Java applet or application, capturing video with Web camera and storing the data in a supported format, transmitting audio and video in real-time on the Internet [10].

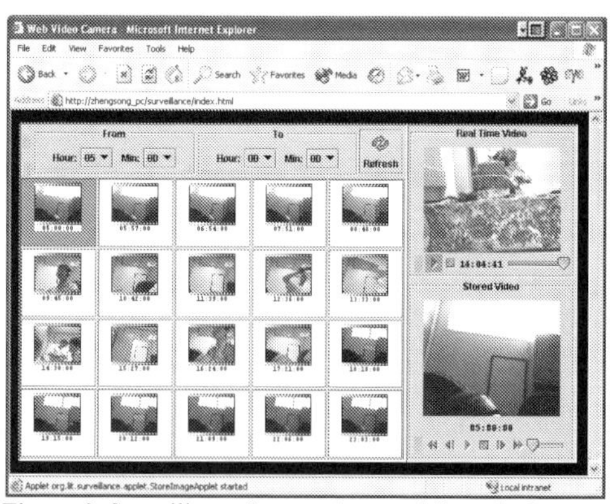

Figure 2. Surveillance System Accessed from the Internet

2. System Architecture

As shown in Figure 1, three custom OSGi bundles, namely camera service bundle, storage service bundle and surveillance service bundle, are included in the proposed home surveillance system. When they work together upon the OSGi framework, real-time video and 24-hour stored video are provided to the Internet, as shown in Figure 2.

2.1 The Camera Service

The camera service implements the JMF to capture real-time video images from a Web camera with a rate of 20 frames per second. The real-time images have a format of raw data and a resolution of 176×144. Thus the size of a frame is 176×144×3=76,032 bytes. Since raw video images consume a large amount of media space when they are saved and bandwidth when they are transmitted from the RG to the client, the camera service further imposes compression computation with the Joint Photographic Experts Group (JPEG) standard on the real-time images to improve the efficiency. JPEG is gaining wide acceptance due to its support for full 24-bit images and providing sufficiently high compression ratios for transmission of real-time video data across the Internet. The average size of a compressed frame (*Quality Value = 0.5*) is about 3,100 bytes (*Compression Rate = 95.9%*). Although H.261 and MPEG standards are designed for moving images and provide high compression ratio, their application to real-time Web-based surveillance is considered unpractical because they are highly CPU intensive and often require dedicated hardware implementations that increases costs [8]. When the camera service interface is called by the other two services, a real-time compressed image frame is responded. The camera service plays a role of service provider. The task of the camera service is fulfilled in following three steps [11]:

- Accessing capture devices. The capture devices are accessed through the `CaptureDeviceManager` which is the central registry for all of the capture devices available to JMF. Each device is represented by a `CaptureDeviceInfo` object.
- Capturing media data. To capture media data from a particular device, the device's `MediaLocator` should be obtained from its `CaptureDeviceInfo` object. Then the `MediaLocator` is used to constructed a `DataSource` which is the input to a `Processor`. To initiate the capture process, the service starts the `Processor`.
- Storing captured media data. A `DataSink` is used to read media data from the `Processor` object's output data source and render the data to a file.

2.2 The Storage Service

The storage service communicates with the storage server of the surveillance system to continuously store and retrieve media data. The storage server can be resided in the RG if the RG has enough hard disk space. Alternatively, the storage server can be located remotely in a very robust machine and the storage service will communicate with the server via FTP, HTTP or other methods.

The storage service calls the camera service every 6 seconds to retrieve a compressed video frame and save it in the storage server with a time-stamping file name of "*hh.mm.ss*.jpg". From this aspect, it is a service consumer. When the storage service is called by the surveillance service with a parameter of time tag, a corresponding stored video frame is retrieved from the storage server and responded. From this aspect, it is a service provider. The time-stamping file names enable the server to store large amount of data in such a way that retrieval is quick and efficient to reduce delay. The whole sequence of video frames is overwritten every 24 hours.

2.3 The Surveillance Service

The surveillance service consumes the camera service to retrieve real-time video images and consumes the storage service to obtain stored video images. It is a service consumer only. To realize the Web-enabled surveillance, the surveillance service bundle includes two components: a server-side Java servlet and a client-side Java applet. The Java applet is downloaded from the residential gateway to the client by a Web browser and runs in the client system. The Java servlet and the Java applet communicate with each other via the OSGi HTTP service. Under the request of the applet, the Java servlet responds with real-time video frames or stored video frames via HTTP streaming. The applet then presents the frames on the Web browser's GUI. Since the communication between the client and the server is based on HTTP, the surveillance video stream can pass through most firewalls.

The OSGi HTTP service also implements the basic authentication service to enhance the Web security, so that the surveillance video can only be accessed by authorized entities. The basic authentication service provides a very simple but not the highest level of security. Basic authentication is based on a challenge/response, username/password model and is supported by all browsers. When a client makes a request for some URLs which are not open to the public, the service will check if the request has proper authentication information in its request headers. If not, the service provides a challenge to the client. The challenge causes the Web browser to display a dialog box in which the user enters a name and password that are sent back to the service. If a user with the given name and password has been configured on the service, the HTTP service honors the request [9].

3. Intra-stream Synchronization for Video Stream

Although the OSGi HTTP service enables the video stream to penetrate the firewalls, the significant drawback behind this solution is that three phases of a HTTP session, namely connection setup, data transmission and connection release, deteriorate the frame transmission delay. In order to illustrate the transmission delay, a residential gateway is connected to the Internet via V.90 for testing. The reason for not testing under broadband connection is that V.90 demonstrates the delay more significantly. The testing results in Table 1 show that a HTTP connection setup time is even longer than a frame's transmission time under the traditional HTTP request/response communication model and the average per frame transmission delay is about 1772.5 ms.

Table1. Per Frame Transmission Delay Under V.90

Sample	Connection Setup Time (ms)	Per Frame Transmission Time (ms)	Connection Release Time (ms)	Per Frame Transmission Delay (ms)
1	1313	774	2	2089
2	969	745	1	1715
3	984	731	3	1718
4	954	747	2	1703
5	1062	785	1	1848
6	969	729	1	1699
7	969	739	1	1709
8	1000	748	2	1750
9	969	750	2	1721
Ave.	1021	749.8	1.7	1772.5

From the testing results, it can be found that the average per frame transmission delay could be reduced if the number of frames transmitted during each HTTP connection is increased. That means one HTTP session can transmit multiple frames instead of one frame only. For example, if five frames are transmitted during one HTTP connection, then the time for a HTTP session is about $1021+749.8\times5+1.7 = 4771.7$ ms and the average per frame transmission delay is estimated as $4771.7/5 = 954.34$ ms, which is much less than the delay in the previous approach. Though the efficiency of each HTTP connection is improved, the client has to wait for 4771.7 ms to download the whole five frames and present them on the GUI.

To further improve the efficiency of video transmission, it needs to reduce the client waiting time. Thus an enhanced HTTP communication between the servlet and the applet is proposed as Figure 3. The client-side Java applet will present video frames on the GUI while receiving them. When the applet sends a request to the servlet, the servlet continuously responds with "*content-length*" and "*image data*" for each frame. The applet keeps monitoring the received HTTP stream. When the applet receives a "*content-length*", it will transform the following length of "*image data*" into an image and present the image on the GUI immediately. Then the applet continues to receive the next frame's "*content-length*" and "*image data*". Under this approach, the HTTP connection setup time can be ignored and the per frame transmission delay is nearly the same as per frame transmission time if a certain number of frames are transmitted during one HTTP connection.

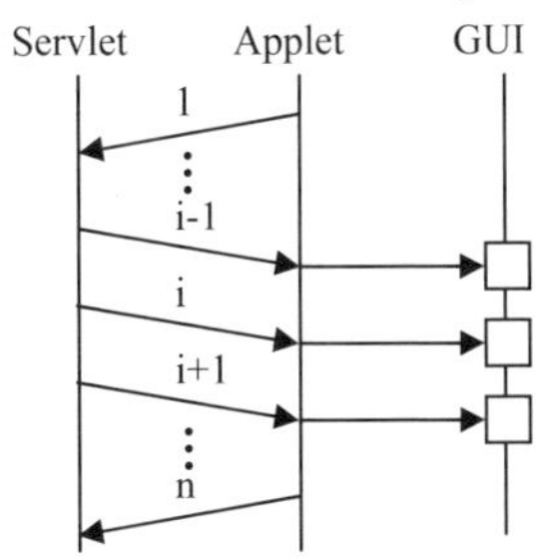

1: Connection setup
i-1: Data of frame (i-1)
i: Data of frame i
i+1: Data of frame (i+1)
n: Connection release

Figure 3. Intra-stream Synchronization

4. The Benefits of the OSGi-based Surveillance Service

Different from most commercial surveillance tools, such as above-mentioned MSN Messenger and JMStudio, the proposed OSGi-based surveillance service has following significant advantages.

- Based on the OSGi platform, a complicated application can be built on multiple service collaboration. Each service brings in new feature to the application. In this paper, three OSGi services, namely camera service, storage service and surveillance service, are collaborated with each other to realize a complicated Web surveillance function. One OSGi service can dynamically discover the other two services and adapt its behavior to the configuration of the environment and other services. The OSGi provides an opportunity to evolve programming model to service-oriented.

- Each OSGi service can come or go without bringing down other services. For example, when the storage service is stopped, the surveillance service and the client side Java applet cannot achieve stored video data from the server. Thus "Service Unavailable" is shown in the stored video area instead of video images, as shown in Figure 4. However, the real-time video is still playing since the camera service is still working. This feature provides service providers a business model which allows end users to access content on a per-use or flat-fee basis [3]. For example, the storage service component could be provided to users on a charge-per-use basis rather than the more conventional sell.

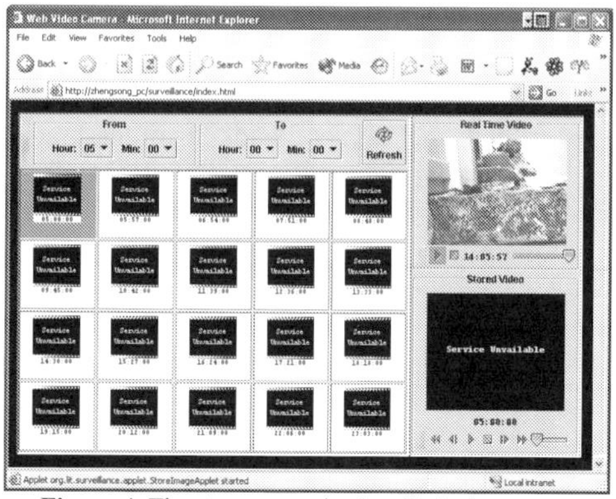

Figure 4. The storage service bundle is down.

- Since the video stream transmission is based on the OSGi HTTP service, the video is able to penetrate most firewalls. The drawback for this mechanism is that it increases video transmission delay due to large HTTP overhead and HTTP connection establishment phases. However, intra-stream synchronization can be introduced to reduce the video transmission delay. As the surveillance service is only for personal use, it is sufficient if the RG can support one or two HTTP simultaneous connections. Compared with Web radio or TV broadcasting server which is connected by huge number of clients, the gateway is not busy and the delay is acceptable.
- The client-side surveillance GUI is embedded on a Web browser instead of depending on any special software. This feature, together with the firewall penetration advantage, enables the surveillance to be carried out on any machines provided a Web browser and Java Virtual Machine (JVM) are installed. Thus the requirement for the client-side software is released and the cost is reduced.
- Since the basic authentication service is implemented by the OSGi HTTP service in the proposed mechanism, the video stream is restricted to be accessed only by authorized entities. The fact that Basic authentication is supported by all browsers also release the requirement for the client-side software.

5. Summary

Leveraging on OSGi HTTP service and Java Media Framework (JMF), this paper presents a home surveillance service which is able to provide real-time video and 24-hour stored video to the Internet. An OSGi camera service is constructed to capture video frames via the implementation of JMF. The OSGi HTTP service is utilized to transmit the video stream, so that the video can penetrate most firewalls which is different from most commercial surveillance tools. Intra-stream synchronization is introduced to reduce the video transmission delay due to large HTTP overhead and HTTP connection establishment phases. Based on the OSGi framework, a complicated application can be built on multiple service support and collaboration. The benefits of building applications upon OSGi framework suggest that OSGi will be a very useful framework in the environment of smart home.

References

[1] http://forum.java.sun.com/thread.jsp?forum=28&thread=436276
[2] Merlin Hughes, et al, "Java Network Programming (2nd Edition)", page 494-495, *Manning Publications Co.*, Oct., 1999.
[3] Dave Marples, Peter Kriens, "The Open Services Gateway Initiative: An Introductory Overview", *IEEE Communication Magazine*, December 2001, pages 110-114.
[4] Pavlin Dobrev, et al, "Device and Service Discovery in Home Networks with OSGi", *IEEE Communication Magazine*, August 2002, pages 86-92.
[5] Kirk Chen, Li Gong, *Programming Open Service Gateways with Java Embedded Server™ Technology*, Sun Microsystem, 2002.
[6] http://www.osgi.org/resources/spec_download.asp
[7] Choonhwa Lee, David Nordstedt, Sumi Helal, "Enabling Smart Spaces with OSGi", *Proc. IEEE Int'l Conf. Pervasive Computing and Communications*, 2003, page 89-94.
[8] A.C.M.Fong, S.C. Hui, "Web-based Intelligent Surveillance System for Detection of Criminal Activities", *Journal of Computing and Control Engineering, Dec. 2001.*
[9] "Java Embedded Server™ Developer Guide", http://www.sun.com/software/embedderserver
[10] Vaida M.-F., Lazar L., "Intruder Detection Considering a Java Platform Application", Proc. *The 24th Int'l Conf. Information Technology Interface*, 2002.
[11] "Java™ Media Framework API Guide", page 78-80.

Toward a Human-Friendly Assistive Environment
D. Zhang and M. Mokhtari (Eds.)
IOS Press, 2004

Quality Based Query Processing for Smart Homes - Some Initial Steps

Jit Biswas, Santos K. Das, Qiu Qiang, Chava V. Saradhi
Institute for Infocomm Research
21 Heng Mui Keng Terrace
Singapore 119613
{biswas, skdas, qiu, saradhi}@i2r.a-star.edu.sg

Abstract

We propose a query based framework for elder care applications in a Smart Home context. Our objective is to feed back assessment parameters of the query result to the source, so that successive query results may be improved. We outline a sketch of a model of quality degradation of a sensor based data source. By incorporating this model into a query framework, it is expected that query refinement will be possible. We propose a methodology to drill through from views and summary data to source data in an iterative fashion, thereby improving the refinement of the data analysis. The application driver is taken from elder care, where activities such as sleeping behavior and gait analysis are taken to be candidate activities for reliable activity identification. This is our first step towards deriving database and data mining techniques that support automatic monitoring of elderly people.

1 Introduction

Like most sensor based applications, elder care applications consist of monitoring activities of the elderly, in order to infer their behavioral patterns. Sometimes these patterns may require remedial actions by care givers and doctors. At other times such patterns may be added to a repository of information either for post-analysis for the person in question, or to add to a compendium of knowledge about aging population. In case of the latter, collections of information will need to be gathered, archived, retrieved and presented appropriately for supporting health-care analysis and applications.

One of the most important aspects of the data that is gathered from sensors is its quality. Poor quality data leads to poor quality analysis. If the data is being used to support elder care applications, it is all the more necessary for the data to be reliable and dependable. Both "Type 1 errors" (failure to report an event) and "Type 2 errors" (reporting an event when it hasn't occurred), are unacceptable. Besides reliability there are several other quality criteria that have been identified in the literature [7], as aspects of data quality (DQ) or information quality (IQ). We use the terms synonymously.

In this paper we discuss our initial ideas on how to model quality issues that arise from sensor based data, how to process the data, extracting useful information by ways of aggregates and summaries, and how to respond to end user queries upon these summaries. We expect that the approach will prove to be useful in the context of a flagship project being undertaken by our institute [6] in the area of elder monitoring and care in homes, and clinics.

The remainder of the paper is organized as follows. In section 2. we briefly discuss why it is important to model sensor quality in an overall framework of query processing [8], differentiating in section 3, our approach from conventional approaches. In section 4. we discuss lineage tracing [2] as a tool to perform interactive drill through and stepwise query refinement. In section 5. we briefly discuss how these ideas can be applied by presenting an example of an activity that is meaningful in the context of elder care. Related work and future work are presented in sections 6. and 7. respectively, with concluding remarks in section 8.

2 Modeling sensor quality degradation

A connected home for elder care is equipped with a variety of sensors for the purpose of gathering state information regarding the elderly who are the focus of observation. The types of sensors may be very simple on-off type sensors such as those that are used to detect the open or close event of doors, windows and drawers. At the other end of the spectrum are sophisticated sensors such as video cameras and microphones that capture visual and audio data. In between are sensors such as motion detectors and infrared and RFID sensors used for a variety of monitoring and control applications within the home.

Our approach is to model the degradation characteristics of sensors using models of physical behaviour of sensors over time, space or some other dimension. Battery power is an obvious aspect to be modelled, focusing on an estimate of the remaining battery lifetime of a sensor, and the non-linear behaviour of sensor output depending on the quantum of remaining battery power. Sensors that are based on mechanical components have to be modelled, taking into account an appropriate model of the wear and tear based on usage pattern of the sensor.

The end goal of modeling degradation behaviour of sensors is to build in the dynamics of sensor failure behaviour into the query processing algorithm and architecture in an integral fashion. Hopefully query optimization could also incorporate sensor degradation models.

Table 1: Typical Sensors and their profiles

Sensor Type	Resolution	Power
RFID	On/Off	low
Motion Detector	mm/cm	medium
Light	intensity	low
On/Off	binary	low
Video	megapixels	high
Audio	sampling rate	medium

3 Difference in our approach

We deal with the problem of data quality from the perspective of the end user, who is assessing the quality of the data. Our approach essentially handles sensor behaviour from a query processing perspective. We approach the problem from a declarative perspective rather than a procedural perspective. Techniques such as sensor network routing and adhoc sensor networking, sensor power conservation, radio layer optimization, sensor instrumentation etc. are isolated individual techniques that do not address the problem from the point of view of the end user.

Our difference is that declaratively we attempt to characterize the problem of data quality from the perspective of the end-user, which is one that is essentially centralized, and abstracted, fused and hopefully coherent. How do we make the transition from this integrated (albeit potentially inconsistent) picture, to a collection of individual distributed states or collections of states?

To enforce declarative design and thinking, we approach the problem from a query processing perspective we start with SQL as the query language. Even though the end user interface may be some object based language, it may be mapped to the relational model in terms of tuple values as snapshots of the real world.

Thus in our approach we assume an underlying model in which all data, whether temporal, spatial, or point data, is stored in relational tables. Quality is modelled as a vector of quality attributes associated with each data value. Quality processing accompanies data processing, whether through data volume reduction techniques, or through inferencing stages, at each step, quality the data is taken explicitly into account while arriving at a query result..

In the next section we discuss lineage tracing, which is a technique employed for scientific databases and data warehousing. Traditional domains of deployment of lineage tracing in scientific data management and heterogeneous database management systems are quite different from the domain of large scale distributed data sources such as are to be found in sensor based systems. Hence the approach of lineage tracing applied to the connected home context is expected to yield many benefits.

4 Lineage Tracing

We envisage a two step process (see Fig 1), whereby data is first captured in a Site Data Base (SDB), and is then summarized and the summaries are transmitted to an Auxiliary Data Base (ADB). A high level query process allows end-users to query the stored summaries. Lineage tracing of views (query results) invariably requires access to data stored in the ADB. However, on occasion, lineage tracing may require the "drill through" operation to go all the way down to the SDB in order to accurately answer the query. In some cases such historical data may not be available at the SDB due to insufficient memory resources. In these cases, approximation and compression techniques may have to be employed. Whenever such functions are used, the quality of data accuracy is invariably compromised.

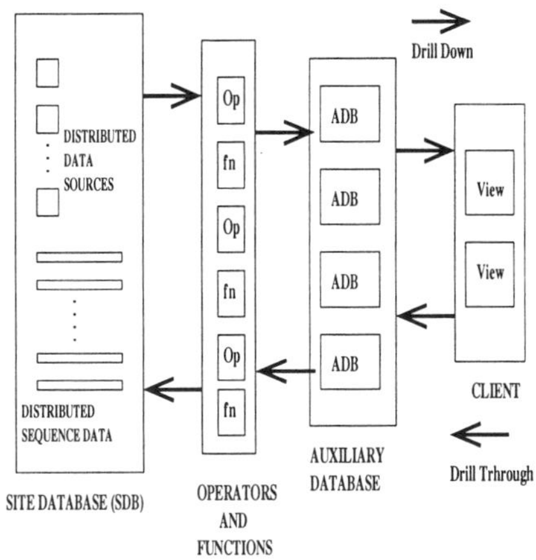

Figure 1: Lineage Tracing Block Model

It is convenient to think of data in sequences passing through functions or unary operators in order to be converted to other sequences of data. Unary operators such as the approximation operator, operate on input sequences in order to produce output sequences. Binary or k-ary operators such as $aggregation$ operate on multiple sequences of input to produce single (or in some cases multiple) output sequences.

Naturally, when we operate on sequences one question of great relevance is how good is the approximation. The goodness of an operator is called the quality of the operator. Operator quality contributes to overall information quality of a system. Sources of error in approximation techniques give rise to sources of error in the overall query result. Thus operator quality is a key ingredient of information quality.

Our objective is to characterize operator quality by the extent to which output sequences faithfully represent input sequences that they originate from. We do this by considering the output sequences as views stored in an Auxiliary Database (ADB). Techniques from lineage tracing [1] allows us to determine the *drilled down* values from the views. We consider the unary operator PLA as a simple unary operator. Characterizing the PLA function as a sequence operator, we characterize its inverse, i.e, the inverse PLA function as an inverse mapping that allows us to create data points in the original sequence that are missing in the view. These inverse functions are either perfect, or they may be some degree of *weakness* as mentioned in [15].

5 Example: Sleep Pattern Behaviour Analysis

To illustrate the use of query processing with quality and lineage tracing, we take an example of activity analysis which is quite important in determining the quality of life and health of elderly people.

Fig 2 illustrates the architecture of the prototype connected home for quality based query processing. In this figure we see a connected home environment where the data is collected from various sensing devices located ubiquitously in the subject's home. We assume that sampled data is stored at a SDB in the connected home and summaries of it are transferred to the ADB which is located at the clinic, to be viewed periodically by the analyst/doctor.

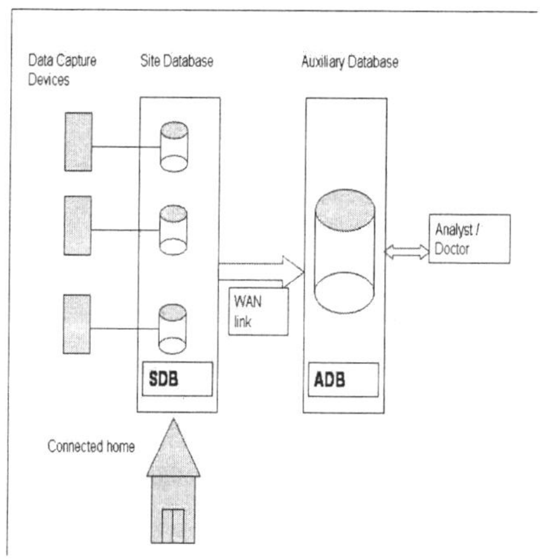

Figure 2: Prototype Connected Home for Quality Based Query Processing

To illustrate function inversion let us consider a sensor that records sensor output amplitudes at a certain sampling rate. Let (X_1, X_2, ... X_n), be the sequence of values of this sensor. The PLA approximation of this sequence would be the set of tuples of the form $((Y_0, f_0), (Y_1, f_1), \ldots (Y_k, f_k))$, where $Y_0 = X_0$ and Y_i is the ith sample of the original sequence, and f_i is the PLA approximating function for the ith segment of the original sequence.

Notice that similar to PLA, the PCA (or Piecewise Constant Approximation) or PSA (Piecewise Spline Approximation) could be used. In these cases the storage requirement at the ADB for the summarized data would be $less$ and $more$ respectively, than that of the PLA. Thus in terms of storage requirement PCA $<$ PLA $<$ PSA; even though in terms of accuracy PSA $>$ PLA $>$ PCA. The choice of which function to use, is best left in the hands of the analyst.

6 Related Work

The application area of elder care is inspired by leading work done in the area of "Context Aware Systems" [5], [13], [11], [12], [3], [17], [9]. Activity tracking and analysis of past behaviour is a subject of great importance and ought to be studied within the framework of techniques which have been developed in the database community. We regard these as the driving applications that invoke operations on back-end databases which monitor and archive the behavioral data pertaining to persons and entities within a system.

7 Future work

The illustration of piecewise linear approximation could be extended to other more powerful functions. There are several other methods besides piecewise approximation functions, such as histograms [14], wavelets [16], and fourier transforms [4], that could be used as approximations in the above example. The key idea here is to illustrate the feasibility of an approach. In our current work we are using this approach to approximate sequences of data arising out of distributed data sources in an elder care prototype demonstrator for a connected home [10] setting.

We expect that our lineage tracing algorithm will allow us to construct source data sequences with quantifiable degree of accuracy which stem from the $weakness$ of the operator. Applications from medical world immediately come to mind, whereby a system of distributed sensors could potentially be used to monitor not only a patient's vital signs such as heart beat and blood pressure, but also could automatically summarize information about personal activities conducted indoors or outdoors.

The techniques we use are a step in the direction of an overall set of tools and techniques for providing information quality in context aware systems.

8 Conclusions

In this paper we have proposed a query based framework for elder care applications that makes explicit, the aspect of quality of information in the data capture and query processing environment. The need for modeling sensor degradation is high-lighted as an important aspect of automatically improving query response. Feedback of quality by way of user provided interaction is examined briefly through a query refinement process. We make use of the concept of drill through from OLAP environments and lineage tracing, in the context of the proposed query processing environment. Our proposal permits mechanisms for supporting drill through at the level of functions in the system. This technique may be used as a tool in OLAP environments whereby powerful visualization capabilities can be made available in the hands of the analyst.

The ideas discussed here are the subject of ongoing work and are still under development. We expect that the result of our research will be used meaningfully in a flagship project of our institute, in the area of elder care.

9 Acknowledgements

The help and guidance of Pang Hwee Hwa are very much appreciated. We would also like to thank Victor Foo for help with sensor data quality modeling.

References

[1] Y. Cui, J. Widom, and J. L. Wiener. Tracing the lineage of view data in warehousing environment. November 1997.

[2] S. Das and J. Biswas. Invertible functions for activity tracking and analysis. June 2004.

[3] A. K. Dey and G. D. Abowd. Cybreminder: A context-aware system for supporting reminders. 2001.

[4] T. D. D. Eric J. Stollnitz and D. H. Salesin. Wavelets for computer graphics. *IEEE Computer Graphics and Applications*, May 1995.

[5] A. G. Hauptmann, J. Gao, R. Yan, Y. Qi, J. Yang, and H. D. Wactlar. Automated analysis of nursing home obervations. *Pervasive Computing*, May-June 2004.

[6] A. H. Kam. I2r flagship project in healthcare. 2004.

[7] L. U. Neumann F. and F. J.C. Quality-driven integration of heterogeneous information system. *VLDB*, 1999.

[8] Q. Qiang and J. Biswas. An information quality adaptation model. June 2004.

[9] J. Reikki, J. Huhtinen, P. Ala-Siuru, P. Alahuhta, J. Kaartinen, and J. Roning. Healthwear: Medical technology becomes wearable. 2002.

[10] V. J. Ritala M., Tieranta T. Context aware user interface system for smart home control. *Proceedings of the Home Oriented Informatics and Telematics 2003, HOIT2003*, April 2003.

[11] D. A. Ross. Cyber crumbs for successful aging with vision loss. *Pervasive Computing*, May-June 2004.

[12] D. Salber, A. K. Dey, and G. D. Abowd. The context toolkit: Aiding the development of context-enabled applications. *Pervasive Computing*, May-June 2004.

[13] A. Sixsmith and N. Johnson. A smart sensor to detect the falls of the elderly. *Pervasive Computing*, May-June 2004.

[14] K. S. Sudipto Guha, Nick Koudas. Data-stream and histograms. *ACM Symposium on Theory of Computing*, July 2001.

[15] A. Woodruff and M. Stonebraker. Supporting fine-grained data lineage in a database visualization environment. In *ICDE*, April 1997.

[16] M. W. Yossi Matias, Jeffrey Scott Vitter. Wavelet-based histograms for selectivity estimation. *Proceedings of the 1998 ACM SIGMOD international conference on Management of data*, June 1998.

[17] D. Zhang, X. Wang, L. Karianto, and W. Huang. Osgi based service infrastructure for context aware connected homes. 2004.

Chapter 4

Communications for Health Telematics

Toward a Human-Friendly Assistive Environment
D. Zhang and M. Mokhtari (Eds.)
IOS Press, 2004

E-Wheelchair: A Communication System Based on IPv6 and NEMO

Thierry Ernst
Keio University, Jun Murai Lab
5322 Endo, Fujisawa-shi, Kanagawa 252-8520, Japan
ernst@sfc.wide.ad.jp

Abstract. The development of Internet technologies based on the IPv6 protocol will allow real-time monitoring of people with health deficiencies and improve the independence of elderly or disabled people. We have designed a communication system based on IPv6 protocols, and we are presently developing an electronic wheelchair to demonstrate the benefit of IPv6 and mobility technologies for health-care usages.

1 Introduction

On the other hand, with the rapid raise of mobile telecommunication technologies, it becomes easier for the active people to keep in touch with peers even while on the move. Most people often traveling generally have a mobile phone, a laptop computer with Internet access and an email address. So, they can exchange text, voice, pictures and videos in a very easy and fashion way. However, although Internet access at office, at home and in hotels is now common, Internet access in the streets and when commuting is still somewhat lacking. With the advent of mobile technologies in IPv6, and particularly network mobility support and multihoming, the time has come to realize the awaited ubiquitous Internet. In order to achieve the ubiquitous Internet, connection to the network must be available everywhere, at anytime, without disruption of service. Thanks to NEtwork MObility (NEMO) support which allows an entire network, referred to as a *mobile network*, to migrate in the Internet topology, anything will soon be connected to the Internet, particularly PANs (Personal Area Networks, i.e. small networks attached to people and composed of Internet appliances like PDAs, mobile phones, digital cameras, etc.), networks of sensors deployed in vehicles (aircrafts, boats, buses, trains), and access networks deployed in public transportation (taxis, trains, aircrafts, trucks and personal cars) to provide Internet access to devices carried by their passengers (laptop, camera, mobile phone, and even PANs).

We think that such mobile telecommunication technologies could highly help the disabled and elderly people to keep in touch and even to improve their independence. Permanent communication between these people with deficiencies and all their peers including family, doctor, nurse, is indeed very important. However, because of the health deficiencies, they have limited means to keep in touch with the people most likely to take care of them. Fashion devices such as mobile phones and laptops connected to the Internet would be useful for them, but these are usually difficult to either understand or manipulate for people with deficiencies. We are therefore defining a communication system based on IPv6 and adapted to the needs of such people. We think that this communication system will be highly beneficial for health-care usages. For the purpose of demonstrating the communication system, we focus on an electronic wheelchair which would allow disabled persons to be monitored and would at the meantime increase their independence. The communication system is relevant to other usages. This system is being defined within the Nautilus Working Group [2] of the WIDE Project community [19]. This Working Group has been set up to demonstrate and deploy IPv6 mobility technologies.

The present paper is structured as follows: we first briefly describe the Internet and the TCP/IP reference model, then we discuss in section 3 the functional needs of the system. In section 4 we then define a communication system based on IPv6 [3] and NEMO [15, 7] that meets those functional needs. In section 5, we highlight the validation of the communication system in our indoor testbed and the E-wheelchair demonstration testbed currently under development.

2 Internet and TCP/IP

2.1 The Internet

The *Internet* is a collection of heterogeneous networks hierarchically organized and running under distinct administrative policies. Typically, the Internet is partitioned into different administrative *domains*. A domain shall usually correspond to a large organization operating an internal corporate network or an *Internet Service Provider (ISP)* (e.g. *UUNET, MCI, Wanadoo, AOL*). A domain is simply speaking a *network* made of *nodes* and *links*. The Internet terminology distinguishes two kinds of nodes: a *router* is a node that forwards packets not explicitly addressed to itself, whereas a *host* is any node that is not a router. Nodes connected on the same communication link form a *subnetwork* (typically, an *Ethernet* link, or a *802.11b WLAN*). Subnetworks are interconnected by means of routers. The node that initiates or terminates the transmission of a packet is referred to as the *end-node*, i.e. the source or the destination of the packet.

2.2 The TCP/IP reference model

Internetworking is performed by the *TCP/IP* reference model which defines the protocol suite used for data exchange between nodes in the Internet. TCP/IP is a *packet-switched* technology. Unlike *circuit-switched* technologies like telephone networks, TCP/IP relies on the *connectionless* concept: routers cooperate to determine the path toward the destination and carry packets between the two end-nodes. The forwarding decision called *routing* is made on a per-packet basis. The intelligence is put at the edge of the network (i.e. end-nodes), whereas the purpose of the network infrastructure is only to provide internetworking. This allows an easy deployment of new functionalities without need to upgrade the network infrastructure. As a result from this, the Internet is not specific network-technology-dependent, allowing a global network of unlimited scope and reach. This has largely accounted for its success.

TCP/IP is very similar to the *OSI reference model*, but does not map well into the seven layers as defined by *ISO*. It has fewer layers than its OSI counterpart as the use of intermediate abstraction layers between the *transport layer* and the *application layer* was not perceived. As its name stands for, it is named after its two main protocols, *Transport Control Protocol (TCP)* [18] and *Internet Protocol (IP)* [3, 17]. IP corresponds to OSI's network layer. Its role is to interconnect all the subnetworks so that any two nodes can communicate with each other. It defines a number of rules, a packet header format, and an addressing scheme which aims at identifying nodes and determining their position in the network hierarchy. It is assisted by a number of other protocols like routing protocols that determine the path a packet has to take between the source and the destination. There presently exists two versions of IP, the getting old IPv4, and the new generation IPv6 [3]. IPv6 is meant to replace IPv4 and to address its shortcomings. IPv6 has built-in features that allow to support the new services requested by recent applications. This includes embedded security and support for mobility, extension headers to specify additional information, native multicast, provisions for traffic reservation, etc. IPv6 also offers a generous number of addresses compared to IPv4. IPv6 addresses are 128-bits large. In theory, this would allow to allocate an address to billions of nodes on every square meter on Earth. In practice, it is much less due to allocation rules but still enough to embed an IPv6 stack in every computer, camera, phone, watch, sensor, etc, ever produced on Earth. For the novice reader, we advice [9, 13].

2.3 *Mobility in the Internet*

Mobility in the Internet arises when a portion of the network changes its point of attachment to the overall topology. However, the Internet is hardly tuned to allow mobility in the midst of data transfers because protocols have not been conceived for devices that change their point of attachment in the topology. Each device is identified by a unique IPv6 address with a prefix which shows the location of the devices in the Internet topology. There is typically a change of this physical IPv6 address each time a *mobile node* (*MN*) changes its point of attachment and thus its reachability in the Internet topology. Support mechanisms are then necessary to maintain open connections. In some cases, the mobile node may indeed be a *mobile router* with a number of nodes (*MNNs*) attached behind it. This forms what we refer to as a *mobile network*. Only the MR changes its physical point of attachment and thus its address. However, this changes of address has an impact on routing to the entire mobile network. This results in losing packets in transit and breaking transport protocols connections if mobility is not handled by specific services.

3 Functional Needs

In this section, we elaborate the requirements for the communication system from a functional point of view. Basically, the system must allow permanent communication between the patient and the peers, real-time monitoring, and improve the dependence of disabled and elderly people.

- Ubiquity: to ensure the system is reachable at any time, any place, with anyone.
- Permanent Connectivity: to maintain connectivity between the patient and its peers while moving.
- Reliability: to guarantee against loss of access coverage of a particular wireless technology and against failure of equipments
- Scalability: to guarantee an expanding number of equipments and users
- Safety: to ensure a proper operation of the system with no risk for the user and to prevent intruders from breaking or disrupting the data communication flows.
- Privacy/Confidentiality: mechanism to prevent intruders from accessing personal information of individuals
- Multimedia Applications: given his deficiencies in using all his senses, the user needs enhanced means to communicate with peers. The overall system must be able to combine data originated or intended to different kinds of senses: vision (images and video, through digital camera, camera, web camera, displays), voice (through microphone and amplifier), touch (through movement detector, blood pressure) and environmental data (humidity, temperature, air pressure, location).
- Real-Time Monitoring: to perform a permanent health check and to guarantee that proper action would be taken in a timely manner and the most effective way in case of health troubles.
- Ease of Use: users of the system may not have knowledge in the underlying technologies and may have limited physical and intellectual abilities. The usage of the system must be as simple as turning the light on.

4 The Communication System

In this section, we elaborate the networking features required to meet the functional needs.

4.1 IPv6

IP is the de-facto protocol to unify the different technologies. A number of reasons drive us to favor IPv6 over IPv4. First, IPv6 has built-in features that allow to support more effectively the new services requested by new demanding applications. This includes support for mobility, multicast, traffic reservation, security, etc. A second reason is that IPv6 offers a generous number of addresses compared to IPv4. As the number of devices connected to the Internet is grooving to millions, it is necessary to have a sufficiently large number of addresses. Not to say, it is also necessary to ensure that the system under development will be compatible with future devices. Basically, any kind of device, like a mobile phone or a watch will ultimately be connected to the Internet, and this will be IPv6, not IPv4. Lastly, deploying IPv6 devices should make application development costs cheaper since these applications and devices wouldn't only be developed for telematics.

4.2 Network Mobility Support

In order to achieve the ubiquitous Internet, connection to the network must be available everywhere, at anytime, without disruption of service, even when a device moves. A mechanism is required to manage the mobility of the equipment within the Internet topology. Mobile IPv6 [11] is usually sought to manage mobility of a single IPv6 device. The disadvantage of this approach is that all embedded devices must be designed to operate this protocol. The IETF NEMO working group [15, 7] has thus been set up recently in an effort to address issues related to network mobility, i.e. entire IPv6 networks that change their point of attachment to the Internet topology. Such work allow to set up network of sensors and exchange data between those sensors and remote computers, while on the move, and transparently to the sensors. The protocol to manage the mobility of entire networks, i.e. NEMO Basic Support [4] is surely a better approach than Mobile IPv6 because it allows to bring an unlimited number of usual IPv6 devices behind a mobile router.

The first task of the working group was to define a terminology [7] which we use in this paper. A MR has at least two interfaces, the *egress interface* is first attached to the home link, and later to a visited link. The *ingress interface* is attached to an *internal link* in the mobile network. All nodes (MR and *MNNs*) attached to a given internal link have their addresses taken from the same mobile network prefixes advertised on this link. *MNNs* are either *fixed nodes* or *mobile nodes*. Fixed nodes are unable to change their point of attachment while keeping their connections open, whereas mobile nodes have this ability, presumably using Mobile IPv6. If such a mobile node is indeed a MR with a number of nodes behind it, a sub-NEMO is getting attached to a root-NEMO. In this former case, the aggregated network is said to be *nested*.

The working group is working on a solution termed *NEMO Basic Support* [4]. The primary objective is to preserve session continuity between CNs and all MNNs behind the MR while the MR changes its point of attachment. This protocol associates each egress interface of a MR with two distinct addresses, much like what is done in Mobile IPv6. The *home address* (HoA) serves as a permanent location invariant identifier whereas the *care-of address* (CoA) serves as a routing directive to the current point of attachment. The permanent HoA is obtained in the home network and has the same prefix as the home link. The temporary CoA is obtained in the visited network and formed based on the prefix advertised on the visited link. The purpose of the protocol is to establish bi-directional tunnels between the home links and the mobile network for each couple HoA/CoA.

4.3 *Multihoming*

To ensure safety and reliability, a continuous connectivity to the Internet must be provided, at anytime, any place. For doing so, the mobile network is preferably best connected via several interfaces, several access technologies and to distinct access networks [8], which we refer to as *multihomed mobile network*. Distinct interfaces may indeed be active simultaneously. As a result, the system must be able to deal with both *horizontal handovers* (between access points using the same communication medium) and *vertical handovers* (between distinct communication medium). As a wide coverage nor a lack of failure cannot be ensured by a single *Internet Service Provider* (ISP), handovers may need to be performed between distinct administrative domains and thus topologically distant parts of the Internet (*global mobility*). This may occur, for instance, when access is offered by different ISPs. The latter is effective to keep communication costs low from a user's point of view. Having multiple points of attachment is also effective to avoid disruption of service when either a particular technology is not available in the geographic area or when one is experiencing some sort of failure. Besides this, provided simultaneous access are available, data must be sent on the most efficient available media according to the type of flow. A number of issues must still be solved first to multihomed mobile networks. Such issues are presently discussed at the IETF within the NEMO working group [16].

4.4 *Seamless Mobility and Adaptive Applications*

Smooth handoffs from one access point to another are necessary to avoid abrupt degradation of the connectivity. This could be provided by FMIPv6, HMIPv6, CARD and other protocols. On the other hand, vertical handoffs between distinct access technologies will necessary result into changes of network conditions. Applications must thus be able to dynamically adapt to the available bandwidth. For instance, transmitting video over a GSM link is not possible, so the application has to switch to a less bandwidth-consuming mode (e.g. refreshing a picture every ten seconds).

4.5 *Security and Other Features*

IPSec and AAA are protocols that can provide for the necessary security, authentication, and confidentiality. Auto-configuration mechanisms allow the system to set up by itself without human intervention.

5 The E-Wheelchair Testbed

We are setting up various IPv6 equipments on an electrical wheelchair. The intend is not to develop an effective prototype at the time being, but to demonstrate and validate the underlying IPv6 technologies. We are currently validating our protocol implementations and communication system on our indoor validation testbed and we are purchasing equipment for our outdoor demonstration testbed.

5.1 *The E-Wheelchair Communication System*

We are relying on NEMO Basic Support (see section **??**) to manage the mobility of the mobile network and provide permanent monitoring. A permanent connectivity and reliability is ensured from multihoming abilities of the system. We will use several wireless technologies to connect to the Internet. Applications sit on other CPUs in the mobile network; a protocol is being designed to exchange preference settings and network quality between demanding applications and the mobile router. The mobile router connecting the mobile network to the Internet will thus be able to choose the most effective available link, according to the need of the application. Demanding applications will thus be able to adapt their flow according to the network conditions. Security between the mobile router and the home agent is provided by IPSec, while authentication and confidentiality will be ensured by proper AAA and encryption mechanisms.

5.2 The Indoor Validation Testbed

The current testbed allows multiple configurations of mobile networks, including nested and multihomed mobile networks. It is composed of two mobile routers and two home agents, each running NetBSD 1.6.1 and NEMO Basic Support. The mobile router is actually connected to a PC which emulates interface switching. Network conditions are thus changing periodically. This allows to performed our tests automatically, as if the mobile router was switching its egress interface between the mobile router's home network and four foreign networks.

Several IPv6 nodes are located behind the mobile router. This includes an IPv6 sensor, and an IPv6 camera. The IPv6 sensor is a prototype designed by the WIDE for the InternetCAR project [10]. It is queried by SNMP-v2 and provides the temperature and the humidity (values are indeed estimated by a number of measures taken over a short period of time). Power can be provided by a power-over-Ethernet hub. The IPv6 camera is a commercial product, and can be manipulated remotely. One can presently monitor the current temperature and manipulate the camera from the web (see http://www.nautilus6.org/show.html, but access to the IPv6 camera is of course restricted for obvious reasons).

Our implementation of NEMO Basic Support [14] is based on the second version of the NEMO Basic Support specification and is presented as an extension of KAME MIPv6 [1] for NetBSD 1.6.1. It supports MR and HA functionalities and both explicit and implicit modes. The HA supports both modes whereas MR can switch from one mode to the other. The implementation also supports DHAAD and IPSec protection between HA and MR. The MR can have multiple interfaces, each with a specific preference. The NEMO Basic Support implementation works fine on a regular basis as it can be seen by monitoring the temperature and humidity provided by the IPv6 sensor located behind the MR and the emulator. We are currently testing multihoming configurations, following the classification provided in [16] and [6]. The results of tests already performed are published in [12].

5.3 The Outdoor Demonstration Testbed

For the demonstration, we have investigated several equipments as for the mobile router, including a PDA running linux, a Soekris mother card, and a laptop. After a few tests and purchases, we end up nowhere with the PDA (hardware limitations), while we are faced with battery issues with the Soekris mother card. We have thus finally selected a new tiny laptop from SONY (VAIO type U50/U70), for its convenience of use (compact size, the display can be shut down, and the keyboard can be removed, battery life time), the numerous potential interfaces, and the possibility to use it under linux or BSD. It can thus easily be used as a mobile router. The heartbeat sensor remains to be designed, whereas the other are already available.

The mobile router will be connected to the Internet via WLAN 802.11 series (native IPv6), cellular phone (using PPP) and AirH (using L2TP because this technology doesn't yet support IPv6). Others communication medium such like a satellite (possibly one-way only, using UDLR) could be envisioned.

We are investigating the purchase of an electric wheelchair. The electrical power of the wheelchair will in essence give power to some of the various IPv6 equipments, though most of them could actually rely on their own batteries, as far the demonstration of the sole communication technologies is concerned. The wheelchair will be equipped with various IPv6 sensors: an IPv6 GPS sensor to determine the location of the wheelchair, an IPv6 sensor to monitor the health of the person (heart-beat sensor) and an IPv6 environmental sensor (temperature and humidity sensor). An IPv6 camera, with remote movement control facilities restricted to a limited number of peers will transmit video of the surrounding scene or of the disabled person. The flow of video will depend on the available wireless technology and may be limited to a single picture refreshed from time to time.

6 Related Projects

The E-Care Town Project [5] aims at creating a town in which people of all ages: young and old, healthy and disabled, can feel comfortable, safe and enjoy living in. Six types of monitoring programs have been defined (e-Health Up Program, e-Family Care Program, e-Nursing Care Program, e-Professional Skill Up Course Program, e-Resident Health Course Program and e-Care Information Security Program). IPv6 equipments and data communication methods are being used, but the project currently doesn't consider IPv6 mobility support mechanisms such as Mobile IP, NEMO, FMIP, etc.

7 Conclusion

The purpose of this paper is to demonstrate how cutting-edge Internet technologies based on IPv6 and network mobility will allow to improve mobility and independence of people with health deficiencies. We have defined the necessary communication system, based on IPv6 and NEMO and we are actively involved at the IETF in the specification of the required protocols. E-Wheelchair is only one of the potential usages of the proposed system. Our E-Wheelchair demonstration testbed is under development while IPv6 implementations are being validated. More in-depth performance evaluation of the system will be performed once the complete system is fully set-up.

Acknowledgments

We are thankful to the members of the Nautilus6 team for all the fruitful discussion that led to set up this demonstration testbed and to the members of the InternetCAR team for providing equipments and advices. As for the current realization of the experiment, we are particularly indebted to Koshiro Mitsuya (testbed set up, NEMO implementation), Romain Kuntz (tests of the equipment), and Francois Leiber (applications).

References

[1] The IPv6 KAME Project, As of 2004. http://www.kame.net.

[2] WIDE Nautilus6 Working Group Web Page, As of July 2004. http://www.nautilus6.org.

[3] S. Deering and R. Hinden. Internet Protocol Version 6 (IPv6) Specification. Request For Comments 2460, December 1998.

[4] Vijay Devarapalli, Ryuji Wakikawa, Alexandru Petrescu, and Pascal Thubert. NEMO Basic Support Protocol. Internet Draft draft-ietf-nemo-basic-support-03.txt, IETF, June 2004. Work in progress.

[5] E-Care. e-Care Town Fujisawa Project Consortium, As of 2004. http://www.e-care-project.jp/english/index.html.

[6] Thierry Ernst and Julien Charbon. Multihoming with NEMO Basic Support. In *First International Conference on Mobile Computing and Ubiquitous Computing (ICMU)*, Yokosuka, Japan, January 2004.

[7] Thierry Ernst and Hong-Yon Lach. Network Mobility Support Terminology. Internet Draft draft-ietf-nemo-terminology-01.txt, IETF, February 2004. Work in progress.

[8] Thierry Ernst, Nicolas Montavont, and Ryuji Wakikawa. Goals and Benefits of Multihoming. Internet Draft draft-multihoming-generic-goals-and-benefits-01, IETF, April 2004. Work in progress.

[9] Christian Huitema. *IPv6 The New Internet Protocol*. Prentice Hall, 2nd edition, 1998.

[10] InternetCAR. WIDE InternetCAR Working Group Web Page, May 2002. http://www.sfc.wide.ad.jp/InternetCAR.

[11] David B. Johnson, C. Perkins, and Jari Arkko. Mobility Support in IPv6. Request For Comments 3775, IETF, June 2004.

[12] Romain Kuntz, EunKyoung Paik, Manabu Tsukada, Thierrry Ernst, and Koshiro Mitsuya. Evaluating Multiple Mobile Routers and Multiple NEMO-Prefixes in NEMO Basic Support. Internet-Draft draft-kuntz-nemo-multihoming-test-00.txt, IETF, July 2004.

[13] David C. Lee, Daniel L. Lough, Scott F. Midkiff, Nathaniel J. Davis, and Phillip E. Benchoff. The Next Generation of the Internet: Aspects of the Internet Protocol Version 6. *IEEE Network*, January 1998. Virginia Polytechnic and State University.

[14] Koshiro Mitsuya. Nautilus6 NEMO Basic Support Implementation. Technical Report ir-nemo-bs-20040712-MitsuyaK.pdf, WIDE at Keio University, April 2004. http://www.nautilus6.org/doc/ir-nemo-bs-20040712-MitsuyaK.pdf.

[15] NEMO. IETF Network Mobility Working Group Web Page, October 2002. http://www.ietf.org/html.charters/nemo-charter.html.

[16] C.W Ng, Eun Kyoung Paik, and Thierry Ernst. Analysis of Multihoming in Network Mobility Support. Internet Draft draft-ietf-nemo-multihoming-issues-00, IETF, July 2004. Work in progress.

[17] Postel. Internet Protocol DARPA Internet Program Protocol Specification. Request For Comments 791, IETF, September 1981.

[18] Postel. Transmission Control Protocol DARPA Internet Program Protocol Specification. Request For Comments 793, IETF, September 1981.

[19] WIDE. WIDE Project: Widely Integrated Distributed Environment, June 2002. http://www.wide.ad.jp.

A New Service Delivery and Provisioning Architecture for Home Appliances

Daqing Zhang, Zhengning Dai, Xiaohang Wang, Xiao Ni, Song Zheng
{daqing, zhengning, xwang, nixiao, szheng}@i2r.a-star.edu.sg
Institute for Infocomm Research, 21 Heng Mui Keng Terrace, Singapore 119613

Abstract. This paper presents a new service delivery and provisioning architecture for home appliances. The basic idea is to subtly incorporate SIP (Session Initiation Protocol) Internet telephony signalling architecture into the OSGi (Open Service Gateway Initiative) service delivery and provisioning framework. Thus the strengths of OSGi and SIP are unified so that wide range of services and devices can be supported. A prototype system is implemented to show the feasibility of the novel architecture.

1. Introduction

Nowadays the number of networked homes and the number of networked appliances are proliferating at an accelerated pace. Although there is an expanding list of home networking technologies (e.g. Bluetooth, IEEE 802.11, HPNA, Jini, UPnP, HAVi, X-10 [1]) to interconnect home appliances, none of them provide necessary support for wide area communication. In order to provide an open and flexible solution to wide area access and management of home appliances, the Open Service Gateway Initiative (OSGi) was founded in 1999. OSGi developed a service-oriented architecture and defined open specifications for delivery and provisioning of software services over wide area network to local devices [2]. OSGi uses a service gateway to bridge the Internet and all the home appliances [3], a service framework is embedded in each gateway to facilitate service delivery and life-cycle management. The service gateway serves as a central point to coordinate home appliances and enable compound services across different home networking standards.

Session Initiation Protocol (SIP) was initially proposed as a signaling protocol in Internet Telephony domain [4]; it was soon found to be applicable to remote access of home appliances across Internet [5]. SIP is a lightweight protocol that fits especially well in mobile devices and small appliances with limited processing power; it supports mobility and asynchronous communication inherently.

While most of the research on OSGi lies in accommodating home networking technologies [6][7], no work has questioned the capability of underlying application layer communication protocol HTTP which OSGi relies on to deliver services. Whereas reference [8] has given a preliminary solution to hook SIP to OSGi platform, its focus is more on the evaluation of SIP as an access solution. It didn't make any attempt to propose a general service-oriented architecture to combine the benefits of SIP and OSGi. In this paper, we propose a new service delivery and provisioning architecture by incorporating the SIP into the OSGi. In such a way, the features of both SIP and OSGi are inherited, much wider range of services and devices are supported.

The rest of the paper is organized as follows. Section 2 and Section 3 give an overview of the OSGi and SIP for home appliance access, respectively. Based on the OSGi and SIP system architecture, the new system architecture is presented in Section 4. The prototype system is described in Section 5. The conclusions of this work are drawn in Section 6.

2. OSGi and Service Delivery

OSGi aims to define open specifications for the delivery and provisioning of services over wide area network to local devices in homes, cars and other intelligent environments.

2.1 OSGi Architectural Framework

The OSGi architectural framework was formulated based on the requirements from several new markets. Fig. 1 shows a typical OSGi architectural framework for end-to-end service delivery and provisioning. The major components of the complete OSGi architectural framework include:

- **OSGi service gateway**: The central component of OSGi is the service gateway. The service gateway mainly handles two separate tasks: a). managing communications to and from local area networks. b). hosting the service platform which includes the OSGi framework and services. The typical communication functionality of a service gateway includes IP traffic forwarding, firewall and Network Address Translation (NAT). The common service supporting functionality includes service life cycle management and service collaboration. The service framework can be viewed as an embedded server augmented with services; it is based on JAVA to make it platform independent.

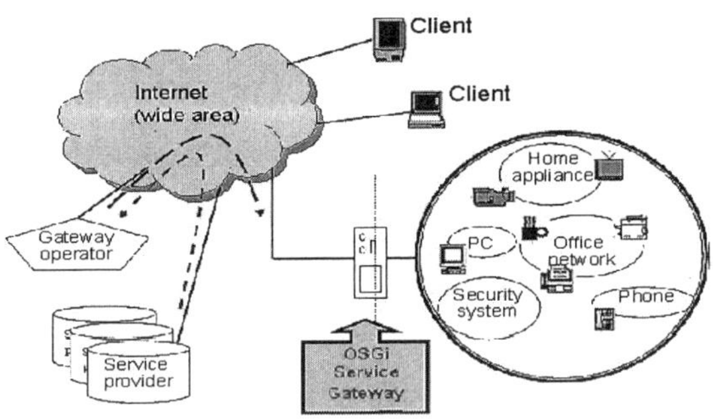

OSGi Service Gateway in the Big Picture

Fig. 1 OSGi architectural framework

- **Service provider:** The service provider provides a range of services such as energy management, safety and security, health care, home automation etc. to consumers. The services are delivered to the OSGi service gateway through HTTP and can be accessed either inside the home network or in the Internet.
- **Gateway operator:** The gateway operator's role is to manage and maintain the service gateway and its services. Functions of a typical gateway operator range from starting, stopping, updating, and removing services to managing the status of the service gateways.
- **Wide Area Network:** The Internet provides the necessary communications between the service gateway, the end user, the gateway operator and the service provider.
- **Local Area Network and devices:** The last major piece of the OSGi is the local area network and the devices connected to the OSGi service gateway.

OSGi provides a service-oriented model to access home appliances. Deploying new features of any device would be translated into putting new services in the OSGi. In such a way, the complexity of the home network technologies is hidden from the end users. Only the required services are made available to them in a friendly manner.

2.2 OSGi Framework

OSGi Framework provides an execution environment for services. The framework includes a Java runtime environment extended with service life cycle management, persistent data storage, version management, and a service registry. Whereas basic services like device access control, log service, http service etc. are integrated with the framework, application services need to be developed using the basic services. Fig. 2 shows the software architecture of the OSGi service gateway.

The life cycle management provided by the framework allows application developers to divide their applications into small self-installable components, called bundles. Bundles are software components implemented in Java that can be downloaded, installed, and activated in a framework. When activated, bundles may register services in the service registry, to provide services to other bundles in the framework. When a service is no longer needed it can easily be removed from the framework, without affecting other bundles. Bundles can be installed and updated in a dynamic and scalable fashion. New bundles can be installed for added features, and existing bundles can be modified and updated, without having to restart the entire system. The service registry is used to find and use other services in a secure and controlled manner. The service gateway operator has full control over the platform and it decides which service bundles are allowed to use.

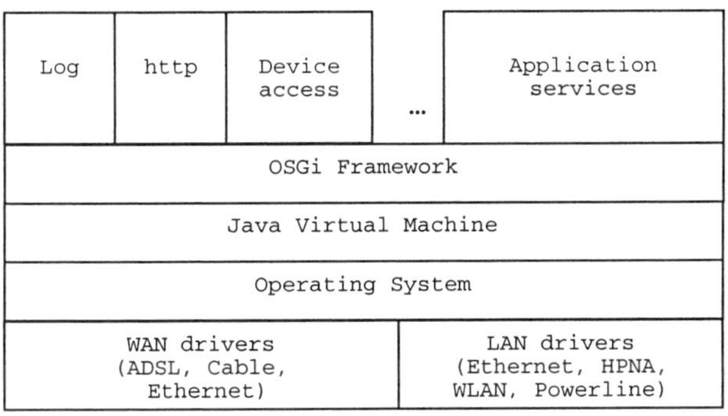

Fig. 2 Software architecture of OSGi service gateway

2.3 OSGi Bundles

In OSGi, bundles are the only software entities for deploying applications. A bundle is a Java ARchive (JAR) file that comprises classes and other resources. The bundle typically contains Java class files and non-executable resources such as HTML presentation and help files. A bundle also contains a manifest file, describing the contents of a JAR file and providing information about the bundle. The manifest file contains special headers to describe the bundle to the framework and states the bundle's dependencies on external Java classes. Furthermore, the manifest file designates a special class to be used as the bundle activator. The framework must use this class and invoke its start and stop methods to start or stop the bundle respectively.

2.4 Key Features of OSGi

The key characteristics of the OSGi include:

- **Platform independence**: Any platform supports Java can run OSGi service framework.

- **Service provider independence**: Common foundation for different service providers to deliver wide range of services.
- **Service collaboration support**: OSGi framework allows services deployed to be discovered and used by other services.
- **Multiple device access protocol coexistence**: OSGi can inter-operate with all existing device access protocols.
- **Security and simplicity**: an OSGi environment reduces the complexity of managing services and guarantees the access to services from different service providers.

2.5 Main Limitations of OSGi

However, OSGi also has the following limitations:

- HTTP is a heavy weight protocol which needs considerable amount of processing power and memory.
- HTTP cannot address the home appliances behind NAT, thus home appliances cannot be accessed directly by a remote HTTP terminal.
- HTTP is connection oriented and does not support multimedia service delivery efficiently.
- HTTP does not support asynchronous communication.

3. SIP for Home Appliance Access

SIP was initially proposed as a signaling protocol in Internet Telephony domain, it has been identified as one of the most promising ways for multimedia communication over today's data networks [9][10]. SIP is designed to work independently of the underlying protocol, so the message in SIP can be sent using either TCP or UDP. SIP provides a flexible way for devices in the WAN to exchange information in a peer-to-peer manner.

3.1 SIP Architecture

There are different entities defined in SIP: User Agent (UA), Proxy Servers, Redirect Servers and Location Servers. SIP UA can take either a client or server role, it initiates request while serving as a client and reacts to request while acting as a server. Proxies fulfill the tasks of application-layer routers, they forward SIP request and response messages. Unlike Proxies, Redirect Servers do not forward messages directly but return the address of a SIP User agent or proxy server. Location Servers contain location information for all the registered devices. A typical SIP request originates from a user agent, passes through a number of proxies and redirect servers until it terminates at the remote user agent.

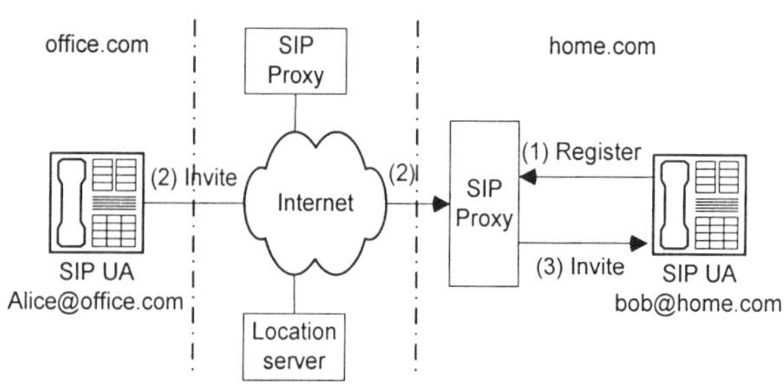

Fig. 3 SIP architecture and call flow

Fig.3 shows the SIP architecture and the steps involved when a user Alice in the office wants to call another user Bob at home. When Bob's SIP phone (UA) powers up, it registers with the home proxy server home.com and the location server, indicating that Bob can be reached at bob@home.com. To initiate the IP call to sip:bob@home.com, Alice's SIP phone, which registers with the office SIP proxy server office.com, sends an Invite message to a nearby SIP proxy. The SIP proxy will then try to resolve the destination address by consulting the location servers and forward the message to Bob's home proxy home.com which will finally pass the message to Bob' SIP phone. The session description protocol (SDP), carried in SIP requests and responses, describes the list of supported features and the transport addresses to receive them. The communication between Alice and Bob then takes place according to the parameters agreed by both devices.

3.2 SIP for Home Appliance Access

SIP was extended to access and control the networked appliances in the home by Tsang etc. [5]. The basic idea is to extend SIP so that the control message and other information can be exchanged between the remote access terminal and the home appliances in a peer-to-peer manner. Fig. 4 shows the SIP architecture for home appliances access.

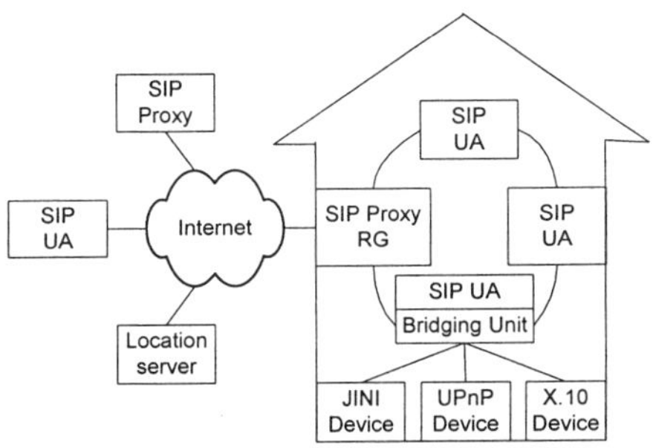

Fig. 4 SIP architecture for home appliance access

Home appliances are connected through various home networks to the Residential Gateway (RG), and the RG also bridges the home network to Internet. RG is usually equipped with firewall and Network Address Translation capability, which provides protection from unauthorised access to the home appliances. If each appliance or appliance controller assumes SIP UA functionality and the RG assumes SIP proxy functionality, then the SIP UA attached in either Internet or home network can access the home appliances using SIP. It is important to note that the appliance controller needs to function as both a SIP UA and a bridging unit; it receives the SIP message from originating SIP UA, retrieves the information and passes it to the controlled devices. The SIP extensions and modifications include [11, 12]:

- URLs are extended to address all the appliances.
- A new method, DO, is defined to issue command instead of setting up sessions.
- A new payload type is specified.
- SUBSCRIBE and NOTIFY methods of SIP are used to support asynchronous communication of devices.

3.3 The Features of SIP

In summary, SIP has the following features:

- **Scalability**: SIP suits for both LAN and WAN, it works with UDP as well as TCP.
- **Simplicity and Flexibility**: SIP is a light weight and text based protocol. It is very simple to add extensions to support new features.
- **Mobility**: a SIP device can REGISTER its current location to a local SIP-proxy. So a calling device does not need to know where the called device is exactly located. The proxy will resolve the address and ensure the message will arrive at the right destination.
- **Service Convergence**: In addition to VoIP, SIP can support wide range of services (e.g. Instant Messaging) through simple extensions, whereas infrastructure remains the same.

4. New Service Delivery Architecture

As described in Section 2, OSGi specifies an ideal service oriented framework for remote home appliance access and management; the main problems of OSGi are all related to the limitations of HTTP. More specifically, these problems are caused by the connection-oriented nature of TCP. If connectionless transport protocol like UDP is also supported for service delivery and access, then the problems like effective multimedia support and asynchronous notification will be alleviated. Fortunately, we have noticed that SIP is such an application level protocol which can complement with HTTP.

Whereas SIP is mainly designed for multimedia service, it also provides interesting services such as instant messaging and presence. However, SIP itself is more for signalling, it is not designed for general service delivery and management requested in the home. Thus a natural way of thinking is: can we find a cost effective way to combine the benefits of the OSGi based service delivery system and SIP based Internet telephony system. In this section, we propose a new service delivery and access approach by incorporating the SIP architecture into the OSGi service delivery and access system. The basic idea is:

- Preserve the OSGi service delivery and provisioning architectural framework.
- Make use of the SIP based Internet telephony signalling architecture.
- Extend SIP with new methods and payload types for home appliances access.
- Incoroperate the SIP proxy in the residential gateway, design a SIP UA and bridging unit service bundle in the OSGi service gateway platform.

The new service delivery and access architecture can be shown in Fig. 5. The main difference between the new system architecture and the previous two systems lies in the software in RG. In respect to the OSGi service framework, the major effort is to implement the SIP proxy, SIP UA and Bridging Unit in the form of OSGi service bundles. In such a way, the two systems are unified subtly while the development effort is kept quite small. The most straightforward benefit the end users can enjoy from the new system is that they can use either HTTP terminal or SIP terminal to access broader range of services ubiquitously. Further more, not only the centralized way of accessing the home appliances through invoking services in RG is supported via HTTP or SIP, but also the peer-to-peer way of accessing home appliances through SIP is maintained. More interestingly, future services from both OSGi and SIP world can be supported inherently. In summary, the proposed architecture exhibits the following features:

- The capability of OSGi in remotely managing the life cycle of services, in unifying all home networking technologies as well as in supporting a common development environment is maintained.
- The rich services of SIP based telephony system like instant messaging, presence, VoIP etc. are inherited. When 3G or 4G multimedia devices become popular, SIP will be crucial for enabling mobile and ubiquitous Internet services.

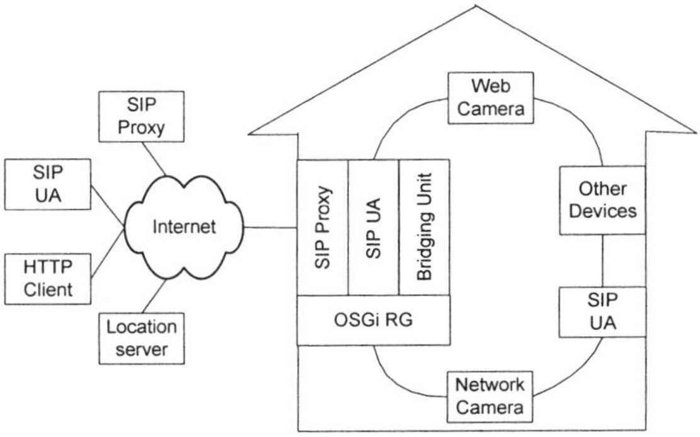

Figure 5 New service delivery and access architecture

- Both HTTP and SIP terminals can be used to access the service, wider range of home appliances and services are supported.
- The strengths of OSGi and SIP based service framework are unified while the development effort is kept to designing reusable service bundles which bridge SIP and other protocols.

5. Implementation Prototype

In order to verify the feasibility of the new architecture, a prototype system has been implemented as shown in Fig. 6. The prototype consists of one client PC connected to Internet, a residential gateway connecting Internet to home network, one web camera connected to the USB port of RG, one AXIS 2100 network camera and one SIP enabled IP telephone connected to RG through Ethernet. Whereas the client PC has both a web browser and SIP user agent, it's used to access the services in RG, aiming to simulate the functionality of remote HTTP and SIP terminals. The RG hosts the OSGi framework, HTTP services, device control services, UPnP service as well as SIP service bundles. It provides a service repository which allows access from either HTTP or SIP terminal; it also serves as an access point interconnecting home appliances in the local network. The web camera and network camera are two devices used to demonstrate the suveillance service. The SIP enabled IP telephone set is used to show the audio/video delivery capability to the remote SIP UA.

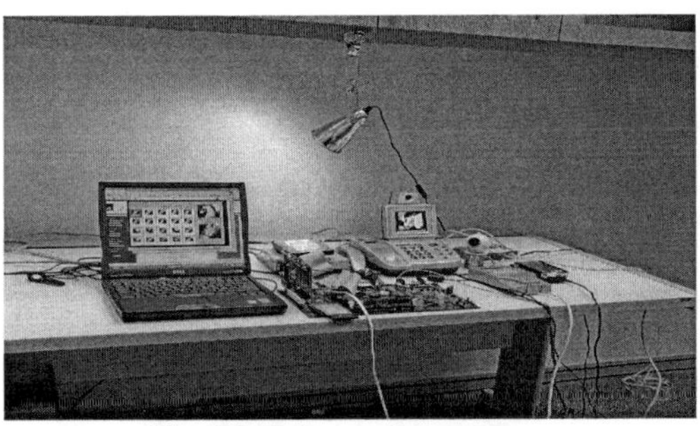

Fig. 6 Prototype system set-up

The RG is Intel Celeron based with embedded Linux (kernel 2.4.17). The OSGi framework adopted is GateSpace OSGi Platform. The SIP Proxy and SIP UA are implemented using Vovida SIP stack. The AXIS camera is an UPnP enabled device and its services are registered in OSGi when the camera is attached to the network. The UPnP services can then be used by other services in the OSGi framework. Using the prototype, three usage scenarios are tested: (1) services on top of OSGi framework in RG delivered to web browser of a HTTP terminal outside home; (2) services on top of OSGi framework in RG delivered to SIP UA of a SIP terminal outside home; and (3) IP enabled devices in home communicate with SIP UA of SIP terminal outside home.

The first scenario corresponds to the original OSGI service delivery and access usage model, where users can control home appliances and stream video through HTTP. The second scenario corresponds to the usage model where SIP is used to convey control message as well as data in the case of applying SIP for remote access of home appliances. The third scenario corresponds to the typical usage model where SIP is used as a signalling protocol for Intenet telephony services and RTP is used to stream multimedia. Fig. 7 (a) and (b) show the results of delivering home monitoring services to the HTTP and SIP terminals, respectively.

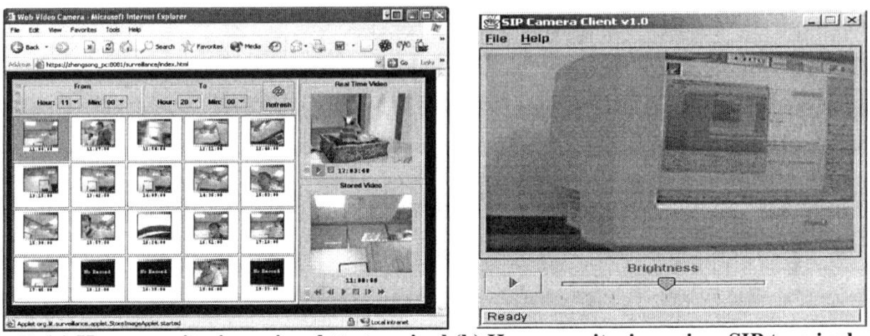

Fig. 7 (a) Home monitoring using http terminal (b) Home monitoring using SIP terminal

6. Conclusion

In this paper, a new service delivery and provisioning architecture for home appliances by incorporating SIP into OSGi is proposed and implemented. The novel system inherits the features of both OSGi and, it provides users with the flexibility to use either HTTP or SIP terminals to access much broader range of services and home appliances. The new architecture successfully unifies the two major and promising wide area access technolgies and can potentially enhance the value of OSGi in the service market. Future work will be on turning the idea of this paper into part of the OSGi specifications.

References

[1] B. Rose, "Home Networks: A Standards Perspective," *IEEE Commun. Mag.*, pp 78-85, Dec. 2001.

[2] OSGi Specification v. 2.0, Nov. 2001. http://www.osgi.org

[3] K. Chen and L. Gong, *Programming Open Service Gateways with Java Embedded Server Technology*, Addison-Wesley, 2001.

[4] M. Handley, H. Schulzrinne, E. Schooler, and J. Rosenberg,, "SIP: Session Initiation Protocol", *IETF RFC 2543*, March 1999.

[5] S. Tsang, S. Moyer, D. Marples, H. Schulzrinne, and A. Roychowdhury, "SIP Extensions for Networked Appliance Communications", *IETF Internet Draft*, draft-tsang-sip-appliances-do-00.txt, Nov. 2000.

[6] P. Dobrev, D. Famolari, C. Kurzke, and B.A. Miller, "Device and Service Discovery in Home Networks with OSGi," *IEEE Comm. Mag.*, pp 86-92, Aug. 2002.

[7] D. Marples and P. Kriens, "The Open Services Gateway Initiative: An Introductory Overview," *IEEE Commun. Mag.*, pp 110-114, Dec. 2001.

[8] H. Wessung, Home Access Technology, MS Thesis, Umea University, Sweden, 2001.

[9] H. Schulzrinne and J. Rosenberg,, "The Session Initiation Protocol: Internet-Centric Signaling", *IEEE Commun. Mag.*, pp 2-9, Oct. 2000.

[10] J. Rosenberg, Distributed Algorithms and Protocols for Scalable Internet Telephony, PhD Dissertation, Columbia University, USA, 2001.

[11] S. Moyer, D. Marples, S. Tsang, and A. Ghosh, "Service Portability of Networked Appliances" *IEEE Comm. Mag.*, pp 116-121, Jan. 2002.

[12] S. Moyer, D. Marples, S. Tsang, J. Katz, P. Gurung, T. Cheng, A. Dutta, H. Schulzrinne, and A. Roychowdhury, "Framework Draft for Networked Appliances using SIP", *IETF Internet Draft*, draft-moyer-sip-appliances-framework-02.ps, June 2001.

Toward a Human-Friendly Assistive Environment
D. Zhang and M. Mokhtari (Eds.)
IOS Press, 2004

Location-Aided On-Demand (LAOD) Routing Protocol for Hybrid Wired-Wireless Networks

M.T. Wu
National University of Singapore
4 Engineering Drive 3
Singapore 117576
Email: stuwumt@i2r.a-star.edu.sg

Winston K.G. Seah & W.C. Wong
Institute for Infocomm Research
21 Heng Mui Keng Terrace
Singapore 119613
Email: {winston, lwong}@i2r.a-star.edu.sg

Abstract. We present the Location-Aided On-Demand (LAOD) routing protocol aimed to achieve better routing performance in a hybrid wired and wireless multi-hop network environment by exploiting the location information of the mobile nodes. This routing protocol is designed to provide wireless multi-hop paths, which can be wireless routing path or wireless-cum-wired routing path. A key concern of our routing protocol design is how to utilize the gateways without congesting them with excessive communication. We use simulation to evaluate the performance of our routing protocol and the results show that it achieves higher packet delivery ratio at the expense of higher routing overhead and average end-to-end delay.

1 Introduction

A mobile ad hoc network (MANET) [1] is a dynamic multi-hop wireless network without any established infrastructure. Each mobile node can communicate with other mobile nodes, which may be multi-hops away, using intermediate nodes as routers. Therefore, each mobile node in the network can act both as a host and as a router.

An autonomous MANET may not be very meaningful as the users can communicate only among themselves, since Internet access is almost indispensable to users. Users expect to have Internet access whenever they are connected to a network. For example, sending and receiving email has become a part of daily life for people to keep in touch with each other. Therefore, it is desirable to integrate the ad hoc network with the fixed-wired Internet into a wired-wireless hybrid network.

One possible useful application for this hybrid network is the inter-vehicle hybrid network [2, 3, 4, 5]. Vehicles in the network form an ad hoc network in order to share the information between them. At the same time, passengers in vehicles can access the Internet through the connection between vehicles and access routers, or gateway, deployed along the roads.

Research effort has been carried out on such hybrid networks [7, 8] and most uses traditional reactive routing protocols like Ad-hoc On Demand Distance Vector Routing (AODV) for multi-hop communication. Motivated by research [6] on pure ad hoc network environments, which makes use of geographical information for routing, it is worth studying routing performance for multi-hop communications complemented with the additional geographical information in this hybrid network environment.

We propose a routing protocol, called Location-Aided On-Demand (LAOD) routing protocol, which aims to achieve better routing performance with the help of geographical information in a hybrid wired-wireless network environment, and study the performance of our proposed LAOD routing protocol through simulations.

The paper is organized as follows. Section 2 gives a brief introduction of the related work on position-based routing protocols and hybrid networks. Section 3 presents the design of our gateway discovery algorithm and LAOD routing protocol. Section 4 presents and discusses the simulation results. Concluding remarks are made in Section 5.

2 Related Work

Position-based routing protocols [6] in MANET make use of location information to forward data packets. They require information about the location of the participating nodes to be available. The means to obtain location information is via a location service. Location service provides source mobile node the current location information of the destination nodes. More details on location service can be found in [6].In these position-based routing protocols, each mobile node maintains a location table that records the location of all other mobile nodes and the time at which that location information is received. The source node then uses this information to improve the efficiency in the transmission of packets. A review of some of these protocols is available in [6]. Most results on position-based routing protocols show that use of location information in MANET significantly improves routing performance.

One of the forwarding strategies used in position-based routing protocols is the greedy packet forwarding. When an intermediate node receives a packet, it forwards the packet to a neighbor closest to the destination. This strategy tries to minimize the number of hops a packet has to traverse in order to reach the destination. However, this greedy packet forwarding strategy may fail to find a path between sender and destination, even though one does exist. This is known as the local maximum problem. If the network is dense enough, such a problem will be less likely to occur.

There has been research on the hybrid wired-wireless networks [7, 8] where traditional reactive routing protocols are used to route the data packets. Improvement may be obtained by making use of location information. Recently, [2, 3, 4, 5] have developed position-based routing protocols for hybrid network environments. However, all these assume the existence of a separate idealized location service, which means that the source node always knows the current location information of the destination node.

3 Location-Aided On-Demand Routing Protocol in Hybrid Network

The LAOD routing protocol aims to achieve better routing performance with the help of geographical location information in a hybrid wired-wireless network environment. Unlike most of the location-based routing protocols, which assume the presence of a separate ideal location service to provide location information of all mobile nodes in the network readily [5], we propose a more practical approach based on gateway nodes, which connected to the wired backbone, together with a gateway discovery algorithm to provide such information.

As the main concern of our routing design is to avoid congesting the gateways with excessive communication, LAOD tries not to use the gateway as long as it can find a path from the source node to the destination node. Therefore, LAOD uses greedy packet forwarding when the destination location information is available. Greedy packet forwarding is used because of its simplicity and efficiency in dense network.

The data packets delivered by LAOD follow either the wireless routing path (Figure 1) or the wireless-cum-wired routing path (Figure 2). Wireless routing path is wireless multi-hops directly from source to destination. Wireless-cum-wired routing path is wireless multi-hops from source to destination via gateways.

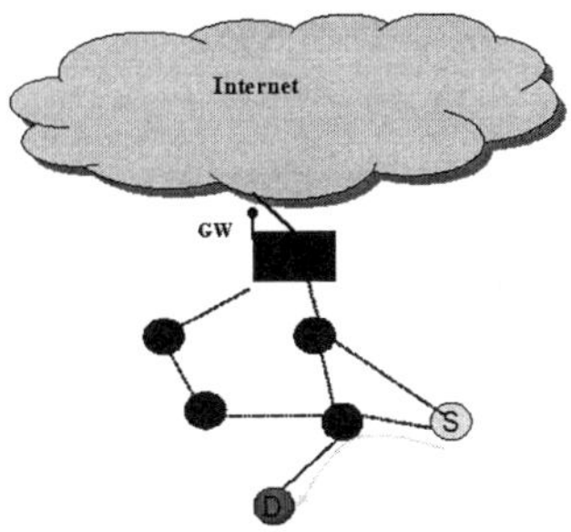

Figure 1: Wireless routing path

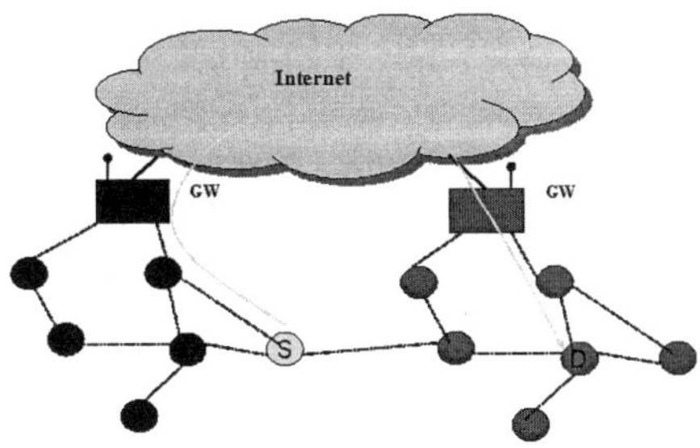

Figure 2: Wireless-cum-wired routing path

3.1 Gateway Discovery Algorithm

The objective of the gateway discovery algorithm is to provide both centralized location service and connectivity between gateways and mobile nodes: a gateway keeps track of the mobile node's address, current geographical location information, and next-hop to this mobile node, while a mobile node keeps track of the gateway's address, geographical location information, next-hop to this gateway, and the number of hops from this particular gateway. This gateway discovery algorithm is integrated together with LAOD into a routing system for this hybrid network. The proposed gateway discovery algorithm consists of a gateway selection mechanism and a location update mechanism.

3.1.1 Gateway Selection Mechanism

Each gateway periodically broadcasts Gateway Advertisement messages. This Gateway Advertisement message is only propagated up to a pre-defined number of hops away from the originating gateway. A mobile node selects its attached gateway based on the hop count, and/or geographical distance from the gateway. The mobile node then sends back a Gateway Acknowledgement message to inform the selected gateway which it intends to be attached to.

3.1.2 Location Update Mechanism

In order to keep location information up-to-date, a mobile node employs two methods. First, a mobile node periodically sends out location update messages to the current attached gateway. Second, a mobile node sends out a location update message when it observes that, due to its movement, a new neighbor is found. A mobile node becomes aware of the existence of new neighbors by checking the received hello beacons. However, in the case when a mobile node stays at a certain location for some period, sending location updates during this interval is unnecessary and wastes network resource. To avoid unnecessary updates, a mobile node keeps track of the location where it did the last update.

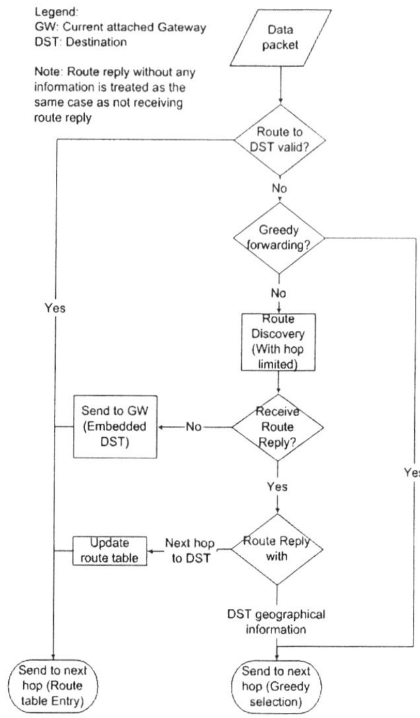

Figure 3: Algorithm Flow Chart for Mobile Node

3.2 LAOD Routing Protocol

With the gateway discovery algorithm, information about the mobile nodes is collected and stored at the gateways. This is then utilized by the routing algorithm in the following manner. Whenever a source mobile node has a data packet to send, it firstly checks its routing table to determine whether it has a current route to that node. If none exists, it initiates the route discovery process similar to that of AODV. But, unlike AODV, the route request message is broadcasted only to nodes in the region within a few hops away from the source instead of the whole network. This region should include the current attached gateway of the source node. Depending on the route reply received, the source node makes the routing decision accordingly (as shown in Figure 3).

- If the route reply is from the destination or an intermediate node, with up-to-date route to the destination, the source node sends packets using the returned route information.
- If route reply is from the gateway with destination geographical information of the destination node, which means the destination is within the same subnet as the source, packets are sent towards the destination by the greedy packet forwarding.
- If route reply is from the gateway but without destination geographical information, or no reply to the route request, the source node sends the packet towards current attached gateway with the destination information.

An intermediate node follows the routing decision made by the source node. Whenever an intermediate node fails to find a next hop, due to a broken route or a local maximum [2], it will send the packet to its attached gateway as last resort, since the gateway might be able to find an alternative route to the destination. If this still fails, it broadcasts a route error message back to the source.

If there is a route reply from the destination or an intermediate node with up-to-date route to the destination, and a route reply from gateways, source node prefers the former route reply.

Data packets are delivered to destination by one of the following mechanisms in LAOD:

- Direct Route Forwarding, which uses route obtained by the route reply from the destination or an intermediate node with up-to-date route to the destination.
- Greedy Packet Forwarding, which uses destination location information.
- Gateway Packet Forwarding, which uses route via gateway.

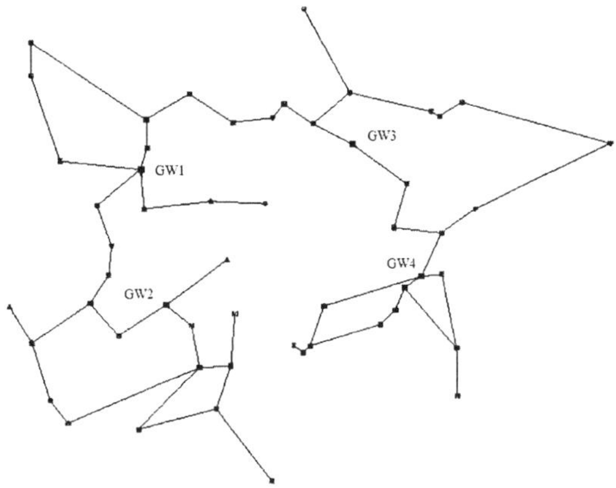

Figure 4: The city area graph used in the simulation

Parameter	Value
Transmission Range	250 m
Simulation Time	900 s
Topology Size	2800 X 1500 m^2
Traffic Type	UDP
Packet Size	512 bytes
Maximum Concurrent Connection	20
Packet Generating Rate	4 packets/s
Number of Gateways	4
Number of Mobile Nodes	150
Advertisement Zone	6 hops
Advertisement Interval	5s
Periodical Update Interval	5s
Hello Beacon Interval	1s
Average Speed	1, 5, 10, 15, 20 m/s
Min Pause Time	10 s
Max Pause Time	20 s

Table 1: Simulation input parameters

4 SIMULATION

4.1 Simulation Environment

The simulations were done using the Network Simulator (NS2) [9] to evaluate the performance of LAOD. We compared the performance of LAOD with AODV.

The scenario chosen for the simulations is based on the graph-based mobility model [10]. To describe the movement of vehicles moving around city area, the city area is modeled as a graph shown in Figure 4. The graph used for the simulations contains 54 vertices representing significant places and 59 edges referring to road segments interconnecting them, covering an area of approximately 2500m by 1800m.

For the simulation, each node moves from one randomly chosen location to the next on a shortest path along the edges. After reaching the destination, a node pauses for 5 to 10 seconds, and then moves to another randomly selected vertex.

In all simulations, the number of nodes is fixed at 150, with the average moving speed varying from 1m/s to 20 m/s. There are four gateways deployed in the region as shown in Figure 4. Each simulation lasts for 900 seconds of simulation time. We simulate 20 Constant Bit Rate (CBR) traffic flows with sources and destination chosen randomly. Each CBR flow sends at a rate of 4 data packet per second, with packet size of 512 bytes. The IEEE 802.11 Medium Access Control (MAC) protocol is used. Both gateways and mobile nodes have the same transmission range of 250m. All the key parameters of our simulations are shown in Table 1.

The following metrics are used to evaluate the performance of the protocol:

- *Packet Delivery Ratio*: The fraction of sent data packets that are successfully delivered to their destination
- *Average End-to-End Delay*: The average time interval between a data packet sent by a source node and its arrival at its destination. Average End-to-End delay is only measured for packets that are successfully delivered to their destination.
- *Normalized Routing Overhead:* The number of routing packets transmitted per data packet delivered at the destination. Each hop-wise transmission of a routing packet is counted as one transmission.

4.2 Simulation Result and Discussion

We simulated LAOD and AODV at each average speed with ten different randomly generated movement patterns. Figure 5 presents the distribution of successful data packets delivery by LAOD. In Figure 5, *Data packets delivered by greedy forwarding* refers to those data packets delivered by greedy packet forwarding while *Data packets delivered NOT by greedy forwarding* refers to those data packets delivered by direct route packet forwarding and gateway packet forwarding. As we can see, in general, around 5% of data packets are delivered by the greedy packet forwarding mechanism. Greedy packet forwarding is mainly affected by the network density. Varying the speed of the mobile nodes does not vary the overall network density, and with the network density unchanged, the performance of greedy packet forwarding does not differ much.

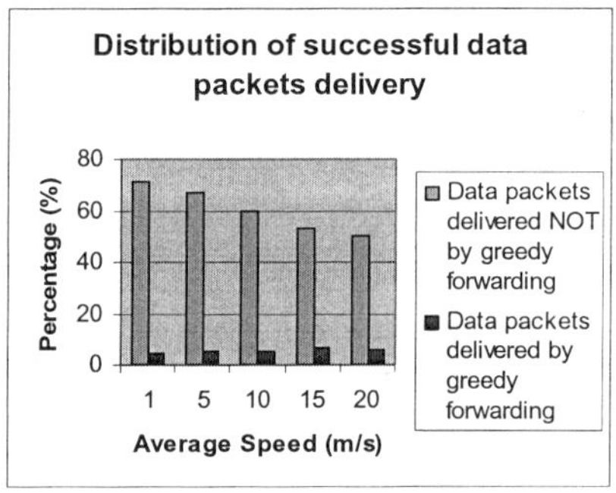

Figure 5: Distribution of successful data packets delivery by and NOT by greedy packet forwarding

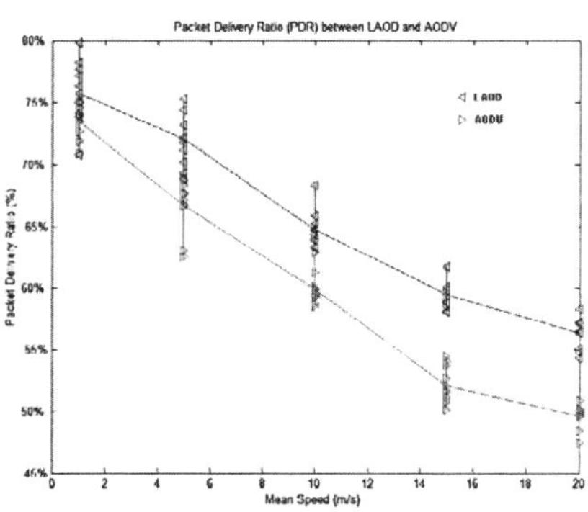

Figure 6: Packet Delivery Ratio (PDR) comparison between LAOD and AODV

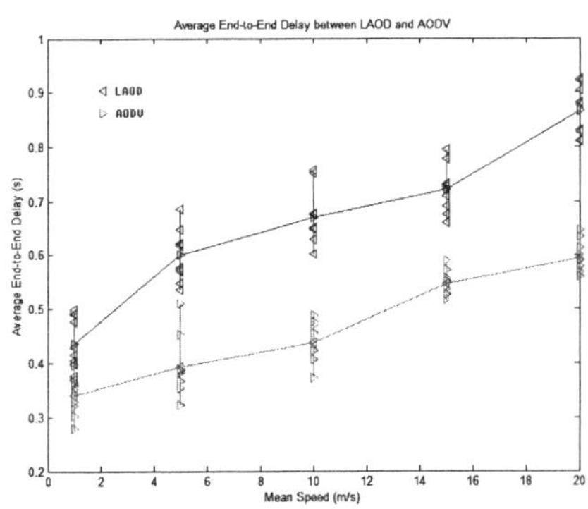

Figure 7: Average End-to-End Delay comparison between LAOD and AODV

Figure 6 presents the packet delivery ratio of both LAOD and AODV. As shown, LAOD achieves packet delivery ratio similar to AODV, with an improvement of around 4% to 5% when mobile nodes are moving faster. As expected, both routing protocols deliver less data packets with mobile nodes' speed increase. As mobility of nodes increase, the probability of link broken increases, which means that the probability of packet drop increases. Without alternate means like greedy packet forwarding, AODV drops more data packets than LAOD does. LAOD, on the other hand, drops slightly less data packets, since greedy packet forwarding does not suffer serious performance degradation as mobile nodes move faster.

Figure 7 shows the average end-to-end delay of these two protocols. As we can see, LAOD has longer delay than AODV. This can easily happen in a network topology, as shown in Figure 8. When data packets, which are forwarded by greedy packet forwarding mechanism from S to D, fail at A due to the local maximum problem, LAOD then tries to counter this problem by forwarding the packets via the gateway from A. A certain portion of such data packets do reach the destination node eventually. In this case, with reference to Figure 8, LAOD forwards data packets following the path S-B-A-B-C-GW-C-E-F-D, while AODV forwards data packets following S-B-C-E-F-D. Therefore, data packets delivered by LAOD travel almost twice the number of hops than those by AODV and thus incur extra delay. The average percentage of such cases in the simulation is shown in Figure 9.

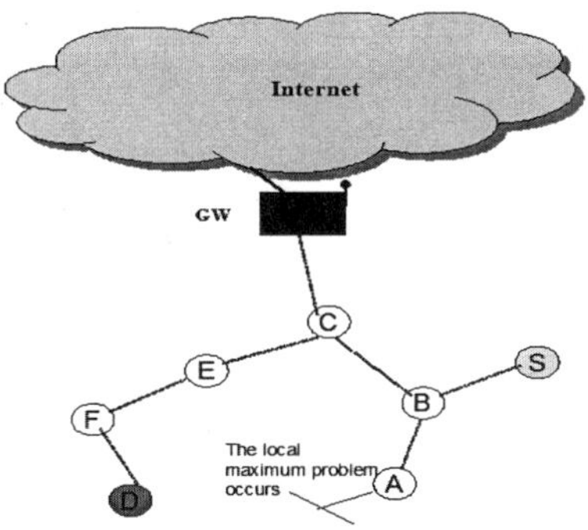

Figure 8: Scenario when greedy packet forwarding fails but gateway packet forwarding succeeds

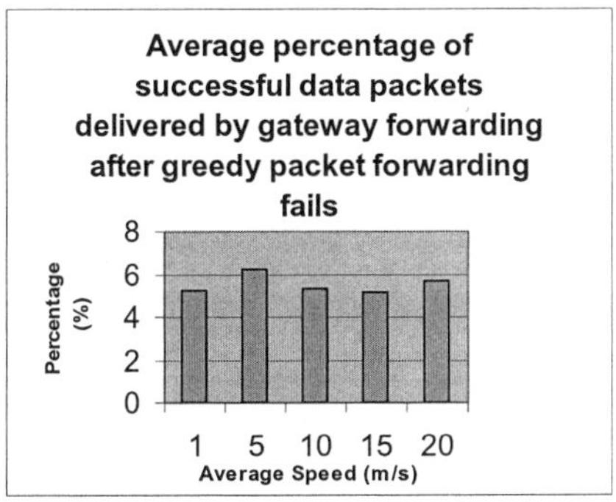

Figure 9: Average percentage of successful data packets delivered by gateway packet forwarding after greedy packet forwarding fails

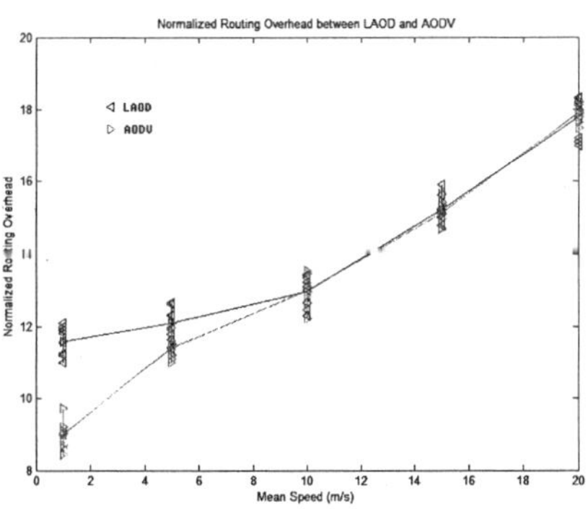

Figure 10: Normalized routing overhead comparison between LAOD and AODV

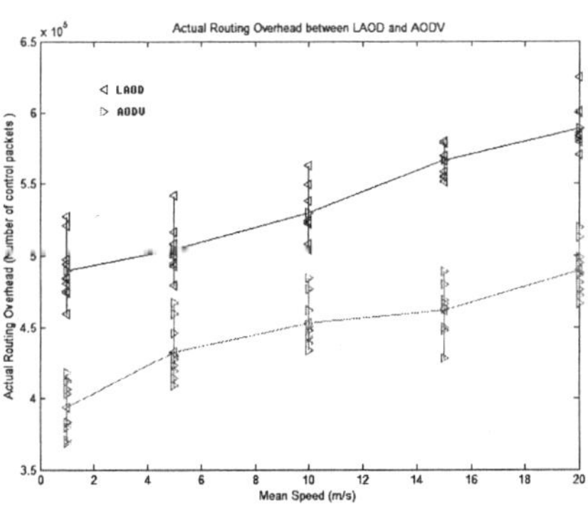

Figure 11: Actual routing overhead comparison between LAOD and AODV

Figure 10 shows the normalized routing overhead of these two protocols while Figure 11 shows the corresponding actual routing overhead. Overhead here includes all the control messages used during the simulation. These are the gateway discovery algorithm's control messages and routing control messages. Gateway discovery algorithm control messages consist of gateway advertisement message, gateway acknowledgement message, and location update message. Routing control messages consist of route request message, route reply message, route error message and hello beacon message. Overall LAOD has higher actual routing overhead than AODV, although AODV has created more route request overhead. By normalizing the overall routing overhead with the number of data packet successfully delivered, LAOD has similar normalized routing overhead as AODV at faster speed, since LAOD delivers slightly more data packets at faster speed which is a key advantage of LAOD when used in vehicular ad hoc networks with fast moving nodes.

5 Conclusion

In this paper, we proposed a new routing protocol, Location-Aided On-Demand (LAOD), together with the supporting gateway discovery algorithm, for hybrid wired-wireless network environments. This routing protocol aims to achieve better routing performance for multi-hop communications between mobile nodes with the help of geographical information. The performance evaluation and comparison has been done through simulation, which showed that LAOD achieves higher packet delivery at the expense of longer average end-to-end delay.

References

[1] IETF, Mobile ad hoc networks working group, http://www.ietf.org/html.charters/manetcharter.html.

[2] W. Franz, H. Hartenstein, and B. Bochow, *"Internet on the Road via Inter-Vehicle Communications"*, GI Workshop ,Communication over Wireless LANs', Vienna, Austria, September 26-28, 2001.

[3] J. Tian, L. Han, K. Rothermel, and C. Cseh, *"Spatially Aware Packet Routing for Mobile Ad Hoc Inter-Vehicle Radio Networks"*, Proceedings of the IEEE 6th International Conference on Intelligent Transportation Systems (ITSC), Shanghai, China, October 12-15, 2003.

[4] Christian Lochert, Hannes Hartenstein, Jing Tian, Holger Füßler, Dagmar Hermann, Martin Mauve, *"A Routing Strategy for Vehicular Ad Hoc Networks in City Environments"*, Proceedings of the IEEE Intelligent Vehicles Symposium, Columbus, OH, USA, June 9-11, 2003.

[5] H. Hartenstein, B. Bochow, A. Ebner, M. Lott, M. Radimirsch, and D. Vollmer, *"Position-aware ad hoc wireless networks for inter-vehicle communications: the fleetnet project"*, Proceedings of the 2001 ACM International Symposium on Mobile Ad Hoc Networking & Computing (MobiHoc 2001), Long Beach, CA, USA, October 4-5, 2001.

[6] M. Mauve, J. Widmer and H. Hartenstein, "*A Survey on Position-Based Routing in Mobile Ad-Hoc Networks*", IEEE Network Magazine, 15(6): pp 30– 39, 2001.

[7] Jorjeta G. Jetcheva, Yih-Chun Hu, Santashil PalChaudhuri, Amit Kumar Saha, and David B. Johnson, *"Design and Evaluation of a Metropolitan Area Multitier Wireless Ad Hoc Network Architecture"*, Proceedings of the 5th IEEE Workshop on Mobile Computing Systems and Applications (WMCSA 2003), Monterey, CA, October 9-10, 2003.

[8] P. Ratanchandani and R. Kravets, "*A Hybrid Approach to Internet Connectivity for Mobile Ad Hoc Networks*", Proceedings of the IEEE Wireless Communications and Networking Conference (WCNC 2003), New Orleans, Louisiana, March 16-20, 2003.

[9] Network Simulator (ns-2), http://www.isi.edu/nsnam/ns/.

[10] Tian Jing, Hähner Jörg, Becker Christian, Stepanov Illya, and Rothermel Kurt, *"Graph-Based Mobility Model for Mobile Ad Hoc Network Simulation"*, Proceedings of the 35th Annual Simulation Symposium, San Diego, California, April 14-18, 2002.

Comparative Performance Analysis of ECG Coding for 3G Wireless Telecardiology System

Alvaro ALESANCO[#], Robert S. H. ISTEPANIAN[*], Salvador OLMOS[#], José GARCÍA[#]
[#] *Communications Technologies Group (GTC). Aragón Institute of Engineering Research. University of Zaragoza, SPAIN.*
[*] *Mobile Information and Network Technologies Research Centre (MINT@K), School of Computing and Information Systems, Kingston University, London, UK.*

Abstract. This paper provides a comparative analysis of two different new ECG wavelet coding methods suitable for real-time wireless telecardiology systems over GPRS and 3G. The methods are based on the transmission of the most significant wavelet coefficients of every segmented ECG block. Two different operational modes can be used in both methods: Constant Bit Rate and Variable Bit Rate. Comparative performance of the two different coding methods under different channel errors conditions is presented.

Introduction

m-health is a new and evolving area of wireless telemedicine that deals with emerging mobile communications and network technologies for healthcare.

The convergence of information and telecommunications infrastructures around telemedicine and mobile telecare systems is fostering a diversity of cost-effective and efficient m-health applications. It is well known that Telecardiology is one of the most mature and successful areas in telemedicine. The most popular field in telecardiology deals with the transmission of electrocardiographic (ECG) signals over different networks and the inclusion of wireless networks opens a wide range of possibilities for it. One of the main challenges in telecardiology is found on patient monitoring and early diagnosis in the area of emergency telemedicine, where real-time ECG transmission is required. Wireless networks have evolved from technologies such as Global System for Mobile communication (GSM) or General Packet Radio Service (GPRS) to the recently developed Third Generation (3G) Universal Mobile Telecommunications System (UMTS), thus permitting wider use of new mobile telemedicine services [1][2]. Emergency telemedicine is synonym of mobile telemedicine since the only way to communicate an ambulance with a hospital is through a wireless channel. Although wireless telemedicine has been applied successfully in recent years, one of the major challenges that remain for effective and accurate real time ECG wireless transmission is the selection of the appropriate robust coding method suitable for such critical medical data. For wireless systems these selection is specially critical regarding the resilience of the coding method for issues such as bit error rate (BER) and bandwidth limitations. Although 3G wireless networks increase considerably the available bandwidth, an efficient coding method is still required, especially when the ECG shares the bandwidth with other clinical information and other users within the mobile network.

Working with pre-recorded telecardiology, the errors produced during transmission yield the retransmission of the data until the information in the receiver is exactly the same as in the transmitter. In data-packet networks such as GPRS or 3G systems, the retransmission of information implies the retransmission of the corrupted or lost packets.

The higher the BER, the higher the number of packets with errors, therefore leading to a higher number of retransmissions and transfer time. Working in real-time telecardiology, when the conditions of the channel are poor the number of packets suffering transmission errors will be large. If the transmission delay is high, the retransmission of information may not be useful because the retransmitted information may be out-dated when it arrives at the receiver. In this case, an efficient ECG coding strategy that detects these errors and endeavour to recover some information from the corrupted packets may be a better strategy than the retransmission.

In recent years, the application of wavelet ECG compression has drawn major attention within the biomedical and e-health research. The focus of most of this work was on improving the coding for store-and-forward strategies. However, most of this research is not reported for recent packetized mobile systems. To the best of our knowledge, no ECG error resilience coding method that can adapt to channel conditions has been reported.

The aim of this paper is two fold. First, we present different ECG wavelet coding strategies suitable for real-time wireless applications based on the transmission of the most significant wavelet coefficients of every segmented ECG block. Secondly, these coding strategies are analyzed through an extensive study carried out under different simulated 3G channel conditions.

1. Real-time wavelet ECG coding

In this section we present a new wavelet ECG coding approach. The method is based on the estimation and coding of the ECG wavelet transform coefficients. The aim of any transformation being used for compression purposes is to concentrate the signal energy into a small number of transform coefficients. It is this energy concentration what leads to the coding gain. Compression is then achieved by selecting a subset of the most relevant coefficients which afterwards are efficiently coded.

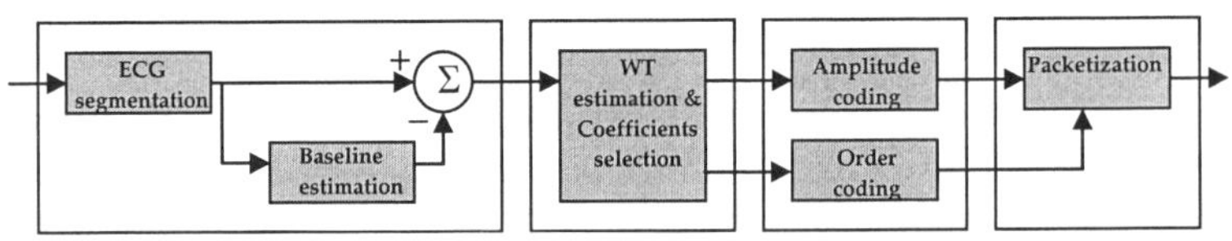

Figure 1. Block diagram of the resilient ECG coding scheme.

To achieve real-time functionality requirements, the ECG signal is segmented into blocks whose coding results are then packetized for transmission. In some network scenarios it is very important to have control over the amount of information transmitted through the channels, that is to say, to control the transmitted bandwidth. To accomplish with this task a Constant Bit Rate (CBR) operational mode has been implemented. However, when the available network bandwidth is large enough, sometimes one would like to guarantee the ECG signal quality instead of the output bit rate. Since the amount of information varies block to block, the bandwidth required to guarantee a reconstruction error is not constant. Hence, this yields a Variable Bit Rate (VBR) transmission mode, which has been also implemented in the proposed method.

In our approach, the ECG coding method is divided into the following stages:

- Pre-processing
- Wavelet transform estimation and coefficients coding

- Packetization

The block diagram of the resilient ECG coding method is show in Figure 1, where the different stages are represented.

1.1 Pre-processing

The ECG data stream is divided into fixed length blocks and every block is coded as an independent entity. Each lead in the block is treated independently through all the coding process. Then the baseline of the acquired ECG signal is removed. As real-time operation is necessary, a fast baseline estimation method is required. A third-order Butterworth filter, which filters the ECG blocks in both directions to avoid phase distortion, was considered.

1.2 Wavelet transform estimation and coefficients coding

After baseline wandering subtraction, a wavelet transform is applied to the ECG block. A *Coiflet* wavelet was used as mother function [3] due to its improved performance on ECG compression [4]. For each block, the wavelet coefficients are estimated. Figure 2 shows a typical wavelet coefficients distribution and their decreasing order arrangement.

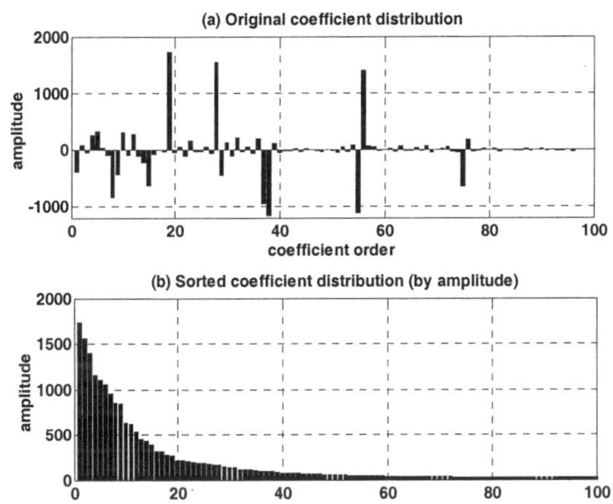

Figure 2. Wavelet coefficients for one ECG block (Block length = 512 samples).

The wavelet coefficients are sorted by decreasing amplitude (see Figure 2 (b)) and the number of coefficients to be transmitted is selected according to a threshold, which depends on the operational mode (CBR or VBR). When operating in VBR mode, the threshold is set up to achieve a fixed Root Mean Squared (RMS) reconstruction error by rejecting the smallest coefficients until their accumulated power reaches the threshold value. Hence, in this mode the threshold is defined in μV units. A variable number of coefficients are needed to achieve the fixed RMS error since the coefficient distribution varies from block to block. However, if the operation mode is CBR, then the threshold is set up to achieve a constant bit rate and then it can be defined in bits per second. The number of coefficients is selected (beginning with those of largest energy) to fulfil the desired transmission bit rate.

After threshold operation, a wavelet coefficients set is preserved for transmission. For each preserved coefficient, its order and amplitude need to be coded and transmitted. Since the relevance of one particular coefficient changes block to block, both order and amplitude of the selected coefficient must be coded in every block. Two different coding strategies are proposed for order and amplitude information in the next sub-sections.

1.2.1 Huffman coder for orders and Pulse Code Modulation (PCM) coder for amplitudes: Strategy A

If the first difference is performed to the orders of the preserved coefficients, advantage can be taken from the fact that relevant wavelet coefficients appears in groups (see Figure 2 (a)). In this way, the histogram of the values obtained after perform the first difference (denoted as order jumps) will be concentrated if small values and among them, value 1 will acquire a high weight (above 40 %) [Ale03]. In this way, a Variable Length Coder (VLC) can be used to take advantage of this property. A Huffman coder has been considered for the implementation of the VLC. On the other hand, in order to code the coefficients amplitudes, a PCM coder which has been implemented.

1.2.2 PCM for orders and Adaptive PCM (APCM) coder for amplitudes: Strategy B

If the amplitudes of the wavelet coefficients are sorted in decreasing order (see Figure 2 (b)), advantage can be taken from the fact that a rapidly amplitude decrease is produced. In this way, an APCM coder that maintains the quantization step and varies the number of bits to code the coefficients amplitudes can be used. After studying many ECG signal blocks the conclusion was that if wavelet coefficients were grouped in subsets of 10 coefficients, the number of bits needed to code their amplitudes can decrease in one bit (starting from the minimum number of bits to code the highest coefficient amplitude) from each subset. On the other hand, in order to code the coefficients orders, a PCM coder was considered.

1.3 Packetization

After applying the coding strategy, all the data needed to reconstruct the ECG signal block is sent to the receiver inside the payload field of a transport layer packet. Not only the information about the wavelet coefficients (order and amplitude) need to be sent but also other information important for the reconstruction process in reception. This information includes the following fields:

- The packet length.
- The number of leads coded in the packet.
- The length of the ECG block.
- The number of coefficients per lead.
- The number of bits needed to code the coefficients amplitudes per lead.

All the fields listed above are grouped within the term packet header. In order to add error resilience in the ECG packet transmission (apart of course from those implemented by the protocols used below the transmission layer) a repetition code has been implemented in the header in strategy B.

2. Simulation Results and Discussion

2.1 Compression performance in error-free environments

The MIT-BIH Arrhythmia database [5] has been selected for performance evaluation of the proposed coding strategies. The sampling rate of the two-lead ECG recordings is 360 Hz and the resolution 11 bits per sample. The Rate Distortion (RD) curves obtained using the two proposed coding strategies for channel 1 of record 100 are shown in Figure 3.

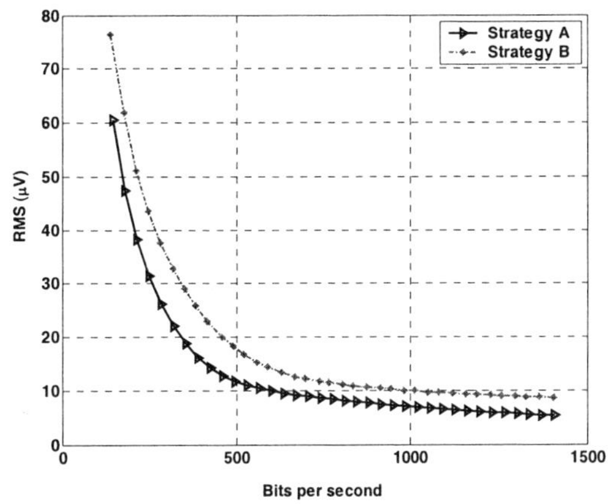

Figure 3. Comparative between the four coding strategies (Block length = 512 samples).

The best performance is obtained for strategy A, as it was expected since strategy A does not use header redundancies. These conclusions are independent of the type of the ECG signal being coded because the effect is produced by the coders used and not by the way the coefficients are selected and the jumps are obtained. Coding strategy A was applied to the signals from the MIT-BIH database when no transmission errors are present. Since the method permits two operational modes (VBR and CBR), results for both modes were obtained and some are shown in Table 1 and Table 2, respectively. In VBR mode (see Table 1), the target reconstruction error is achieved with a high level of accuracy (not only in mean but also with a low standard deviation). On the other hand, the data rate achieved presents a large standard deviation indicating that the number of bits needed to guarantee a constant reconstruction error may vary largely block to block due to the different number of transmitted coefficients.

Table 1. VBR mode compression performance (mean ± sd).

	Target RMS (μV)					
	10		30		50	
Record	Achieved RMS	Achieved data rate	Achieved RMS	Achieved data rate	Achieved RMS	Achieved data rate
100	10 ± 0.04	586 ± 81	29.4 ± 0.4	259 ± 43	48.6 ± 0.9	173 ± 37
119	10 ± 0.04	898 ± 101	29.4 ± 0.4	404 ± 81	48.7 ± 0.9	300 ± 68

Like in VBR mode, when working in CBR mode the target bit rate is achieved in an accurate way, both in mean and standard deviation (see Table 2). On the other hand, the reconstruction error presents a large standard deviation (compared with the value obtained in VBR), indicating that the reconstruction error may vary largely block to block, depending on the ECG signal block waveform. These conclusions are the same for all the records in the MIT database.

Table 2. CBR mode compression performance (mean ± sd).

	Target Data Rate (bps)					
	300		500		700	
Record	**Achieved RMS**	**Achieved data rate**	**Achieved RMS**	**Achieved data rate**	**Achieved RMS**	**Achieved data rate**
100	24 ± 5.3	300 ± 3	12 ± 1.4	500 ± 3	9 ± 0.8	700 ± 3
119	51 ± 18	301 ± 3	22 ± 6.2	501 ± 3	13 ± 2.3	701 ± 3

2.2 Compression performance in error prone environments

Real-time ECG transmission through wireless channels involves bit errors in reception. In order to simulate the performance of the system in different 3G wireless channel conditions, a 3G channel simulator previously developed in the University of Zaragoza has been used. The transmission rate selected for simulation was 64 Kbps and the mobile speed 120 Km/h. Further details of the channel and UMTS simulator can be found in [6] .

When receiving a transmitted ECG signal, there are two quantities that contribute to the total RMS error ($RMS_{received}$). There is a reconstruction error due to lossy compression (RMS_{codec}). Additionally there exists an error introduced by the channel ($RMS_{channel}$) due to transmission errors. In strategy A, packets with transmission errors are discarded. In order to calculate the RMS error index [7], this block of data is replaced by a constant value equal to zero representing that no signal information is available. In strategy B the packet information is tried to be recovered. Nevertheless if an inconsistence is found in the decoding process, then the packet is discarded and a constant value of zero is placed instead. Since $RMS_{channel}$ error does not depend on the ECG signal being transmitted and general tendencies in the results on RMS_{codec} error (regarding coding strategies) are similar no matter the ECG signal being compressed, the analysis of the performance results presented for record 100 in the next sub-sections is valid to any ECG signal.

Values of transmission rate are given now through PDU length, which is the length of the transmitted packet. The relation between PDU length and transmission rate is given in Eq. 1,

$$R = PDU_{length} \cdot \frac{f}{N} \tag{1}$$

where R is the transmission rate, f is the sampling frequency (360 samples per second) and N is the number of samples per ECG block (512 in this case). The distortion-BER curves for each coding strategy when transmitting record 100 (first minute) are shown in Figure 4. The graphics have been obtained averaging 40 runs in CBR mode with a block length of

512 samples. The results correspond to the coding strategies when working in CBR mode (target PDU length 500 and 700 bits).

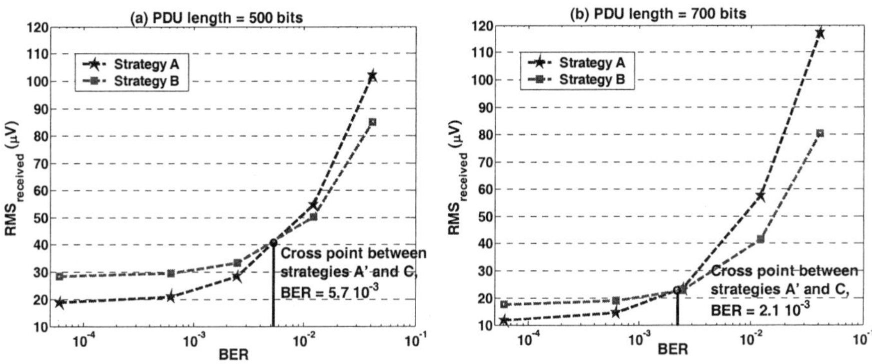

Figure 4. Average $RMS_{received}$ values showing the performance of the coding methods when using in transmission over a simulated UMTS channel (CBR mode. Block length = 512).

Strategy C presents the best performance as the BER increases but it presents the worst efficiency for low BERs (see Figure 4). Header redundancies and robust wavelet coefficient coding make the PDU increase to maintain the same RMS_{codec} error compared with strategy A. The combination of header redundancies, PCM coders (robust in wireless environments) and error amplitude detection makes this strategy the best option when the channel BER increases. The cross point (in BER) between strategy A and C depends on the PDU length (and thus on the transmission rate). This effect can be explained considering that the differences in RMS_{codec} error between strategy A and C decrease as the transmission rate increases (see Figure 3). Hence, the approach of RMS_{codec} error values as the PDU length gets higher (see Figure 3) leads to a cross point located in lower BERs values.

3. Conclusions

In this paper, we described a new resilient ECG coding technique based on the wavelet transform suitable for real-time wireless telecardiology applications. The codec can work on two operational modes: VBR and CBR thus enabling the control of the reconstructed signal error or the transmission rate respectively. We have proposed and tested two coding strategies to code the relevant amplitude and order (or jump) wavelet coefficients: strategy A, which uses Huffman coder for jumps and PCM coder for amplitudes, and strategy B which uses a PCM coder for orders and an APCM coder for amplitudes and header redundancies.

The simulation results on error-free environments suggest that the proposed coding method (strategy A for transmission in error-free environments) presents a good performance for compressing the ECG signals with high compression ratios and acceptable clinical data for further diagnosis.

The simulations results in 3G wireless channels (UMTS) suggest that the selection between A and B depends on the channel BER and the transmission rate. As the BER increases, strategy B takes advantage over strategy A. The cross point between both strategies depends on the transmission rate.

Ongoing work is currently underway to test the system in this real-time transmission 3G wireless environment between selected patient population and specialist medical centre, both in U.K and Spain.

References

[1] Pattichis, C.S., Kyriacou, E., Voskarides, S., Pattichis, M.S., Istepanian, R.S.H., Chizas, C.N., 2002, Wireless telemedicine systems: an overview, *IEEE Anten. Prop. Mag.*, vol. 44 (2), pp. 143.153.

[2] Tachakra, S., Wang, X.H., Istepanian, R.S.H., Song, Y.H., 2003, Mobile e-health: the unwired evolution of telemedicine, *Telemed. J. and e-Health*, vol. 9 (3), pp. 247.257.

[3] Cooklev, T., Nishihara, A., 1999, Biorthogonal Coiflets, IEEE Trans. Sig. Proc., vol. 47(9), pp. 2582.2588.

[4] Bradie, B., 1996, Wavelet packet-based compression of single lead ECG, IEEE Trans. Biomed. Eng., vol. 43(5), pp. 493.501.

[5] MIT-BIH arrhythmia database CD-ROM, 1997, Third ed. Cambridge, MI: Harvard-MIT Division of Health Sciences and Technology.

[6] Gállego, J.R., Hernández, A., Canales, M., Valdovinos, A., 2004, Adaptive multimedia traffic multiplexing for dedicated channels in the UMTS system, *The Ninth IEEE Symp. on Computers and Comm.,* Alexandria (Egypt).

[7] A. Alesanco, S. Olmos, R.S.H. Istepanian, J. García, "A novel real-time multilead ECG compression and de-noising method based on the wavelet transform" *Computers in Cardiology*, 2003, pp. 593–596, Sept., Thessaloniki (Greece) 2003.

Chapter 5

Personal Assistive Devices and Robotics

Toward a Human-Friendly Assistive Environment
D. Zhang and M. Mokhtari (Eds.)
IOS Press, 2004

Six-DoF Force-Torque Wheelchair Control by Means of the Body Motion

Milan KVASNICA
Institute of Information Technologies, Tomas Bata University in Zlin
Nam. T.G. Masaryka 275, CZ-76272 Zlin, Czech Republic
E-mail kvasnica@ft.utb.cz, mkva@grasp.cis.upenn.edu

Abstract. The paper introduces the human-robot, respectively human-computer interfaces for the control of the wheelchair for people with various types of disabilities and elderly people. The first control system is based on a set of instructions derived from the body motion and sampled by means of the six component force-torque transducer inserted between the saddle and the chassis of the wheelchair. The second control system is based on a set of instructions derived from the head movement. On the head are fastened five laser diodes radiating light rays with following scanning of the light spots configuration on the floor by means of the CCD camera. Presented here is assignment of geometrical configuration of the light spots position for the control of the wheelchair. The activity of the force-torque transducer is based on axial shiftings and angular displacements caused by the human body motion.

Introduction

Significant progress in communication on human-robot interface, oriented on people with various types of disabilities and elderly people was presented in last years. An eye-gaze respectively eye-mouse tracking system oriented on people with motor disabilities was introduced in [1], [3] and [7]. A system using hand gesture, respectively face gesture was presented in [2], [4] and [6]. The head controller was described in [12] and the head joystick was described in [8]. Human-robot shoulder interface for the wheelchair control based on the body motion was presented in [5].

The aim of this paper is to introduce sensory system for communication on human-robot interface for people with paralyzed motion coordination, but with the ability to do the incline of the body. This control system is based on a set of instructions derived from the body motion and sampled by means of the six component force-torque transducer inserted between the saddle and the chassis of the wheelchair. The six-component force-torque transducer is used for the control of the wheelchair by means of the instruction set. Simultaneously is used for the active compliant assistance, see Figure 1.

The second control system is based on a set of instructions derived from the head movement. On the head are fastened five laser diodes radiating the configuration of the light rays with following scanning of the light spots configuration on the floor by means of the CCD camera, see Figure 1, Figure 3.

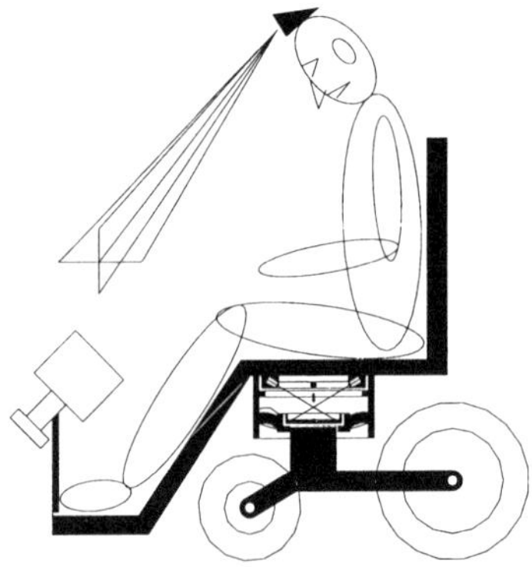

Figure 1. The force-torque transducer inserted between the saddle and the chassis of the wheelchair and the CCD camera for the sampling of the head joystick light spots configuration on the floor.

1. The force-torque transducer

The explanation of the activity is introduced on a simple modification of the six-component force-torque transducer. An example of the six-component force-torque transducer with the acting force -Fz is depicted in Figure 2. Laser diodes 1 emit crossing light rays 2 creating the edges of a pyramid, intersecting the 2-D CCD array 4 in light spots 3. The beginning of the 3D rectangular pyramid coordinate frame x,y,z is chosen in the crossing point of the light rays (the apex of a pyramid shape). Unique light spots configuration on the 2-D CCD array changes under the force-torque acting between the flanges 5 and 6 connected by means of elastic deformable medium 7. The beginning of a floating 2D coordinates frame x_{CCD},y_{CCD} is chosen in the geometrical center of the 2-D CCD array. An even number of four light rays simplifies and enhances the accuracy of the algorithm for the evaluation of three axial shiftings and three angular displacements. In addition removes the ambiguity of the imagination at the rotation of the 2-D CCD array around the straight line passing through two light spots, where for two different angles belongs one position of the third light spot.

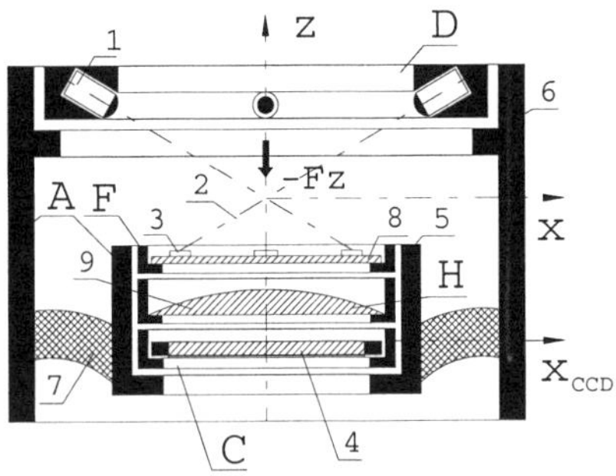

Figure 2. Six-component force-torque transducer.

2. Human-robot interface for the wheelchair control by means of the body motion

Many people with limited mobility like to enjoy life and they ride a wheelchair on popular tourist spots with typical leisure activities to high adventures and wilderness expeditions. These expeditions are oriented on long trips where is useful the active compliant assistance by means of the feedback control based on the damping device with a shock absorber. This active compliant assistance is able to overcome some barriers and to predict some hazard in unexpected situation like the quick halt on the stone or the raid on sharp slope. Basic part of compliant assistance is the six component force-torque transducer inserted between the saddle and the chassis see Figure 1. Force-torque transducer used for dynamic weighing of the user and the load on the wheelchair improves the dynamic stability at maneuvering and the comfort for enjoy from the ride.

In addition this force-torque transducer is possible to use for the scanning of the instruction set based on the body incline.

The module of five laser diodes is fastened on the outer flange of the force-torque sensor and the rays are intersecting the translucent screen in light spots A,B,C,D. The intersection of the abscises AB and CD is the point S. The length of the abscises AS, SB, CS, SD is u_1,u_2,u_3,u_4. The light spots configuration is analyzed and processed for the navigation and positioning of the wheelchair.

Purposeful body incline against the saddle is represented by the light spots 3 configuration in the 2-D CCD array 4, of the force-torque transducer; see Figure 2, which is analyzed like the force-torque acting in six components. Following commands are used for two-degrees-of-freedom control of the wheelchair; see Figure 2 and Figure 3.

- **Start** - the body incline in chosen direction outwards the light spots dead zone position.
- **Stop** - the body incline inwards the light spots dead zone position.
- The **Dead Zone** is defined for the dividing ratio u_1/u_2 for example by the interval <0.8;1.2>, u_3/u_4 is symmetric <0.8; 1.2>.
- **Forwards, Backwards** for the first DOF - the dividing ratio of diagonals $u_1/u_2 > 1.2$ respectively $u_1/u_2 < 0.8$.
- **Turn to the Left – Turn to the Right** is similar for the u_3/u_4. Final direction of the wheelchair motion is the vector sum of mutual perpendicular components u_1/u_2 and u_3/u_4.
- The **Magnitude** of the dividing ratio u_1/u_2, u_3/u_4 is assigned to the velocity of the wheel chair motion for two degrees of freedom (DOF).
- The **Motion Control System of the Wheelchair** enables parallel control of two degrees-of-freedom.
- The **Light Spot A is oriented** in front direction. This is needed for the orientation of the wheelchair against the basic light spot position.

Some applications of the signal filtering for the elimination of the body incline are needed for users with muscular trembling at neurological diseases and on rough surface.

3. Human-robot interface for the wheelchair control by means of the head motion

The sensory system is based on a set of instructions derived from the possibilities of the head movement. On the head are fastened five laser diodes radiating light rays with following scanning of the light spots configuration on the floor by means of the CCD camera, see Figure 1 and Figure 3.

The module of five laser diodes is fastened on the head of a wheelchair user and the rays are intersecting the floor plain in light spots A,B,C,D. The intersection of the abscises AB and CD is the point S. The length of the abscises AS, SB, CS, SD is u_1,u_2,u_3,u_4. The light spots configuration is analyzed and processed for the navigation and positioning of the wheelchair.

Purposeful head motion of the five laser diodes module is represented by the light spots configuration and is scanned by means of the CCD camera. Following commands are used for two-degrees-of-freedom control of the wheelchair on the floor:

- **Start** - the head movement with the module outwards the light spots dead zone position.
- **Stop** - the head movement with the module inwards the light spots dead zone position.
- The **Dead Zone** is defined for the dividing ratio u_1/u_2 and u_3/u_4 for example by the interval <0.4; 1.2>, u_3/u_4 is symmetric <0.8; 1.2> for the angle Ω by the interval $<-5^0;+15^0>$.
- **Forwards, Backwards** for the first DOF - the dividing ratio of diagonals $u_1/u_2 > 1.2$, respectively $u_1/u_2 < 0.4$.
- **Turn to the Left – Turn to the Right** - last increment of the angle Ω is positively $\Omega > +15^0$, respectively negatively $\Omega < -15^0$ oriented, or alternatively ratio of diagonals $u_3/u_4 > 1.2$ respectively $u_3/u_4 < 0.8$.
- The **Magnitude** of the dividing ratio u_1/u_2, u_3/u_4 and the angle Ω is assigned to the velocity of the wheel chair motion for every DOF.
- The **Light Spot A is Recognized** by means of the enhanced intensity, color, respectively shape in contrast with light spots B,C,D. This is needed for the orientation of the wheelchair against the basic light spot position.

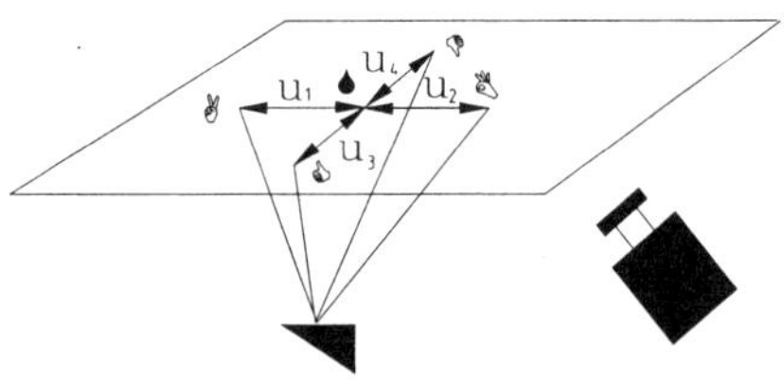

Figure 3. The five light spots configuration on the floor sampled by means of the CCD camera.

4. Experimental Hardware for Experiments with Described Mechatronics Systems

The wheelchair control by means of the body motion and by means of the head motion was implemented by means of following hardware, see [16].

- The Data Translation high-accuracy, programmable, monochrome frame grabber board DT3155 for the PCI bus. It is suitable for both, image analysis and machine vision applications.
- The microprocessor controlled programmable timer PIKRON ZO-CPU2 used for the timing of the light exposure and asynchronous switching of the laser diodes configuration.
- The configuration of miniature laser diodes F-LASER 5mW with focusing optics radiating structured light rays.
- Digital B/W video camera SONY KC-381CG with digital signal processor and high resolution 795Hx596V 1/3" CCD sensor with high sensitivity (0.02lux at F0.75) and interline transfer, digital light level control system for the back-light compensation,

with auto-exposure or manual exposure system, aperture correction and internal or gen-lock/line-lock external transfer.

- Zoom Lens Computar MLH-10X with 10x macro zoom, maximal magnification 0.084~0.84x, maximal aperture 1:5.6, maximal image format 6.4x4.8mm (average 8mm), focus 0.18~0.45m.

The image processing of the light spots from the CCD camera and the control algorithms were developed by means of the MATLAB, see [16], [17], [18] and [19].

Conclusion

Advancements on human-computer interface enabled the development of assistive technologies oriented on the help for disabled people. Described sensory systems help them to perform daily living tasks namely to manage independent mobility of electrical wheelchair or to control a robot manipulator for the use of a feeding utensil or for the moving with other objects. The customization of three universal portable modules and their combination enables convenient implementation in rooms or along corridors, for the comfort of the wheelchair user. The processing of the information from described devices enables low cost design by means of the single cheap micro-controllers.

Many fields could benefit from the use of sensory systems oriented on people with various types of disabilities. Non-standard interfaces are useful namely on workplaces, where an operator is steering the operation in more degrees of freedom, or where is needed to do more parallel operations, as for example a surgeon at neuro-logical operations. The modular design presented here enables easy customizing of wide variety of applications in rehabilitation robotics. In general, this modular design concept allows low cost design, enhanced demands for safety and reliability, maximization of service life because of ease repair and the use of modular components for both types of sensors.

Acknowledgements

The support from the grant Vyzkumne zamery MSM 281100001 "Automatizace vyrobnich procesu a technologii". is gratefully acknowledged.

References

[1] Do-Hyoung Kim, Jae-Hean Kim, Myung Jin Chung. An Eye-Gaze Tracking System for People with Motor Disabilities, Proceedings of the 7th International Conference on Rehabilitation Robotics ICORR'2001, Evry Cedex, France, 2001.

[2] Kawarazaki N., Hoya I., Nishihara K., Yoshidome T. Welfare Robot System Using Hand Gesture Instructions, Proceedings of the 8th International Conference on Rehabilitation Robotics ICORR'2003, Daejeon, Korea, 2003.

[3] Jae-Hean Kim, Bang Rae Lee, Do-Hyoung Kim, Myung Jin Chung. Eye-Mouse System for People with Motor Disabilities, Proceedings of the 8th International Conference on Rehabilitation Robotics ICORR'2003, Daejeon, Korea, 2003.

[4] Inhyuk Moon, Myungjun Lee, Jeicheong Ryu, Kyunghoon Kim, Museong Mun, Intelligent Robotic Wheelchair with Human-Friendly Interfaces for Disabled and the Elderly, Proceedings of the 8th International Conference on Rehabilitation Robotics ICORR'2003, Daejeon, Korea, 2003.

[5] Jae-Woong Min, Kyoobin Lee, Soo-Chul Lim, Dong-Soo Kwon, Human-Robot Interfaces for Wheelchair Control with Body Motion, Proceedings of the 8th International Conference on Rehabilitation Robotics ICORR'2003, Daejeon, Korea, 2003.

[6] Fukuda T., Nakashima M., Arai F., Hasegawa Y., Generalized Facial Expression of Character Face Based on Deformation Model for Human-Robot Communication, 11th IEEE International Workshop on Robot and Human Interactive Communication, RO-MAN'2002, Berlin, Germany, 2002.

[7] Ito Akira, An Approach to the Eye Contact throught the Outstaring Game Nirammekko, 11th IEEE International Workshop on Robot and Human Interactive Communication, RO-MAN'2002, Berlin, Germany, 2002.

[8] Kvasnica M., Six DOF Sensory System for Interactive Positioning and Motion Control in Rehabilitation Robotics, Proceedings of the 8th International Conference on Rehabilitation Robotics ICORR'2003, Daejeon, Korea, 2003.

[9] Kvasnica M., Algorithm for Computing of Information about Six-DOF Motion in 3-D Space Sampled by 2-D CCD Array, Proceedings of the 7th World Multi-Conference SCI'2001-ISAS, Vol. XV, Industrial Systems, Part II, Orlando, Florida, USA, 2001.

[10] Kvasnica M., Six DOF Measurements in Robotics, Engineering Constructions and Space Control, Extension Volume XX of the hard copy conference Proceedings of the 8th World Multi-Conference on Systemics, Cybernetics and Informatics - SCI'2002-ISAS'2002, Orlando, Florida, USA, 2002.

[11] Kvasnica M., Van der Loos M., Six-DOF Modular Sensory System with Haptic Interaction for Robotics and Human-Machine Interaction, Proceedings of the World Automation Congress WAC'2000, ISORA, Maui, Hawaii, USA, 2000.

[12] Kvasnica M.: A Six-DOF Modular Sensory System with Haptic Interface for Rehabilitation Robotics. Proceedings of the ICORR'2001, 7th International Conference on Rehabilitation Robotics, Paris-Evry, April 2001, France.

[13] Kvasnica M.: Modular Force-Torque Transducers for Rehabilitation Robotics, Proceedings of the IEEE International Conference on Rehabilitation Robotics, Stanford University, July 1999, Stanford, California, USA, 1999.

[14] Kvasnica M.: Six-DOF Sensory System for Interactive Positioning and Motion Control in Rehabilitation Robotíce. International Journal of Human-Friendly Welfare Robotic Systems, Volume 4, Number 3, September 2003, Korea, 2003.

[15] Kvasnica M.: Head Joystick and Interactive Positioning for the Wheelchair. Proceedings of the 1st International Conference on Smart Homes and Health Telematics, ICOST'2003, Paris, September 2003, France, 2003.

[16] http://www.neovision.cz

[17] http://www.humusoft.cz

[18] http://www.humusoft.cz/MATLAB/MATLAB.htm

[19] http://www.mathworks.com/

Dynamicity in smart homes concept applied to complex system: The Manus Robot

M. A. Feki[1], M. Ghorbel[1], M. Hariz[1], B. AbdulRazak[1, 2], B. Grandjean[2], M. Mokhtari[1,2]
[1] Handicom Lab, GET/INT, 9 rue Charles Fourier, 91011 Evry, France
[2]INSERM U.483, University Pierre & Marie Curie
mohamedali.fki@int-evry.fr

Abstract:

The use of dynamicity concept applied with multi-modal sensors and complex systems at smart homes concept can potentially enhance people with disabilities' freedom and quality of life. We present ongoing research work aiming in reducing the control complexity while performing daily living tasks by the use of assistive technological aids, such as a robot. Many people, due to a severe disability, may have a loss of strength, control, dexterity or any combination. Manus, which is a wheelchair mounted Robot, can be used to assist such people in daily living tasks or in a vocational settings. We focus on general software architecture of Manus concept and describe its flexibility to carry out different operations, rather than to be dedicated to a single task.

We present three applications: a smart homes project enabling those people to configure and manage their complex environment; A generic dynamic module allowing scan of users environment objects and will be able to extend its interaction to cover all complex system. A software robot system Manus will be exposed underlying the use of standard XML to produce an available module responsible for dynamicity aspect in the context of assistive robotics.

1 Introduction:

There are several characteristics that are commonly found at smart homes: In deed, smart homes consists on acting on the user environment to make it more accessible by adding automated controlled systems used through a common user interface which is defined as an environmental control system. Moreover, smart homes permits to control and coordinate multiple devices indoor or outdoor. To be more comfortable, smart homes dedicated to people with disabilities naturally requires dynamicity/auto configuration, allowing the environment to process information and to adapt to user's requirements and to changing conditions.

Designing and implementing smart homes often requires a breadth of knowledge not limited to a single discipline, but integrating aspects of machine learning, human-machine interfaces, wireless networking, and mobile communications. The purpose of this paper is to underline that those knowledge requires a dynamic module which could serve all those integrated modules especially Manus Robot (Figure 1) in real-time conditions.

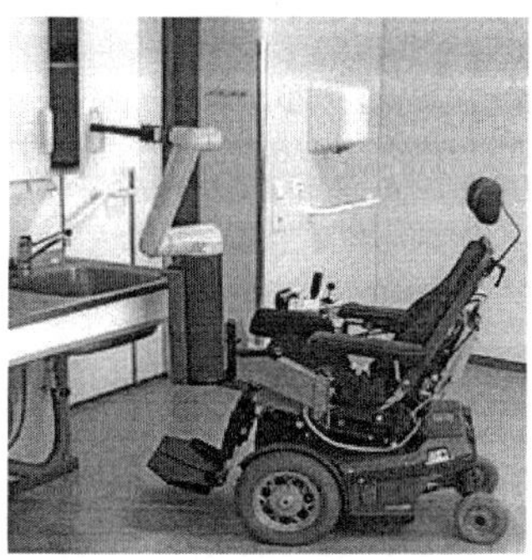

Figure 1: Manus robot

2 Manus robot

MANUS tele-manipulator is a robot mounted on an electric wheelchair. Its objective is to favour the independence of people with disabilities who have lost their superior or inferior members' mobility, by increasing the potential activity and by compensating for prehension motor incapacities. Manus is a robot tele-manipulator with six degrees of freedom, with a gripper in the extremity of the arm which permits the capturing of objects (capacity of 1,5 kg) in all directions, and a display. All are commanded principally by a 4x4 touch keypad and by a joystick with the latest prototype version and soon, a mouse or a tactile screen. The 4x4 keypad gives the user the possibility of handling MANUS, and the show unit (display) gives the information of the state of the MANUS system [1].

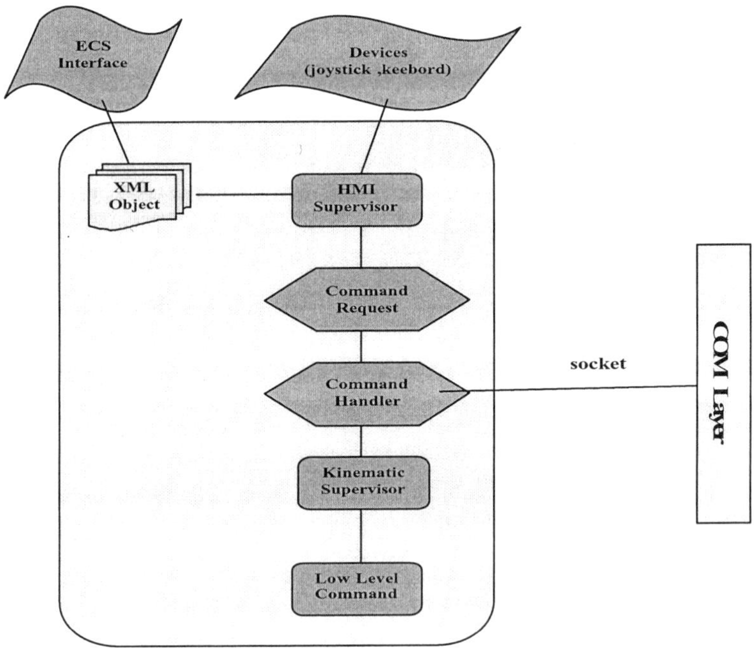

Figure 2: Manus software architecture

During previous works [2], we implemented a software architecture based on oriented object language C++.

- ECS / OT Interface: allows a simple configuration of Manus' actions, parameters and events and provides an XML configuration file.
- Devices: a library of command's interface, this software is part of the user interface layer which enables a management of several plugs drivers.
- HMI supervisor: this layer supervises the work of the system: it converts user events into actions, transmits the information to the low layer modules, manages errors situations and synchronization of modules.
- Command Request: Interface between the HMI layer and Kinematics layer. It sends orders to kinematics handler.

- Command Handler: translates orders and sends them to low layer in order to activate the articulations motors.
- Kinematics Handler: supervises the system states and manages the error's messages.
- COM Layer: In case of connection with smart homes, the Manus Robot is managed directly from an exterior communication module based on Socket TCP/IP mode.

Figure 2 describes the architectural layer and underlines the ability of the user to manage the robot by different manner. In fact, we developed an added extension script into ECS software that specifies if the user would like to choose a keyboard, suitable mouse, adapted joystick or any requested input devices. This implies that the user needs and preferences are a primary key for building the human machine interaction.

3 Dynamicity in smart homes:

The motivation for integrating Dynamicity is to bring computation into the real, physical world. The goal is to allow computers to participate in activities that have never previously involved computation and to allow people to interact with computational systems the same way they do with other people: via gesture, voice, movement, and context.

In human-machine interaction, a great deal of information is conveyed without explicit communication. Gestures, facial expressions, relationship to other people and objects in the vicinity, and shared histories are all used as cues to assist in understanding the explicit communication. [5].

There is also very little shared module between the human and the computer: Dynamic module in human-computer interaction includes any relevant information about the entities in the interaction between the user and computer, including the user and computer themselves and his environment composed of several equipments and objects. We define applications that use dynamicity to provide task-relevant information and/or services to be available when user needs to use it. A major problem has been the lack of uniform support for building and executing these types of applications supporting dynamicity. This paper describes architecture to support dynamicity concept into smart homes application dedicated to people with disabilities. We provide a discussion of how dynamicity has been handled in previous work and why we would like to handle it as a generalized module shared by all layers. Our concept of smart homes allowing us to handle user environment in a standard manner based on XML technologies [6] [7]. In next sessions, we discuss the architectural support necessary for using dynamicity concept and underline the mainly features of extended dynamicity to complex systems.

4 Implementation

In this paper we will be referring to the devices that support our system as "Smart Home Devices". We assume that these household devices have a JVM embedded within and are able to communicate with the surrounding environment using the UPNP protocols allowing covering several kinds of heterogeneous protocols. We announce also the existence of an independent static module allowing our application to have the possibility to run from a static configuration made by the user [8]. Further, each device has an embedded network card allowing it to be easily plugged into the nearest network space. Dynamicity concept in our implementation is mainly based on four components:

✍ **Smart Home Client (HMI)**: The Smart Home Client represents the GUI (Generic User Interface) for all Smart home compliant devices. It is able to detect the devices on the home network dynamically. It also displays the icons of the different devices. Upon clicking on a particular device by the user, the GUI will download the dynamic mobile code and run it. The HMI supervises the whole system: it converts user events into actions according to selected output devices (Manus, TV, VCR, etc.), transmits the information to the feedback module, and manages multimodal aspects, errors situations, the synchronization of modules, etc.

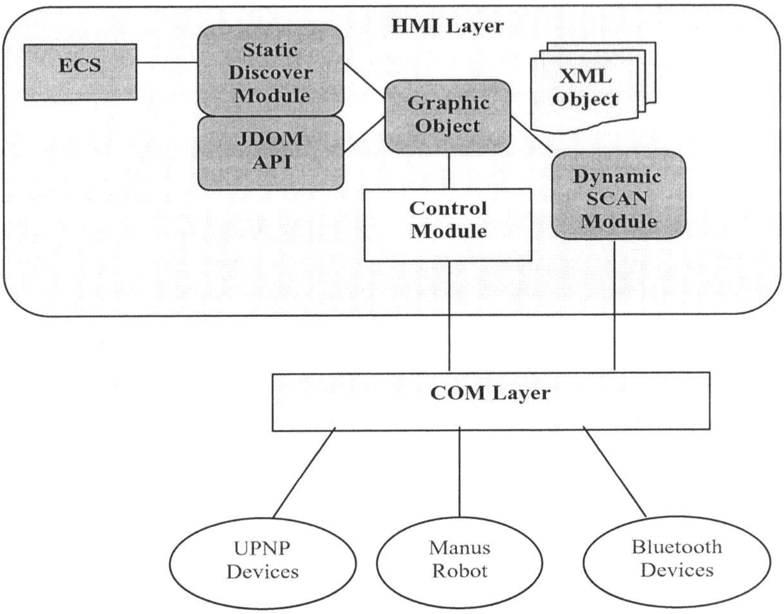

Figure 3: Dynamicity in smart homes architecture

✍ **Dynamic Graphic User Interface**: Since household devices vary significantly in their capabilities and functionality, each device may have a different interface for configuring it. For instance a "door" should provide an interface to open/close/lock the door. But for a VCR the interface should include controls for playback, rewind, eject etc. We would like our devices to be *truly* plug and play. Which means when a new smart device is employed, the user need only to hook it up to the network after which the device is instantaneously detected by the Smart Home supervisor (HMI) *without* the need of loading any device drivers. We use the necessary facilities provided by UPNP coupled with JAVA THREAD technologies for creating "network plug and play" devices, which when connected to a network, they announce their presence and enable network users to remotely exploit these devices.

✍ **Dynamic Discovery Service Code (DDSC)**: To be able to achieve the goals of being a truly and plug and play devices, each of our Smart device's will implement some "Dynamic Discovery Service Code module" that extends Java's "JTHREAD" class and interact with JDOM Parser which is responsible for creating a standard XML Object describing all devices discovered with related services and actions [6]. Here, the smart device programmer can identify what functionality the end user can control and whether features/parameters should be enforced or not. Once the device is detected by the GUI, the

DDSC is transferred over the network using CORBA protocols and is executed on the GUI's location whenever the user desires to configure that particular device. The GUI is capable of running and detecting new smart devices without the need to add any drivers or interfaces to it. We succeed to run an effective and robust DDSC at lower network layer which allow us to discover all devices in dynamic manner. See the figure below for clarification.

✍ **COM Layer (CL)**: Deals with specific characteristics of any output device according to its communication protocol (CAN, infrared, radio protocol, etc.). Indeed, traditional home services are proposed by home devices manufacturers by means of a proprietary control device which may be accessed either directly or from the phone network. Services allowing the (remote) control over lights, heating or shutters are usually proposed and implemented by proprietary means. On the other hand, home services are gaining more and more interest in the computer science community. In particular, several service discovery systems have been proposed that use open and standard Internet communication protocols in order to discover available devices and to send commands to them. Although these solutions are independent from device manufacturers, the lack of home devices understanding Internet protocols has restricted the proliferation of home appliances of such systems, which still restricted to computer applications. In order to ensure the independence from home devices manufacturers, the COM layer is mainly based on the Ametsa service which offers a generic interface allowing clients to be aware of the arrival/removal of devices to/from the network and to send specific commands to devices. Ametsa uses a service discovery system based on UPnP [9]. UPnP functionalities are used to be aware of arrival or removal of devices and to send or receive commands to/from available devices. As many home devices are not able to manage Internet protocols, we have developed gateways which translate UPnP protocols on the corresponding (proprietary) protocol of devices.

5 Extended architecture

5-1: A CORBA based architecture to support dynamicity with complex system:

Last section lets us aware of some components used to support dynamicity. Such dynamicity has to be able to evolve and support new technologies. For this purpose we have attention to integrate also complex systems such as robot or wheelchair applications. First, we succeeded to enable the Manus management using socket technologies. As Manus architecture (Figure 2) don't dispose of a Dynamic Service Discovery code the connection and the management of this object is still static. Current work aims to combine java, CORBA and XML technologies to install an affordable robot mobile code. Synthetics work at COM Layer is needed to integrate all XML object created to be parsed at HMI Layer.

CORBA (Common Object Request Broker Architecture) defines interfaces and services to support interoperability and offers transparency to build distributed applications. It takes advantage of interoperability between different manufacturer platform as hardware and software, and facilities the use of clients and servers in various languages [10]. CORBA was chosen for this purpose. Figure below (Figure 3) shows that Interconnection between com and Manus is easy since CORBA is an open system handling interoperability with different hardware, software and operating systems.

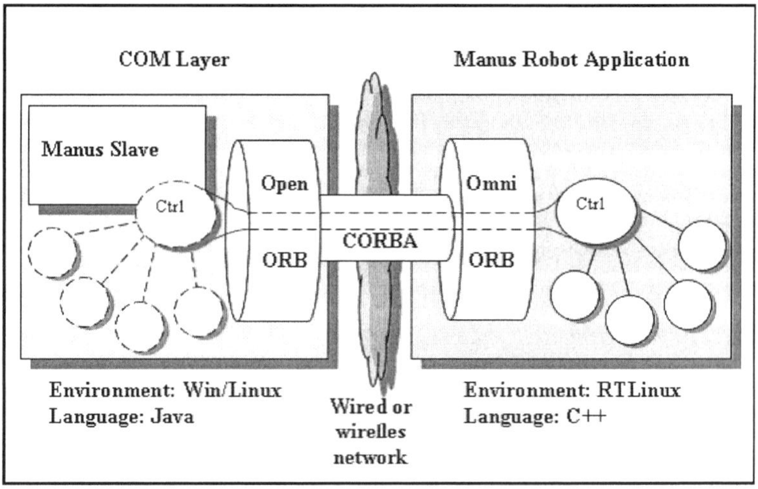

Figure 4: Manus Dynamicity Module based on CORBA

5-2: A visual feedback module to support favour dynamicity:

Among the difficulties encountered by user who have limited movement to percept neared object in "obscure" environment, we implemented a visual feedback module on Manus application (Figure 4).

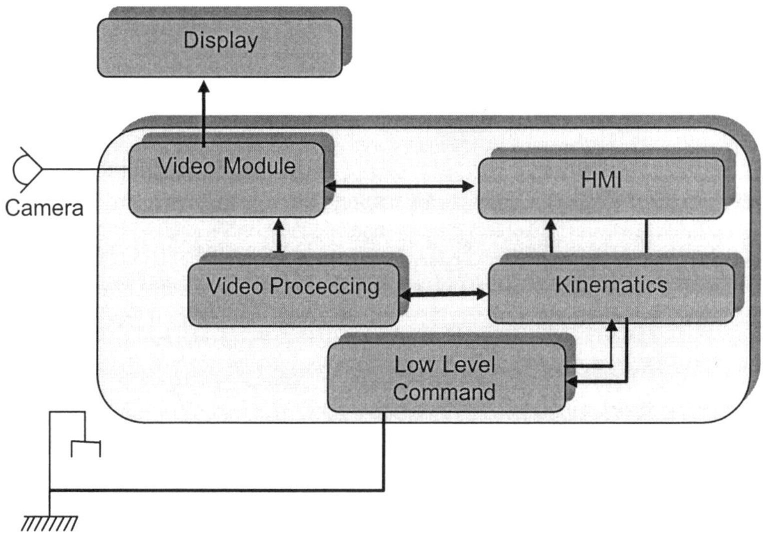

Figure 5: Video severing feedback in Manus system

This module gives simply information about the state of the robot but it is still incapable to describe environment's state. For example, visual feedback allows user who cannot move their hand and so cannot catch an object by ground, to do it very simply. In deed, we can assist the command of the robot: it is enough that the user selects an object in the display screen and choice the suitable actions. The implementation of this module can be either on Manus side, or Client side (PDA, Tablet PC.). It depends on the processing capacity of the machine carrying out the video treatment. Following architecture underlines the integration of video processing and video module into Manus concept. After video flow capture, video module parses useful data and transmits video frames to video processing module. Considering the significant description of those frames, the video processing module is enabling to assist the movement of Manus arm in order to reach the target.

The two previous modules are developed with C++ languages and are easy to integrate in our modular architecture in order to have more pertinent information related to surrounding environment. (Example if the door sounds we can have a visual return allowing the guest identification).

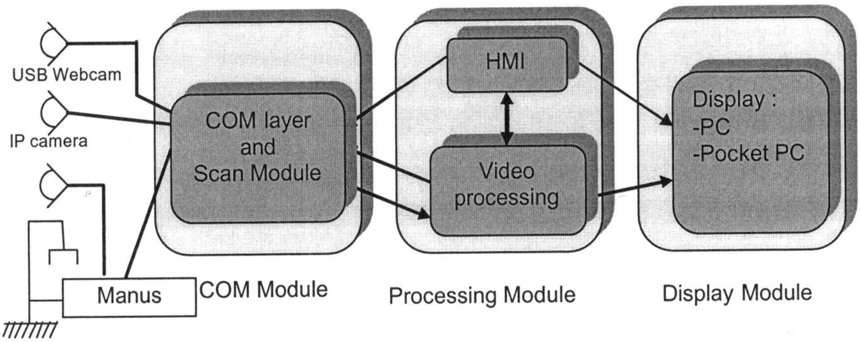

Figure 6: Shared processing module in smart homes concept

6. Conclusion

In this paper we outlined our approach to integrate dynamicity concept into smart homes. We presented evolution of the Robot Manus architecture to take into account supplementary module such as video and dynamicity. Moreover, this paper underlined integration of new Manus evolution into smart homes concept in order to allow a flexible control of Manus.

Dynamicity described in this paper is a key element of future research activity which will focus on "Context Awareness" applied to smart homes, smart devices and originally to complex devices such as Robot or wheelchair.

As results, we aim at testing our prototype with users in real time conditions. For that, we are in phase of mounting an evaluation platform in many public places such as hospital, holiday's accessible location or at living area.

Acknowledgements

The authors would like to thank the people who have participated actively in this presented research activities from INSERM U.483, ENST Bretagne, ENST Paris and INT. Fund for this project are provided by GET and by the Foundation Louis Leprince Ringuet through the smart homes project, and by AFM and European Commission through the AMOR project.

References

[1] Abdulrazak B., MokhtariM., Grandjean B., « Toward a New High Level Controller for Manus Robot: The Commanus Project » Proc ICORR 2001, 7th International Conference on Rehabilitation Robotics, « Integration of assistive technology in the information age », Ed. IOS Press, pp.221-226, INT-Evry, France, April

[2] Mokhtari M., Abdulrazak B., Feki M.A., Rodriguez R., Grandjean B., «Integration of Rehabilitation Robotics in the Context of Smart Homes: Application to Assistive Robotics » HWRS-ERS Journal, An International Journal of Human-friendly Welfare Robotic Systems. Vol. 4, N°2, P29-32. 2003.

[3] Abdulrazak B., Mokhtari M., Grandjean B., Integration of a robotic arm in the environment of Disabled People : The commanus Project. AAATE'2001, Ed. IOS Press. Ljubljana, Slovenia, september 2001, P285-290.

[4] Plessis-Delorme E., Didi N., Mokhtari M., Roby-Brami A. An evaluation of two types of user control interface for the MANUS arm robot. In: Advances in Perception-action coupling. EWEP'5. Editions EDK, 1998. P156-161.

[5] Sumi Helel and all, "Smart Phone Based Cognitive Assistant" available at http://www.healthcare.pervasive.dk/ubicomp2003/papers/Final_Papers/14.pdf.

[6] Feki M.A. , Abdulrazak B., Mokhtari M., « XML Modelisation of Smart home envirement », Proc ICOST 2003, Ed. IOS Press, pp.55-60, Paris, September 2003

[7] Feki M.A., Integration of wireless communication in smart homes for disabled and elderly people. In Proc. AAATE'2003, Ed. IOS Press. Dublin August 2003.

[8] Abdulrazak B., Mokhtari M., Feki M.A., Grandjean B., Rodriguez R.; «Generic user interface for people with Disabilities: Application to smart home concept » Proc ICOST 2003, Ed. IOS Press, pp.45-51, Paris, September 2003.

[9] Segarra, M.T., Thépaut, A., Keryell, R., Poichet, J., Plazaola, A., Peccate, B.: Ametsa a Generic Home Control System Based on UPnP. ICOST proceedings, ISBN 158603 3808 (IOS Press), France (September 2003) 73-80.

[10] Object Management Group. "CORBA Basics". www.omg.org/gettingstarted/corbafaq.htm

Toward a Human-Friendly Assistive Environment
D. Zhang and M. Mokhtari (Eds.)
IOS Press, 2004

Keeping in Touch With Cognitively Impaired People

How Mobile Devices Can Improve Medical and Cognitive Supervision

Hélène Pigot and Sylvain Giroux

Département d'informatique,
Université de Sherbrooke
2500 boul. Université, Sherbrooke, Canada J1K 2R1
{Sylvain.Giroux, Helene.Pigot,}@USherbrooke.ca
http://www.dmi.usherb.ca/~sgiroux/domus/

Abstract: Governments aim at keeping at home and in their community people suffering from cognitive impairments (Alzheimer disease, trauma, schizophrenia...). But resources are scarce. Mobile devices can improve their autonomy and safety. They can also lessen the burden on health professionals and relatives. The services of an Agenda House use PDAs 1) to give cognitive assistance to patients, 2) to help supervisors to monitor activities of daily living (ADL) of patients, 2) to collect ecological data to improve diagnosis and treatments, and 3) to give human assistance on request or in case of emergency exploiting in particular geo-localization services.

1 Introduction

In Canada, the current social and medical politics aim at keeping at home and in their community as most as possible people suffering from cognitive impairments (Alzheimer disease, trauma, schizophrenia...) [4]. But many issues need to be address:

- With respect to in the activities of daily living (ADL) of patients, autonomy must be fostered. If not stimulated, cognitive capacities often deteriorate rapidly.
- Safety and security must be ensured indoors and outdoors.
- Human resources are often too scarce and overworked.

Mobile devices can offer part of the support cognitively impaired people still need. As well, mobile devices can relieve professionals from some of their work.

Furthermore when a patient stays in her community, physicians lack the real data and information they need to cure or assess her health state. Ecological data can dramatically help in modifying or fine-tuning diagnosis and treatments. Indeed medication has often significant side effects —anxiety, sleepiness…— and information provided by the patient are not reliable. Up till now the effects of a change of medication will be known just at the next appointment, which means often one month later in Quebec.

This paper discusses features and implementation of an information system for cognitive assistance and remote supervision: the agenda home (AH). Services are designed especially for mobile devices. They provide practical solutions to the issues above [10]. First we analyze the range of domicile infrastructures where to deploy AH (§2). Then we show how supervision can safely foster autonomy (§3). Next we describe cognitive assistance to patients and remote supervision by professionals or relatives (§4). Once short-term direct and remote assistance is ensured, we go further and gather ecological data to foster better treatments (§5). Finally geo-localization helps to ensure safety and security of patients outdoors (§6). Finally some details of the implementation are presented (§7).

2 Domicile Infrastructures Adapted to Patients Cognitive Profile

"Homes" and "communities" can be classified according to residents' health states, residents' level of autonomy, and services available on-site. We are currently developing a strategy to integrate AH in various domicile infrastructures as a continuum evolving with the patient cognitive profile. These domicile infrastructures are

- Hospitals: of course, the system can be used to monitor activities of patients and lessen the burden put on nurses. But we intend to use it mainly to prepare their deinstitutionalisation, letting them live in a supervised apartment preparing a transition to a move in the community.
- Specialized residences: patient disease is rather severe; medical staff is always available on-site; patients may either live in individual apartments or shared spaces, for instance [11]; many services are available on-site: cafeteria, nurses...
- Family residences: patient disease is not enough severe to impede them to be autonomous, though they cannot live completely alone; one or two unspecialized human resources are available on-site; few cognitively impaired people are supervised; few services are available on-site.
- Supervised apartments: patients are quite autonomous; there is no specialized staff; one person is in charge of the apartments; there are no specific services on-site.
- Houses: this is the least supervised domicile; patients live autonomously without on-site human support [9].

Usually, a person suffering from the Alzheimer disease will slowly move from her house towards the hospital as her cognitive state deteriorates.

3 Supervision: Fostering Autonomy

The very spirit of our work is to foster patient's autonomy in a supervised real-life environment. More concretely, a patient has the charge to manage and perform most of her ADLs. She is also responsible to enter ecological data on the mobile device. Supervisors are there to help in case of need or emergency. A supervisor status may range from health professionals to relatives. They may be present on-site, but not necessarily.

To support the autonomy of patient and to ease the task of supervisors, we implemented and integrated various software components for 1) ADLs monitoring, 2) collecting ecological data, and 3) services based on geo-localization (Fig. 1). The client components run on mobile devices, more precisely personal digital assistants (PDAs) enhanced with wireless network connections and GPS. The server components run on a PC and connect to a database. Data may be transferred either in real-time or in a batch mode, for instance, when a network connection becomes available. Special care was put on user interfaces because, on the one hand, no or few learning could be expected from cognitively impaired people and, on the other hand, supervisors may have to monitor many patients for several activities. So user interface must be intuitive, simple, and effective. In the next sections, we give details on the services implemented with respect to ADLs (§4), ecological data (§5), and geo-localization (§6).

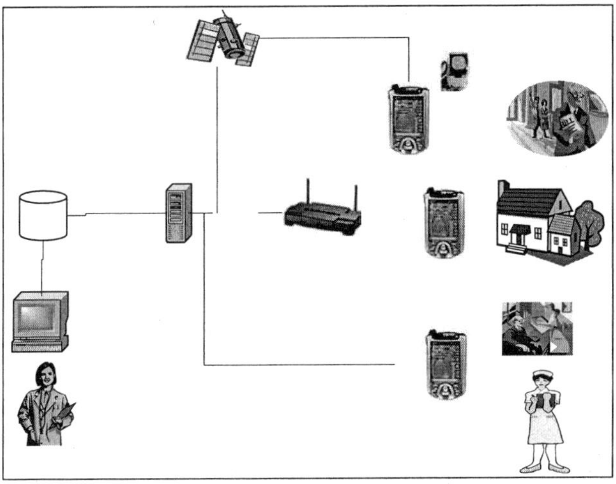

Figure 1 Infrastructure: patients and supervisors use iPAQs to connect to the server through wireless networks. The system is available both indoors and outdoors. Outdoors a GPS provides the user location.

4 Cognitive Assistance for ADLs

In an Agenda House, the aim of software components related to cognitive assistance is primarily to monitor specific ADLs —meals, medication, medical appointments... Supervisors should intervene just in case of failure or emergency. So a patient's PDA and a supervisor's PDA will run different client components. Each client connects periodically to the server. The server saves the data in a database, and synchronizes and distributes the information between patients and supervisors clients. The patient client acts as a cognitive assistant for managing and monitoring ADLs over time. It also informs supervisors of ADL completions (§4.2). The supervisor client enables her to manage the set of ADLs (§4.1), to manage and supervise patients (§4.3), and coordinate supervisors (§4.4).

4.1 Specification of ADLs

Supervisors manage a library of ADLs. They can create, modify and delete ADLs. An ADL is described by a name, a recurrence period of time (hour, day, month, once) (Fig. 2a), time to be completed, duration, start and end date (Fig. 2b). Once defined, ADLs can be assigned to patients on an individual basis (Fig. 2c) in their agenda. Other user interfaces allow to browse this library, for instance to see how much ADLs are effectively used.

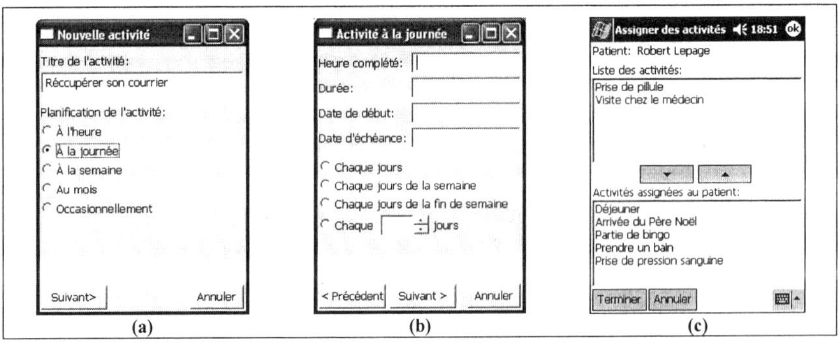

Figure 2 : Using a mobile device, a supervisor can create an ADL (a) (b) and assign it to patients (c).

4.2 An Enhanced Agenda System as a Mean for Cognitive Assistance

An enhanced agenda system is specially tailored to act as a cognitive reminder of ADL for a patient. The client component running on a patient's PDA is kept very simple (Fig. 3a). There is an auto-login procedure to the server. The patient has no user name or password to enter. The user interface displays just one window presenting the ADLs to perform for the next three hours. To not overburden the cognitive capacities of a patient, at most four ADLs are listed[1]. To indicate an ADL completion, the patient just clicks on the button of the ADL[2]. A patient can also request help by clicking a button at the bottom of the screen. Other information such as time of completion is also put in the database (Fig. 3b).

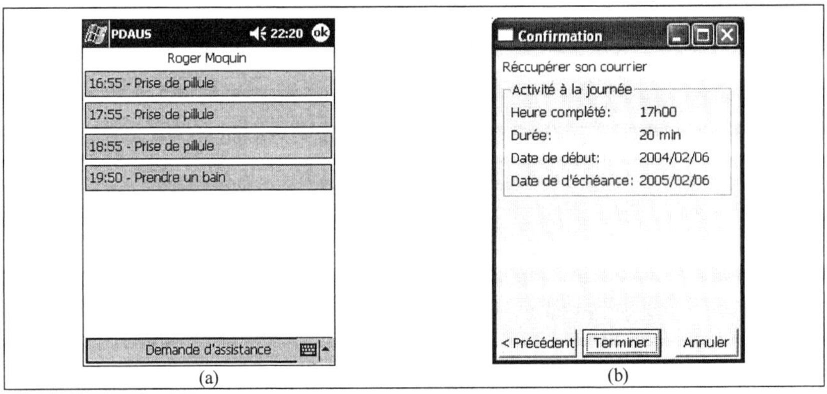

Figure 3 Client component acting as a cognitive assistant on the patient's PDA.

[1] Using a configuration file, we can personalize according to the patient cognitive capacities how many ADLs to display and the ADLs time frame.

[2] To assess an ADL has effectively been done, we intend to use evidence coming from the environment in future releases. For instance, if the ADL is "taking medicine", smart sensors can detect that the medicaments cabin was opened, providing some evidence.

4.3 Keeping in Touch

The AH supports remote cognitive supervision, still preserving the intimacy and safety of patients. Each supervisor owns a PDA running the client component for monitoring ADLs. Supervisors and patients keep in touch through a server. The server collects information, records it in a database, and dispatches changes to supervisors and patients' client PDAs.
The client component of the supervisors' PDAs enables her to monitor at distance her patients' ADLs (Fig. 4). For each patient, a list of ADLs to perform is set by the supervisors; the ADLs can be chosen from a library of ADLs (§4.1). A supervisor usually monitors many patients. Lists of a patient's ADLs and assigned patients can be changed dynamically using PDAs. Supervisors' user interface for monitoring is made of

- The *Residents* panel displays one's list of patients (Fig. 4a); a color code indicates for a patient if intervention is required.
- The *ADLs* panel enables a supervisor to edit her patient's ADLs (Fig. 4b).
- The *ADL* panel enable to see the state of one ADL for a given patient (Fig. 4c).

Color and shape codes enable to see the state of the patients in a glimpse. Red means time to complete the ADL is over and patient did not perform it. Yellow means time to complete the ADL is almost over and patient did not yet perform it. Green means everything is fine. This way, supervisors get a feedback on the realization of the ADLs [1] without having to enquire directly to the patient preserving her privacy and respecting her autonomy.

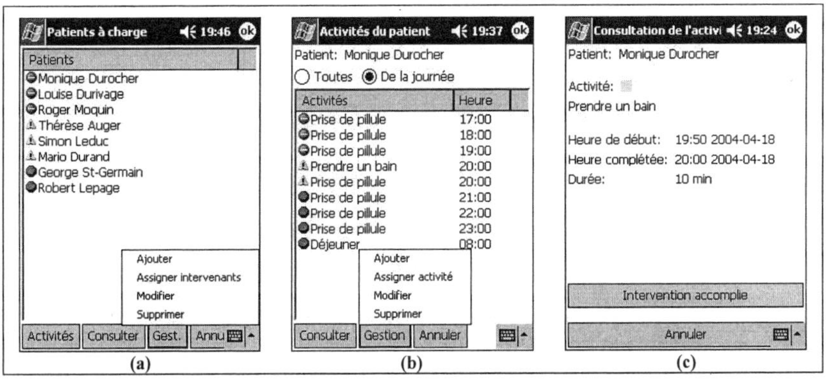

Figure 4 Supervisor's PDA: client component for monitoring ADLs of patients.

4.4 Coordination of supervisors

Synchronisation and coordination of supervisors is imperative. A patient can be supervised by more than one person. Supervisors may change over time. Moreover most of the time supervisors are employees. Working shifts have to be considered. The *Supervisors* panel enables to assign one's patient to another supervisor (Fig. 5). It is useful for synchronisation, e.g. when a supervisor work shift is over or when a supervisor is too busy.

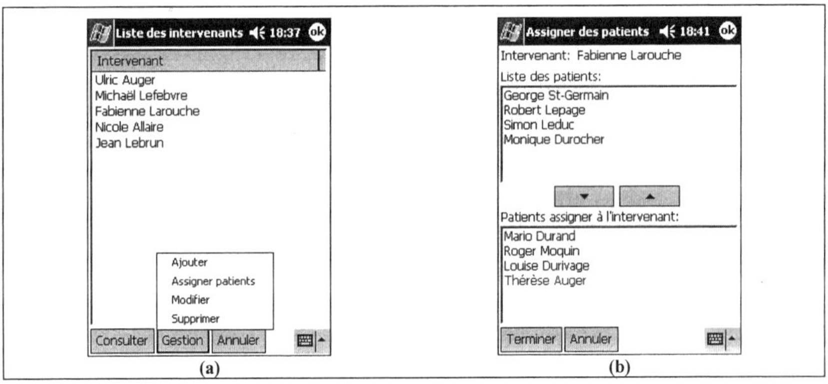

Figure 5 User interfaces for the coordination of supervisors for monitoring patients.

5 Ecological Data: Gathering Information for Better Treatments

Collecting ecological information may be of tremendous value for delivering better treatments. With such a feedback, physicians may fine-tune medication more rapidly and measure disease evolution more precisely [8]. For instance, one may measure the occurrence and intensity of medication side effects —somnolence, anxiety, oblivion, etc. Panels (Fig. 6) on the client PDA are used by a patient to:

- record symptoms and grade their intensity according to a predefined scale (Fig. 6a).
- take useful notes, e.g. when a patient forgot an appointment (Fig. 6b).

Date, time and position are also registered. This information is sent to the server on a batch mode. Data can be later analyzed to improve diagnosis and treatments. In particular, these components will allow schizophrenes to gather ecological data useful for psychiatrists.

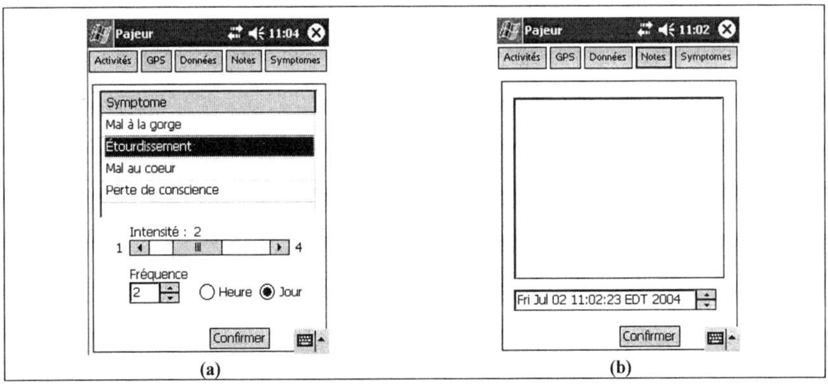

Figure 6 Patient user interface to register the intensity of her symptoms and to take some notes.

6 Geo-localization: Detecting Crisis and Assisting People

Geo-localization is another critical issue. Knowing a patient position may be worthful [6] and even vital in many situations and for a range of purposes:

- to send directly somebody at the patient location if she is in crisis or in danger;
- to forbid specific zones;
- to analyzed paths and detect characteristic pathologic patterns of movement of patients suffering from schizophrenia to detect crisis states;
- to predict the goal of a patient combining path history and analysis [3].

When a patient is outdoors, a GPS connected to her PDA get her position. This position is sent at predefined time interval to the server. Path analysis can then be performed. Currently client and server components are under development to specify and manage forbidden zones. This is a key issue for the deinstitutionalization of patients at the Centre de réadaptation de l'Estrie. They want to ban specific zones to patients that were drug addicts. Next step will be to implement algorithms that detect and recognize pathologic path patterns. It will be applied to schizophrenia. The aim is to detect patterns indicating occurrence of a crisis, more precisely 1) when a patient stands for a long time at specific locations, e.g. in front of a church, and 2) when she walks back and forth along a sidewalk a lot of times. We will also implement means to locate indoors position.

7 Implementation

The implementation is in standard Java (J2SE) for the server part and PersonalJava for the client part on PDAs. On the PDAs, user interfaces were implemented with SWT. On the PDAs, the virtual machine was J9 for PocketPC. The various component were tested on HP iPAQ 4155 and HP iPAQ 1945 running Microsoft PocketPC OS. Indoors the wireless connections to the server use IEEE 802.11b. Outdoors the wireless connection is made through a Sierra Aircard. Each PDA connects to the server through TCP sockets. The server allocates a different thread to each connection. PDAs and server exchange serialized objects, RMI is not used. If the connection is lost, the PDA tries to restore it. We keep the traffic low. For instance, when a patient checks an ADL as done, a message is sent to the server. The server first updates the database, and then it sends a message to the PDAs of supervisors to inform them a change occurred. If the PDA is concerned with the change, it requests more details. For the PDAs, a communication service is under development to manage a generic batch mode, or to keep messages in a queue waiting till a connection is available. Finally a configuration file can be use to personalize the application: auto-login, font, font size, message strings…

8 Conclusion

In this paper we showed how mobile devices can improve the autonomy of cognitively impaired people living in their community. They can also lower the burden of supporting professionals or relatives. We described services enabling 1) supervisors to monitor ADLs of patients, 2) to collect ecological data for improving diagnosis and treatments, and 3) to exploit geo-localization to ensure safety and security of patients outdoors. Next steps are

- to perform in situ experimentation, principally at the CRE;
- to validate the usability of the services for supervisors and patients;

- to assess the fitness of the services to the organisational infrastructures such as the Centre de réadaptation de l'Estrie (CRE) and familial residences;
- to integrate a distributed plan recognition system to validate the completion of ADLs [2] [5]. This service will integrate information coming from multiple sources to get a more accurate idea of the current stage of an ADL. For instance, it will be possible to know if an ADL has begun, is in process, or is completed;
- to optimize traffic and standardize communication between servers and PDAs;
- to implement personalization schemas based on user profile and cognitive capacities, e.g. on the deterioration scale of Alzheimer disease of Reisberg [9];
- to analyze the evolution of cognitive diseases from the evaluation of performance over time of the ADLs.

Agenda Home components will be part of smart homes [7] [2].

9 Acknowledgments

We gratefully thank for the implementation: Jean-Francois Moreau, Michaël Lefebvre, Ulric Auger, Patrick Girard, Ludovic Lebel, Patrick Bélanger, Simon Godard, Yannick Nadeau. We also express gratitude for their feedback and hints to Emmanuel Stipp (Centre de recherche Fernand Séguin), Ghislain Massicotte and Gaston Leroux from the CRE.

10 References

[1] B.R. Bonder, and M. Wagner, *Functional performance in older adults*. 2nd Edition. F.A. Davis. 2000.

[2] S Giroux, et al., *Indoors Pervasive Computing and Outdoors Mobile Computing for Cognitive Assistance and Telemonitoring*, 9th International Conference on Computers Helping People with Special Needs, July 7-9, 2004, Paris, France.

[3] L Liao, et al., *Learning and Inferring Transportation Routines*, Nineteenth National Conference on Artificial Intelligence, San Jose, CA, 2004.

[4] Ministère de la Santé et des Services Sociaux. Direction générale de la planification et de l'évaluation. (1998). *Le virage ambulatoire en santé physique: Enjeux et perspectives*. Coll. Études et analyses. Québec.

[5] Paquette, G., et al., *EpiTalk, generating advisor agents for existing information systems*, J. of AI in Education, AIED Society, AACE, vol. 7, no 3-4, 1996.

[6] D. Patterson, et al. *The ActivityCompass*, First International Workshop on Ubiquitous Computing for Cognitive Aids, Gothenberg, Sweden, 2002

[7] H. Pigot, et al., *The intelligent habitat and everyday life activity support*. 5th Intern'l Conf. on Simulations in Biomedicine, April 2-4, 2003, Slovenia, pp.507-516.

[8] B. Reisberg, et al. *Signs, symptoms and course of age-associated cognitive decline*. In S. Corkin, et al., *Aging : Alzheimer's disease : a report of progress*. New York. Raven Press. 1982. pp. 177-182.

[9] V. Rialle, et al. *Health 'smart' home: Information technology for patients at home*. Telemedicine Journal and E-Health. 8 (4), 2002.

[10] M. L. Lange. *Technology and occupation : contemporary viewpoints. The future of electronic aids to daily living. Am. J. of Occupational Therapy*, 56 (1), 2002, 107-109.

[11] V. Stanford, *Using pervasive computing to deliver elder care*. Pervasive Computing, Vol. 1, no 1, Jan-Mar 2002, pp. 10- 13

Toward a Human-Friendly Assistive Environment
D. Zhang and M. Mokhtari (Eds.)
IOS Press, 2004

Controlling Smart Spaces by Blind and Low Vision Individuals Using Technology Available in 2004

Christian D. Hofstader
Vice President / Softwhere Engineering
Freedom Scientific, St. Petersburg, Florida, USA

Sheena Iype
Research Assistant
FCS Corporation, Noida, India

Abstract. Many common devices found around the modern household are completely or partially inaccessible to blind people and those with diminished vision. This paper surveys a number of emerging standards, devices designed for blind and low vision people and the increasing popularity of home networks, that will drastically improve accessibility for be LV people in the coming years.

1 Introduction

Many common devices found around the modern household are completely or partially inaccessible to blind people and those with diminished vision. Some of the most *modern* devices actually make accessibility for blind and low vision (BLV) individuals more difficult to use. Flat-panel displays, on screen displays and other techniques used to control and configure consumer-electronics and household appliances are virtually impossible for a be LV person to use it all. Fortunately, there are a number of emerging standards, devices designed for blind and low vision people and the increasing popularity of home networks that will drastically improve accessibility for be LV people in the coming years.

Already, however, in 2004 there are a variety of consumer devices as well as assistive technologies available for the be LV person to enjoy the use of today. Thus, the topic of this paper is the solutions that the BLV individual can start using immediately.

2 Needs and Use Scenarios of the BLV Individual

Each blind or low vision individual will have his or her own specific needs for access to a wide array of different items in their household, educational and professional environments. This section will describe, in brief, some of the most common needs for and use scenarios of a smart space for a BLV person.

2.1 Access to Communication Devices

Perhaps the single most important class of devices that a BLV individual must be able to access are those that are used to communicate with others. Telecommunications devices, which are required by US law to be accessible, are becoming increasingly complex and exposing interfaces on touch screens which are, for all practical purposes, impossible for a BLV user to access. The typical modern telephone still has push buttons with which a BLV individual can dial the phone but features ranging from caller ID to speed dialing address books are unavailable, making these conveniences impossible for the BLV individual to use.

Communications devices are a cornerstone of personal safety as well as a method of delivering and retrieving a vast array of different types of information. As telecommunications devices have added features which make them more powerful for the mainstream user, they have become increasingly difficult for the BLV users to access. Features like speed dialing which, in older technology, merely required the user to remember a series of button presses are now, more frequently, accessed through an inaccessible menu system. Thus, instead of needing to remember a handful of numbers for emergency needs, family and friends, health care providers, etc., the BLV person can no longer access this feature at all.

If the telecommunications device also exposes its interface through one of the protocols listed later in this document, the BLV individual can access all of the features and functionality through the interface exposed on the user agent of their choice.

2.2 Access to Appliances

Like telecommunications products, home appliances are increasingly exposing their interfaces via touch screen and flat panel displays. Such interfaces are impossible for a BLV individual to access. It is possible, with the addition of tactile markers, for a BLV person to make limited use of such appliances but they are effectively prohibited from using the majority of features on the appliance. If the appliance has a menu system that changes, the tactile markers will be rendered useless and, as this is an increasingly common practice, the BLV individual is effectively prevented from using the appliance at all.

In a recent survey of consumer appliance retail outlets in St. Petersburg, Florida, the author found that there was only one washing machine (among hundreds of models observed) that still had mechanical controls and would, therefore, be accessible. There were zero microwave ovens, zero dryers, three stoves and very few other items that could be fully controlled by a blind person. The stores surveyed were: Walmart, Sam's Club, Home Depot and Circuit City. Over 300 different products were observed.

Controlling home appliances is important to the health, safety and happiness of virtually all individuals. If a BLV individual can only use a limited set of features on their appliances, they are also limited to what they can eat, drink and how they might dress. They may also be jeopardizing their safety if they cannot tell whether or not a stove has been left on, how long an item has been in the microwave or other details which can cause a fire or injury by touching an exposed hazard.

2.3 Access to Consumer Electronics

Entertainment is important to a fulfilling lifestyle. For years, audio equipment like stereos and recording studio devices have been very popular among blind and low vision people. Increasingly, though, newer products are replacing the traditional mechanical controls, which with a little training were fairly simple for a blind person to access, with touch screens, flat panel displays and "on screen" menus which use one's television to display information which can be manipulated via a remote control.

As the trend toward these modern controls continues, the BLV population is left with fewer functions of their consumer appliances that they can use. Memorization of the button locations on a remote control is a tactic used by many BLV individuals (including the author) but, as more functions are added to consumer electronics devices, the meaning of the buttons on a remote can changed based upon the state of the device and said state is, in no way, reported in a manner that a BLV person can access.

2.4 Greater Independence

The unifying use case for pervasive accessibility to all devices is that as accessibility increases, so does the independence of the individual with special needs. In the case of BLV adults, they will, given increased accessibility, be more productive, safer, healthier and less of a burden on others who may today need to perform simple tasks because of the lack of accessibility to electronic and information technologies in the home, educational and employment environments.

3 The current state-of-the-art in Devices Available for Blind People

This section describes, in brief, the assistive technology devices currently available for BLV users that can be employed to control *Smart* devices in their homes and other places.

3.1 PAC mate from Freedom Scientific

The most sophisticated of the products available to BLV consumers today is the PAC mate line of products from Freedom Scientific. The author is employed by Freedom Scientific and, therefore, may have a bias toward this product. The major difference, however, between the PAC mate and the other portable devices available for blind and low vision users is that it can support all of the major networking technologies currently being used to control Smart devices. Many current PAC mate users, of which there are over 3000, use wireless networks, blue tooth and Ethernet. Because of its open design, the PAC mate will be able to support new technologies as they enter the market as long as they are supported with drivers for the Microsoft Pocket PC platform.

Freedom Scientific made the decision to use an off-the-shelf operating system in order that their customers can leverage the technology developed for mainstream users. While the main PAC Mate unit is priced for the niche, blindness market, the peripherals and third party software is both ubiquitous and relatively inexpensive.

3.2 Elba by Papenmeier

The Elba is an interesting device in that it is a portable product designed for blind and low vision users that runs the entire GNU/Linux terminal based system. Hence, with appropriate drivers written for this platform for a broad enough array of peripherals, the Elba, theoretically, should be able to provide the blind and low vision user with access to many Smart devices.

3.3 BrailleNote Family of Products by PDI.

The BrailleNote family of products from Pulse Data, Inc. can be used to control some Smart devices as long as the communication only requires Ethernet today, PDI has announced a new device that will support wireless technology that is due to release later in 2004. The Pulse Data family of products are not capable, at this time, of supporting 802.11, Blue Tooth or many of the other technologies required to control Smart devices.

The Pulse Data products are also based entirely upon KeySoft, a proprietary software system written specifically for their devices. As the PDI products are closed systems, it is unknown if they will be compliant with emerging standards.

3.4 Others

It is possible and even sometimes convenient for a blind or low vision person to use an off-the-shelf laptop computer to perform many of the functions detailed in the sections describing the devices specifically designed for the BLV community. These are often less optimal because of their size, relatively short battery life and difficulty attaching to a refreshable Braille device. The positive side of using a consumer device for controlling smart spaces is that they tend to be considerably less expensive than products designed specifically for BLV consumers.

4 Networking Standards Available for Communicating with Smart Devices

There are currently a number of different standards available to communicate with Smart devices. At the current moment, these different standards cannot communicate directly with each other. Thus, there is some level of Chaos and a high level of technical sophistication required by an individual who wants to increase the level of automation within their household.

4.1 WiFi/802.11

The most common wireless home networking protocol is known as 802.11 and it is commonly called WiFi. There are three WiFi standards: 802.11 A, B and G. The primary differences between the three is the speed with which they can transfer data. As of this writing, 802.11 B (11 megabits per second) and 802.11 G (1 gigabits per second) are dominating the marketplace. 802.11 A was a poorly defined standard and, as a result, devices supporting it were superfluously incompatible with each other and with the B & G versions of the wireless protocol.

4.2 Blue Tooth

One of the radiofrequency base standards is called Blue Tooth. It is popular in PDAs, cell phones and in some newer laptops. It is available as a peripheral on the PAC mate but, as of the writing of this paper, not available on any of the other devices designed specifically for the blindness and low vision market.

4.3 LonWorks

LonWorks is a networking technology designed to connect legacy devices to current networking technologies. As of the writing of this paper, no device designed specifically for the BLV user can communicate directly with a LonWorks system. Fortunately, there are a number of gateway devices available that convert LonWorks to Ethernet and/or 802.11 which can solve the protocol problem.

4.4 Ethernet

Ethernet is the oldest of the still commonly used networking technologies. There are numerous devices available that can be attached to a home network via Ethernet. Virtually all of the advanced assistive technology products mentioned above can communicate using Ethernet. There are also a number of bridge products that will convert from Ethernet to other networking systems and vice versa, thus, a system needn't be entirely based upon this standard.

4.5 Radio Frequency ID (RFID)

Another emerging standard is that of the RFID tags. If an RFID reader is attached to one of the devices mentioned above, the BLV individual can use the technology to perform activities ranging from some orientation and mobility and way finding tasks to identifying products, reading embedded instructions for a product and virtually anything else that may be stored on an RFID tag.

5 Standards for controlling Smart Devices

There are a number of data standards competing to dominate the Smart Space market. This section describes, in brief, a few of the more popular emerging standards.

5.1 Universal Plug and Play (Upnp)

As of the writing of this document, in June 2004, there have been more than 200 products that support the UP&P protocol introduced to the consumer market. This may not sound like many when compared to the entire population of consumer-electronics products, high technology products and home appliances but, when put into the context of the fact that they were fewer than a dozen UP&P ready products available one year ago, the growth in the adoption of the standard by mainstream product manufacturers is very promising. As of today, it appears as though UP&P will emerge as the most successful of the standards now competing for market share.

5.2 Java/Jini

Java/Jini is a protocol similar to UP&P that is being developed by an entirely separate standards body. It is intended to provide similar services to UP&P. The Java/Genie protocol, however, has not been adopted by any consumer-electronics products, technology products or home appliances as of the writing of this paper. There is, however, a lot of research in universities and other laboratories going into this standard so It deserves to be mentioned as an emerging protocol.

5.3 HTML/XML

A number of consumer electronics products have been introduced that attach to a home network via 802.11 or Ethernet that expose their interface through an HTML based web page placed on the home intranet. If these web pages are compliant with the accessibility standards set forth by the World Wide Web Consortium Web Accessibility Initiative (W3C/WAI) or equivalent, they can be conveniently used by a BLV individual using one of the devices mentioned above.

5.4 Proprietary Standards

During our research for this paper, we discovered that there are a variety of additional networking standards proprietary to the organizations who manufacture them. As far as the author knows, none of these are accessible to blind or low vision people. Some of these include garage door openers and other popular home appliances.

6 Converging Technologies

To make a world that is truly universally accessible, the Chaos the currently exists among the differing standards for networking in the home, will need to have technical bridges built to unify the system for the user. Currently, the V2 (http://:www..myurc.org) is working on such a project. It is unlikely, however, that the work being done by V2 will start to appear in consumer products of a reasonable price within the next three years.

6.1 Network Agnostic Standards

V2 and some other projects, however, are taking the steps to separate the data standard from the networking standard. Thus, and assistive technology that understands the V2 protocol will be able to operate any device connected to the network that speaks V2 and understands the network technology supported by the assistive technology. This alone will be a major step forward in providing Universal excess ability as, today, the data formats tend to be bound to the networking technologies.

6.2 Permitting the Market to Select Its Own Standard

Any group of people can gather together and call itself a committee. This committee, if it so chooses, can declare the results of its work to be a standard. If, however, neither assistive technology nor mainstream product adopts the standard it is, in effect, not actually a standard at all. Over the next few years, various standards will be proposed, some will succeed and others will fail. The reasons for their success or failure have more to do with decisions being made by the large manufacturers of consumer products and, to a lesser extent, the manufacturers of assistive technologies. Economics will play an important role in whether or not a standard is adopted; the one thing we can be certain of though is that as technologies improve Smart Spaces will become more accessible for blind and low vision individuals.

7 Challenges for the Future

As different technologies emerge as standards and user agents become increasingly available to BLV individuals, there will be many challenges remaining before smart systems become available to the majority of BLV individuals in the world.

7.1 Cost of Smart Technology

The first hurdle to deploying smart, accessible technologies to the majority of the BLV population will be the combined cost of the accessible mainstream products and the user agents produced by the assistive technology companies. Some governments, most of which are in Europe, provide different levels of subsidies for assistive technologies but no where in the world does a national health system or private health insurance arrangement provide reimbursement for the purchase of consumer appliances or electronics devices.

In the US alone, approximately 70% of all blind people are unemployed. In a nation like India, where there are 20 million blind people, virtually none have jobs. Thus, out of pocket expenses for blind people must be restricted to what they can afford.

Fortunately, smart devices of all kinds will be produced for the mass market instead of being specialized for BLV users. Thus, the prices of smart appliances will be similar to those of the current, *dumb* generation. Replacing all of the appliances in one's home will not occur immediately as this will be cost prohibitive but as the BLV population replaces or upgrades electronic devices in their home, educational and work environments, they can now start, at a reasonable price point, to choose accessible, smart products.

7.2 Training the User Population

One of the most difficult challenges in providing for a BLV audience is finding the individuals and teaching them about the availability of accessible products. Once the BLV individuals learn about the products, it will then be necessary to teach them how to access them via the user agent of their choice. A well designed user agent will make the interfaces to a wide array of different devices as similar as possible which will minimize training costs but this will remain one of the most difficult challenges for years to come.

7.3 Enforcing Adherence to Standards

The lifecycle of an assistive technology for BLV users is far longer than that of a mainstream consumer product. Thus, as standards emerge, they must be made to adhere, with backward compatibility, to those with the largest number of user agents which have been deployed. The mainstream user agents will be considerably less expensive than those specialized for people with special needs so they may be viewed as disposable. It will also be incumbent upon the assistive technology manufacturers to ensure that their devices are designed with enough flexibility so they can be adapted with software upgrades so they can communicate with different devices as the standards evolve.

8 Conclusions

This paper describes a lot of different technologies in brief. The one conclusion that can be drawn from this effort is that there are a lot of people working on and money being spent on smart technologies. The fact that the majority are being targeted toward the mainstream market will drive the economics of the next generation of consumer products and, as a result, blind and low vision people, with the user agents of their choice, will be able to enjoy far greater control of their environments than ever before.

9 More Information

A number of companies and standards are mentioned in this document. The following is an incomplete list of places where additional information can be found about these products and topics.

9.1 Freedom Scientific, Inc.

Freedom Scientific, manufacturers of the PAC Mate line of products, can be found at http://www.freedomscientific.com.

9.2 Pulse Data, Inc.

Additional information about Pulse Data and its line of BrailleNote products can be found at http://www.pulsedata.com.

9.3 Papenmeier

The Elba, the only GNU/Linux based device for blind users, can be found at: http://www.papenmeier.de.

9.4 Universal Plug and Play

The Universal Plug and Play consortium can be found at: http://www.upnp.org.

9.5 V2

The publicly available information about the work being done by the V2 committee can be found at:
http://www.myurc.org.

9.6 LonWorks

Information about the LonWorks networking system can be found at: http://www.lonworks.com.

9.7 Others

There are numerous other technologies mentioned in this paper. They can be found in numerous locations on the Internet and some can be found in consumer electronics stores and catalogues. For a list of the products that the authors reviewed for this paper, please feel free to write to Chris Hofstader at chrish@freedomscientific.com and he will gladly provide you with an Excel spreadsheet containing the products studied for this effort.

Toward a Human-Friendly Assistive Environment
D. Zhang and M. Mokhtari (Eds.)
IOS Press, 2004

Application of Mobile Phone Technology in the Elderly – A Simple Telecare System for Home Rehabilitation

Toshiyo TAMURA, Yasushi MASUDA*, Mitsuyoshi SEKIMOTO**, Yuji HIGASHI** and Toshiro FUMOTO **

Department of Biomedical Engineering, Chiba University

**Nara Institute of Science and Technology* *

Fujimoto Hayasuzu Hospital

Abstract: This study examined the use of mobile phone for home health care and described an alternative telemedicine framework. The framework aims to transmit small but sufficient amounts of data for daily monitoring of residential subjects' basic health status. We tested the remote monitoring of heart rate and respiration. The system was tested in real home-visit rehabilitation environments and was found to be useful both for the therapist and the patients in planning and evaluating daily rehabilitation training.

1 Introduction

Advances in Information Technology and Telecommunications (ITT) have played a catalytic role in recent developments within the field of Assistive (Rehabilitation) Technology, facilitating the introduction of new products and services. The importance of ITT to elderly people cannot be over-stated. As well as everything else that a personal computer (PC) user takes for granted in this electronic age (communications and health information through the internet, smart houses and other applications.), a elderly person must also handle the PC as an ordinary telephone or mobile phone. To avoid a complex handling of PC resulted in very restricted access to today's services and facilities, we have been developed a tele-health care for home rehabilitation without PC.

2. Methods

2.1 System configuration

The system consists of a monitoring system in the home and a viewer system for the therapist. A

TCP/IP network using various physical communication infrastructures connects the sub-systems (Fig.1).

The home-side system consists of an air-filled mat, a sensory and analysis unit, and a bridge unit that handles connections. When a subject lies on the mat, the mat senses pressure from the subject's respiration or heartbeat. The analysis unit (Bio-Sensor Node BN-6, Yokogawa Electric Corp.) continuously monitors pressure perturbations with a pressure sensor and estimates rates for predefined timeframes. Estimates are stored in a built-in web server system in HTML format, accessible via an integrated Ethernet interface. The analysis unit originally constructed a direct connection between household products, air-filled mat with amplifier in our case and Internet. However, we need another converter to transfer data to the currently available communication tool such as a mobile phone. An embedded microserver unit (OpenBlockSS, Plat Home Inc.) serves as the bridge unit. Since the unit is integrated in a fanless microcomputer module, it conforms to the silence requirement. A mobile phone modem (MobileDP 2496P, NTT DoCoMo Corp.) connects the bridge unit and a mobile phone (Fig.2a).

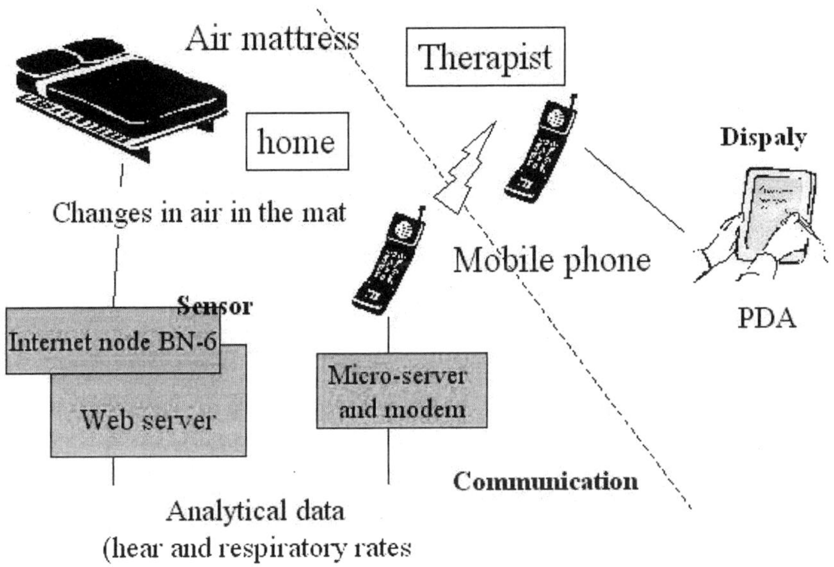

Figure 1 System configuration

Therapists would access the home-side sensor node to browse a subject's status and could quickly check various patients shown in Fig.2(b). To track or record long-term transitions in health status, the system would have to store and arrange acquired information. In addition, if signs of emergency arise, the hospital side would have to contact the home side immediately. Since therapists do not necessarily have expert computer knowledge, the viewer system should have a simple interface that does not require special knowledge for setup, browsing, or reporting.

We therefore developed a viewer system using a personal digital assistant (PDA) and a mobile telephone. PDAs have web access via popular web-browser interfaces, as well as simple text-editor functions suitable for making reports. An infrared modem links the PDA and the mobile phone.

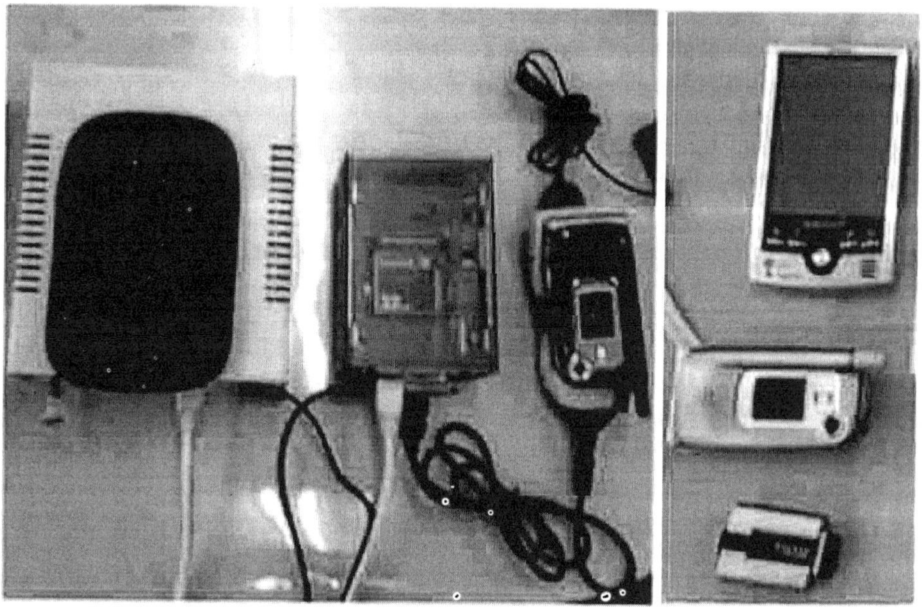

(a) (b)

Figure 2 (a) The system in the home fro, left Bio-sensor node, micro-server, and mobile phone. (b) The system using therapist. Form top PDA, mobile phone and connector

The connection between the sensor and the viewer system should be carefully balanced between performance and cost. Our system requires information on estimated heart rate and respiratory rate at several points after exercise. Such data use a few kilobytes of space at most, even when formatted in HTML text. If formatted as HTML, on-request rather than permanent connections should be designed. To ensure the subject's privacy, protection of measured data is very important when connecting the sensor and viewer terminals through a public communication infrastructure such as the Internet. Thus, privileged access or encryption should protect the data. Our system limits access to the phone number for incoming calls to the bridge unit. Additionally, password authentication is requested when connecting.

2.2 Subject and experimental set-up

We operated the system in real patients' homes to evaluate its potential. We conducted the testing in Miyazaki Prefecture, Japan. A therapist from Fujimoto Hayasuzu Hospital and two residential patients joined in the experiment. Prior to the experiment, the hospital's ethics committee ensured that the patients and their families had given both oral and written informed consent.

The system was placed in a briefcase for easy installation. Prior to the experiments, the therapist was given brief instructions on system installation and use. After the brief explanation, the therapist could install the system in five minutes.

The therapist used the PDA system to measure heart and respiratory rates under the following three conditions:

1. At the hospital, 30-60 minutes before training,
2. At the patient's home, at the beginning and end of the training,
3. At an outdoor location, remote from both the home and hospital, 30-60 minutes after training.

Figure 3 shows the measurement points of the experiments. A is the hospital where the therapist works, C and D are the patients home. On a way to a patient home, the therapist tried to contact the patient's record at the point of B.

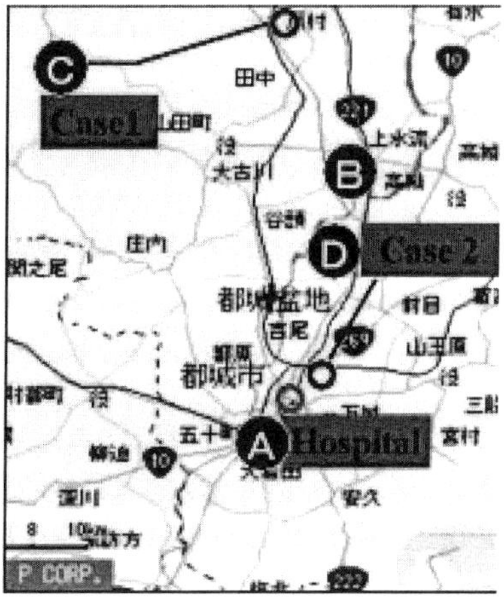

Figure 3 Measurement points

3. Results

Each operation took approximately 2 minutes, including about 40 seconds for HTTP data transmission. Although radio wave malfunctions caused several lost connections, the system recovered easily by reloading via the web browser. The therapist used each measurement to check the patient's stability. Although heart and respiratory rates increased immediately after training, the increased rates were considered safe and the subject recovered in 30 minutes. Figure 4 shows the results of the experiment. In a patient (case 1) who lives 30 km apart from the hospital, the heart and respiratory rate were obtained at hospital one hour before rehabilitation training. Those were obtained on a way to the patient home pointed at B, then before and after rehabilitation training at patient home. After 30 min of rehabilitation training, the therapist visited next patient (case 2) and the heart and respiratory rates were obtained both patients.

The result of case 1 indicates the higher heart and respiratory rates were observed after rehabilitation training but those were down after 30 min. However, there is no tendency for case 2.

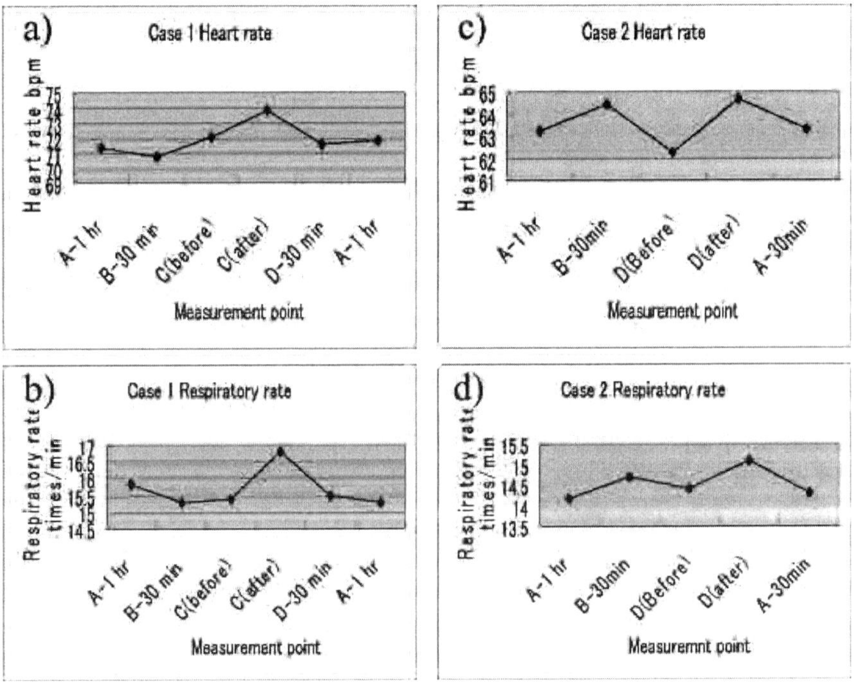

Figure 4. Results

4. Discussion

The system successfully obtained data on patient status. Because we simplified the system structure so that the therapist needed only to plug in to start or stop the system, the time and cost for installation and maintenance were appropriate for our needs. Patients also approved of the system's compact, silent, and non-constraining nature.

Acknowledgements

This work was partly supported by Longevity Sciences (10-3), NEDO (NEDOH14-0603001) and Pfizer Health Research Foundation

Author Index